# VITAMIN D AND CHOLESTEROL

# VITAMIN D AND CHOLESTEROL

## THE IMPORTANCE OF THE SUN

Dr David S Grimes MD FRCP

Barbara & Mike,

Best wishes,

David

© David Grimes, 2009

Published by Tennison Publishing

May 2009

ISBN 978-0-9562132-0-4

Cover design by Clare Brayshaw

Prepared and printed by:
York Publishing Services Ltd
64 Hallfield Road
Layerthorpe
York YO31 7ZQ
Tel: 01904 431213
Website: www.yps-publishing.co.uk

# CONTENTS

*Dove non va il sole, va il medico*
(Where the sun does not go, the doctor goes)


*Sunlight is the only disinfectant which sustains the man while it kills the microbe*
James Burn Russell (1837–1904)


*Many older people remember when sunshine, milk, bread, butter, and meat were good for you and were recommended by physicians*
Faith T. Fitzgerald, 1994


*To be accepted as a paradigm, a theory must seem better than its competitors, but it need not, and in fact it never does, explain all the facts with which it can be confronted.*
Thomas Kuhn, 1996

# ACKNOWLEDGEMENTS

I would like to thank the international medical community for the vast amount of information that I have been able to read during the past 40 years, much of which has contributed to the story that this book unfolds. I also thank the editors of a wide range of excellent medical journals that are the way in which information travels.

The accumulation of information to produce this book would not have been possible without the help of the library staff of the Royal Blackburn Hospital, Linda Riley, Clare Morton, Sarah Glover and Margaret Webster. I would also thank Susan Rogers for her dedication in typing the manuscript.

I must thank my wife Jenny for allowing me to be perhaps negligent of domestic responsibilities during the 40 years of reading and the time spent writing this book. She has been a great strength and support.

Within the text I acknowledge those teachers of medicine who have given me stimulus and ideas, and my present colleagues who have provided me with an environment of learning. Also I am indebted to the legion of patients from whom I have learnt most of all. We will meet Abdul, Frank, Rachel and Alan.

# PROLOGUE

Abdul was born on 22 October 1961 in Pakistan, in a village close Rawalpindi. The family was poor. His father worked on the land but his mother did not work outside, staying in the house most of the time. As far as he can remember his mother wore a head-scarf but she did not cover her face. Abdul did not go to school but he would spend his days playing outside with the other boys.

In 1971 the family emigrated to England in search of a better life. They settled in Oswaldtwistle in Lancashire, where his father obtained employment in a textile mill. Abdul went to school in Oswaldtwistle but he did not play out very often. They lived in a terraced house without a garden. The textile mill in which his father worked closed down but he was able to obtain work as a labourer in a cement factory and the family moved, again living in a small terraced house. After leaving school with no qualifications, Abdul worked in a factory as a battery filler. In England two more children were born to the family but they were not as healthy as Abdul was in childhood. One suffered from learning disabilities and the other was congenitally deaf.

Abdul had always been of low weight and small in stature but in 1993, at the age of 32 years, his health deteriorated. He visited his family doctor with symptoms of lethargy. He was 52 kg in weight and initial blood tests showed that he was anaemic, and further investigation showed that he had advanced renal (kidney) failure. He was clearly critically ill and his family doctor therefore arranged for him to be admitted to the hospital as a matter of urgency. Full assessment included an ultrasound scan that showed the kidneys to be small and shrunken, the result of progressive inflammation over a period of perhaps 10 years, usually driven by an immune process. The disease was not reversible. Abdul was started on life-saving dialysis and put on a maintenance programme. In 1996 he received a kidney transplant.

On further investigation he was shown to have a low serum calcium level in the blood and the serum parathyroid hormone (PTH) concentration was very high. The combination of the two indicates biochemical features of osteomalacia, the result of vitamin D deficiency, and he was given the vitamin D supplement that was necessary. However, the vitamin D supplement had to be stopped quite early because his blood calcium level rose to above the normal range; he had developed tertiary hyperparathyroidism, a rare but well-recognised complication of advanced chronic renal failure.

In 1995 Abdul sustained a fracture of the scapula, an unusual fracture that was almost certainly a manifestation of continuing osteomalacia. The next development was in 1997, when he developed enlarged lymph glands in the neck, cervical lymphadenopathy. Chest x-rays showed more enlarged lymph glands within the chest. Biopsy of the neck glands confirmed the clinical suspicion of tuberculosis and he was given a 6-month course of treatment with rifampicin, isoniazid and pyrazinamide.

In 1998 Abdul developed sudden onset of weakness of his left arm; this was because of a cerebral infarction, a stroke. In 2001 he was admitted to hospital as an emergency because of a sudden onset of chest pain. An ECG showed features of myocardial infarction (heart attack). On that admission he was found to have a high blood glucose level and a diagnosis of diabetes was made. He later went on to receive treatment with oral hypoglycaemic agents.

In 2002 his kidney function deteriorated and it appeared that the immunological/inflammatory process (glomerulonephritis) that had damaged his natural kidneys was now damaging the transplanted kidney. In October 2004 he was admitted as an emergency because of a sudden onset of weakness of the right leg. He had sustained a further cerebral infarction, or stroke. Blood tests showed deteriorating renal function. Despite this huge burden of illness during the past 10 years, Abdul remained cheerful and optimistic. This was the last time I saw Abdul.

In December 2004 he developed a staphylococcal septicaemia. Despite full intensive care support, his kidney function deteriorated rapidly and he died. His age was 43 years. The good life that Abdul's parents expected for their children had failed to materialise.

-------------------------------------------------------------

Frank was born in Accrington in 1943, into a household of significant socio-economic deprivation. His father had been born in 1910 but had a great deal of illness. He had spent quite a lot of time as a young man in a sanatorium being treated for tuberculosis. This meant that he was never able to establish regular employment, and at the time Frank was born he was working as a part-time caretaker. Frank's mother did some work as a part-time cleaner.

Frank passed through school without education making much of an impact on him, and he left at the age of 15 without any qualifications. He had a succession of jobs in unskilled work, usually as a storeman. He married at the age of 24 and had two children. The cycle of socio-economic deprivation continued and there was never much money in the family. They lived in a small house close to the centre of Accrington.

In his early 20s, Frank developed dyspepsia and, after a barium x-ray, was found to have a duodenal ulcer. At the age of 31 years, because of worsening symptoms, surgical treatment (vagotomy and pyloroplasty) was undertaken in 1974, shortly before effective medical treatment became available.

He became unemployed in 1980 at the age of 37 and did not work afterwards. By that time ill health had developed, mainly in the form of low-grade bronchitis. He had smoked 20 cigarettes a day during his adult life but did not drink very much alcohol.

At the age of 40 Frank was admitted to hospital as an emergency because of severe chest pain, which was found to be caused by a myocardial infarction. Appropriate medical treatment was given and he made a good immediate recovery but subsequently developed angina. By the age of 48 he was experiencing pain in his calf muscles on walking and peripheral atherosclerotic vascular disease was diagnosed. This progressively worsened, causing quite severe restriction of mobility. He continued to smoke despite advice to stop.

Although he was thin as a child and young adult, his weight increased when he stopped work and this also affected his mobility. In 1996, at the age of 53 years, he had a stroke, a cerebral infarction, causing a right hemiplegia and a severe speech disturbance. He spent 2 months in hospital and recovery was only partial.

In 2002 he was admitted to hospital because of severe chest pain, the result of a further myocardial infarction, but he survived this further development. He was left severely disabled and was unable to go outside. He was not able to manage stairs and slept downstairs.

In 2004 he had a second stroke, which was fatal. His age was 61 years.

-----------------------------------------------------------------

Stuart was a doctor, a director of public health in Lancashire. He was careful about his personal health, not smoking, moderate with alcohol, eating the right food, taking exercise, having normal cholesterol and blood pressure. It came as surprise to him when he developed chest pain at the age of 58 years, but he realised that he was having a heart attack. He was admitted to hospital and a diagnosis of myocardial infarction was made; he went on to make a good recovery. He was so puzzled by this unexpected turn of events that he wrote an article 'Why me?' [1]. He could not understand his predisposition to an illness that he, like others, was taught to be to the result of a faulty lifestyle, and his was faultless. But he remembered, when I was in conversation with him, that as a child he was badly sunburnt and for the rest of his life he was very careful to avoid exposure of his skin to the sun. Stuart died at the age of 70.

-------------------------------------------------------------

*Leila's skin is pale and immaculate, soft as a baby's bottom. The facial colour changes between white, yellow and pale grey. The life she leads is reflected in her childlike skin that never sees the sun, and her hands – rough and worn like an old woman's. For a long time, Leila felt dizzy and weak – when she eventually went to see the doctor, he said she needed sun and vitamin D.*

*Paradoxically Kabul is one of the sunniest towns in the world. The sun shines nearly every day of the year, 1800 metres above sea level. The sun makes cracks in the earth, dries up what were once moist gardens, burns the children's skin. But Leila never sees it. It never reaches the first-floor flat in Mikrorayon, nor in behind her burka. Not one single curative ray gets past the grille. Only when she visits her big sister Mariam, who has a backyard in her village house, does she allow the sun to warm her body. But she goes there only on rare occasions.*

*Aimal is Sultan's youngest son. He is twelve years old and works twelve hours a day. Every day, seven days a week, he is woken up at daybreak. At eight in the morning, Aimal opens the door to a little booth in the dark lobby of one of Kabul's hotels. Here he sells chocolate, biscuits, soft drinks and chewing gum. He counts the money and is bored. He calls the shop 'the dreary room'. His heart bleeds and his tummy churns every time he opens the door. This is where he must sit until he is fetched at eight o'clock in the evening, when it is already dark outside. He goes straight home to eat supper and go to bed.*

Åsne Seierstad, *The Bookseller of Kabul* [2]

# PART 1

# UNDERSTANDING ILLNESS AND DISEASE

# 1
# THE NATURE OF DISEASE

The improved health of the population of the UK and western Europe is quite remarkable compared with what it was 100 or more years ago. There are, of course, many exceptions, and disabling or fatal illness can strike individuals at a time when they should be looking forward to many more years of active life. It is inevitable, however, that we must look at averages and at the population in general, but not forgetting the misfortunes of individual people.

When we use a descriptive term such as average life expectancy, it is good to think that 50% survive beyond that average, but our concern must be with those who die at an age below the average. The approach of public health is to do just that, to improve the average and, in particular, the life expectancy of the young. What we find is that during the past 100 years or more the life expectancy from birth has shown the most dramatic improvement, whereas the life expectancy of someone who has survived to the age of, say, 40 years has improved only a little. It is the prevention of childhood illness that has shown the most success.

But adult health has also improved, mainly in the reduction of illness and disability (that is morbidity) rather than death (mortality). This has been expressed most clearly as 'the compression of morbidity' [1,2], indicating that, whereas in former times illness became a characteristic of many years of late adult life, we find today that adults are remarkably healthy for many years, until things appear to go wrong quite suddenly, leading to a relatively short period of illness before inevitable death. The reasons for this may be medical interventions, such as hip replacement surgery, that maintain activity in the place of previous disability, but there are clearly other factors that are also responsible.

A recent example of the compression of morbidity is the late Alistair Cooke, who died on 30 March 2004 at the age of 95 years. He had been working on his weekly broadcast of *Letter from America* until only about 6 weeks before his death. He fell at home and was confined to bed as a result. His decline in health was then rapid and irreversible.

To be able to form conclusions about the survival of the population and to reach judgements about the health of the population in the distant or near past, we must be aware that the collection of accurate data is vital. This is a fairly recent phenomenon and, at a national level, it requires a high level of government organisation through a high-quality civil service. This inevitably means that comparisons between different countries are not always reliable, and it also means that historical comparisons can have rather uncertain foundations.

It is also important to appreciate that the understanding of illness and disease is not absolute but varies over time and, to a certain extent, can be cultural. This again complicates international comparisons, and we find that descriptions and indeed concepts of illness might be very different. Even within Europe and North America we find some major differences, well described in the book *Medicine and Culture: Notions of Health and Sickness in Britain, the US, France and West Germany* [3].

An example of differing concepts of illness between otherwise similar countries is 'hypotension' (low blood pressure). Gillian Hatt, a social scientist from the University of Bath, UK, noted in a letter to *The Lancet* [4]:

*As someone who is interested in the sociology of medicine I am confused by the debate about the existence of hypotension as a clinical syndrome. This condition seems to be recognised as a serious illness in Germany but Anglo-American physicians do not consider it to be a clinical entity. And when British doctors state that the condition does exist it is often identified as a psychiatric symptom associated predominantly with 'neurotic women'. How can a clinical entity 'exist' in one country but not in another?*

It is possible that differences are diminishing because of the internationalisation of clinical medicine (a result of a move to English as the international language of medicine), more international conferences and multinational collaborative research projects such as MONICA, which we will visit in later chapters.

I have used the words 'illness' and 'disease' and it is important to determine exactly what these words mean. 'Illness' is applicable to an individual and is an expression of a perceived or real disturbance of the physical or psychological state of that individual, bringing him or her to a disadvantage regarding work and enjoyment of life. Illness is effectively a disability but is very much part of the individual person. 'Disease' is something different. Disease is something that is scientific, meaning that it can be measured and is objective, not just the result of the opinion of one person. It is general to the population and not specific to an individual.

Diabetes is a disease. It was first measured in a qualitative way by the recognition of a sweet taste to the urine, associated with severe illness that was usually fatal within a few days or weeks. The diagnostic test was refined by the chemical detection of a sugar (later identified as glucose) in the urine in a semi-quantitative way, using the Fehling's or Benedict's reactions, graded by one to four plus signs. More recently it became possible to measure the glucose content of the blood in a fully quantitative way as milligrams (mg) of glucose per 100 millilitres (mL) of blood, a measurement system still used in the USA, but also as millimols per litre (mmol/L), this being part of the standard international (SI) unit nomenclature used in the UK and other European countries. It is quite clear, therefore, that by random testing an individual can be defined as having diabetes by a simple blood test, even at a time when the individual has no symptoms or perception of illness.

This leads to another issue: at what point is it decided to differentiate those suffering from diabetes from the 'normal' population? In this example we must ask what we accept as a normal blood glucose level and what we regard as abnormal. Because the measurement of blood glucose is scientific and objective, it is not the responsibility of the individual to determine whether or not he or she has the disease, but it is determined by a health professional based on results of blood tests.

The World Health Organization (WHO) determined that 11 mmol/L is the level of blood glucose above which a person is diagnosed as having diabetes. But what if the threshold were to be reduced to 10? There has been discussion of this because there is a feeling that a blood glucose of between 10 and 11 places an individual at a health disadvantage compared with others with a level of less than 10, and those in this marginal range could be included in the disease state. Such a change would immediately increase the proportion of people in the population with diabetes and so it can be seen that redefining a disease can have a major influence when we look at historical comparisons with the present day. An 'epidemic' can be the result of better case finding rather than true incidence of disease.

Increasingly during the 20th century, diseases have become defined by many new methods of biochemical testing that are cheap, rapid and readily available. Indeed, such is the widespread use of routine blood tests that doctors are increasingly detecting disease in people who are not aware that they might be ill.

This brings us back to 'illness', which, as mentioned, is the way in which an individual experiences a health disadvantage. Certain characteristics of the individual combine with the disease to produce the illness, and so it is convenient to think of illness in terms of a simple formula:

$$\text{illness} = \text{disease} \times \text{behaviour}$$

What this means is that the expression of a given disease (for example diabetes or influenza) on the sufferer can be amplified or otherwise modulated by the behaviour or other characteristics of that individual.

There has been a great deal of research into 'illness behaviour', which is related to individuals and has many cultural and ethnic variations. Perhaps the most important work on illness behaviour was undertaken by David Mechanic, from the University of Wisconsin, USA, and a summary of his work was published in 1961 [5]. He studied the ethnic basis of illness behaviour, demonstrating, for example, that 71% of Jewish people in the study and 70% of Episcopalians expressed a high inclination to use medical facilities compared with only 32% of Christian Scientists and 42% of Catholics. He quoted the previous work of Mark Zborowski, which indicated that people of Jewish and Italian extraction tended to exaggerate their pain experience, while those of Irish extraction proved more stoical [6]. These differences indicate that individuals, families and communities respond to illness in socially patterned ways.

There had previously been a study indicating that people from higher income groups tend to report themselves ill more readily than those of lower income groups [7]. This study also pointed out that people from lower socio-economic groups tend to have more symptoms but report themselves to be ill less often than those of higher socio-economic groups, and are less likely to visit a doctor. This ultimately became known as the 'inverse care law', that those with the greatest medical need are least likely to seek or receive it. These issues are of immense importance when we try to look at patterns of disease in different societies and in different countries: are we measuring true disease incidence or perceived incidence?

Although generalisations are interesting when understanding concepts such as illness behaviour, the important part of the medical process is when a patient reports an illness. It is the responsibility of the doctor to identify the disease component of that illness and it is helpful if the doctor has available a method of measurement that allows an objective identification of disease. Measurement removes uncertainty and removes much of the potential error of the doctor. It also improves standardisation and reduces argument and opinion.

Blood tests have made identification of disease readily available to the doctor, with the minimum of discomfort and danger to the patient. However, many blood tests lack sensitivity and it is possible for major disease to be present with blood tests remaining normal. This applies in particular to most forms of cancer.

We therefore need alternative methods of measurement to supplement blood tests. Clinical examination is of limited value because of its low level of sensitivity, which means that disease must become very advanced before it can be detected by the eye, the hand or the stethoscope of the doctor. The invention of X-ray technology in 1895 by Wilhelm Roentgen, at the time Professor of Physics at the University of Würzburg, Bavaria, was an enormous step forward, enabling a doctor to look inside the body of a patient. However, its value is limited, being restricted mainly to bone structures and the lungs, but it was nevertheless an extremely important development.

X-ray technology was improved by a staggering proportion with the invention of computed tomography (CT) in the early 1970s by the English engineer Sir Godfrey Hounsfield (1919–2004), who was working in the laboratories of EMI (Electrical and Musical Industries) in the UK. He shared the Nobel Prize in medicine in 1979 with Allan Cormack, a South African physicist who developed a similar imaging system independently. CT scanning enabled the radiological examination of the soft tissues within the body, in particular those enclosed by the skull. Further remarkable refinements of CT have been developed since, as a result of the increase in computer power that we have seen during the past 30 years.

Further important technological advances have been ultrasound scanning, once again looking at soft tissue structures in the body, particularly within the abdomen. This was first developed in the 1940s by Theodore Dussik at the University of Vienna, Austria, refined in the 1950s by Donald Neal and John Read at the National Cancer Institute of the USA, and introduced as an important clinical tool by Ian Donald, Professor of Obstetrics and Gynaecology at the University of Glasgow, UK. Donald was able to locate and examine the developing foetus, initially to identify its position and also the uterine attachment of the placenta. The most recent advances of ultrasound technology allow the inspection of detailed facial and internal features of the foetus at a remarkably early stage.

Magnetic resonance imaging (MRI) is another modality for looking into the body, based on the physico-biological principles first described by Paul Lauterbur in New York, USA, and Sir Peter Mansfield in Nottingham, UK. Raymond Damadian in the USA built the first MR scanner in 1970, and produced the first human images in 1977.

Another important technology for the determination of internal disease is the electrocardiograph (ECG) for investigating the electrical function of the heart. The first machine was invented by Augustus Waller (1856–1922) in 1887, while he was working at St Mary's Hospital, London, UK, based on the electrometer invented in Germany in 1872 by Gabriel Lippmann (1845–1921), who in 1908 received the Nobel Prize for Physics for the invention of colour photography. However, a much more sensitive machine, using a moving-string galvanometer, was invented in 1901 by the physiologist Willem Einthoven (1860–1927), Professor of Physiology at the University of Leiden, the Netherlands. This technology has enabled the rhythm of the heart to be displayed and the presence of disease of the heart muscle to be identified with very considerable sensitivity and accuracy.

All these technologies are what can be described as non-invasive, which effectively means that nothing is introduced inside the body. Minimally invasive technologies appeared somewhat later. The first gastroscope, an instrument to visualise the inside of the stomach, was introduced by Rudolf Schindler in the early 1920s in Berlin, Germany. With the help of the German instrument maker George Wolf, the initial rigid gastroscope was modified with a flexible tip about 10 years later. The invention of fibre-optic technology in the1950s was the next important breakthrough. Harold Horace Hopkins at the Imperial College of Science and Technology in London, UK, first developed the idea that a fibre-optic bundle could be used as the basis of a scope for viewing the internal parts of the human body (an endoscope). On receipt of a grant from the Royal Society, the development work was undertaken by Narinder Kapany for his doctoral research [8]. Hopkins' and Kapany's crude fibre-optic bundle ultimately transformed the gastroscope into a flexible, technologically advanced and clinically useful instrument, mainly by the large Japanese optical industries. Fibre-optic endoscopes enable internal examination of the body through natural openings (orifices), namely the mouth, nose, anus, vagina and urethra, and also by minimal artificial openings, such as laparoscopy, arthroscopy, thoracoscopy, etc. These technologies are widely used and considerably diminish the dangers to patients compared with traditional surgical exploratory procedures.

The point of all these technologies is to look for pathology, which means visible disease, a structural abnormality of the body that must, by definition, lead to a disadvantage to the individual. One of the most important medical scientific philosophers of all time was Theophrastus Von Hohenheim, born in Zurich, Switzerland, in 1493. He was known as Paracelsus and his thinking became the basis of the medical–scientific enlightenment of the late 17th century. He was the first person to establish the concept of pathology [reviewed by Charles Webster; 9,10]. Paracelsus conceived disease as being a specific entity, with localised abnormalities within the body possessing a distinct natural cause, and he formed the view that the specificity of disease would lead to specific remedies. This was very much in contrast to previous medical thinking based on the writings of Galen, which had no vision of intervention or cure. The views of Paracelsus were also in contrast to the religious concepts of illness as being demonic possession, with people resigning themselves to what was inevitable as God's will. An example of the previous Galenistic teaching was that of hysteria, in which it was said that illness in women was the result of the womb (uterus, hysteros) moving around inside the body and causing mischief. It was this vague and unprovable concept that Paracelsus challenged. An important part of his early work was the identification of mercury poisoning as an occupational disease. Perhaps of even greater importance, he also identified that mercury poisoning could have certain advantages, and this led to the development of mercury treatment for syphilis, a disease that was widespread and feared at that time.

The process of pathology as a scientific and clinical discipline is to look at abnormal tissue using not only the naked eye but also the microscope, a process pioneered in particular by the German pathologist Rudolf Virchow. Once again, we have a system of measurement that ideally should not be subjective. All pathologists must use a common visual 'language' to avoid confusion and to allow communication of standardised clinical information. In practice, however, there is inevitably a grey area, the importance of which is intensified by our present-day insistence on early detection of disease, in particular cancer. A definite diagnosis will inevitably be late in the course of a patient's illness. The pressures upon the pathologist to make the diagnosis early can result in uncertainty, with difficulty in determining whether microscopic appearances are compatible with a normal range or whether they lie outside that range and indicate a disease state. Sometimes the pathologist will honestly express uncertainty and must be applauded in doing so. Pathologists might seek a further opinion, which could be from themselves after an interval of time and the inspection of tissue at a later stage in the patient's illness, or be a second opinion from a colleague. Once again we are faced with uncertainty that could cause data from two locations to be unreliable or incompatible.

Medical processes in Britain, Germany, Scandinavia and North America are strongly based on pathology but things are not necessarily the same in other countries. A striking example is the frequent diagnosis of liver disease in the French population, a diagnosis based on a patient's symptoms and indeed usually a self-diagnosis. In the UK, a diagnosis of liver disease would always be based on abnormal blood tests and possibly a liver biopsy examination (that is, objective evidence of disease). This has not, until recently, been the case in France, where a diagnosis of 'liverish' would appear to represent an illness, the major component of which is likely to be behaviour with only a minor component of disease.

However, we must be careful in making such assertions, as there must be some diseases at present that are not yet measurable. An attribution of symptoms to the liver might be mistaken but there must be patterns of disease that are not yet fully identified.

The process of clinical medicine is thus the process of initially recognising a pattern that different people might have in common. Such a pattern is purely descriptive and is often called a 'syndrome'. Although it hides considerable ignorance of cause, it is an important aid to understanding and an important step towards treatment. The second stage is to describe a structural abnormality, a pathology, and the third step is to identify the cause. An example is epidemic jaundice as the descriptive term, hepatitis as the pathology and the virus hepatitis A as the cause. Another example is heart attack as a general descriptive term and myocardial infarction as the pathology, but in this example there is no identification of the cause of the disease process and so our understanding stops with a pathological description.

Descriptive statistics (data) are generally based on disease, which is measurable, rather than illness, which is not, and this is particularly so when we are dealing with disease that has a fatal outcome. Although a disease might be recognised with adequate accuracy, data collection demands a process continuing from recognition to recording, and this must be in a form that is standardised. It must then be collected and assimilated. Death certification is of immense importance because it feeds these processes nationally, and internationally through WHO. Historically, the accuracy of the death certificate has depended upon autopsy information but in recent years up-to-date imaging techniques have helped in the identification of disease before death.

This means that, at the present time, the recorded causes of death are more accurate than in times gone by. Data collection is improving and comparisons between different locations and different times are becoming more powerful.

# 2
# DISEASE PATTERNS IN THE 18TH AND 19TH CENTURIES

Disease statistics at the turn of the 18th and 19th centuries were collected because of the efforts of inspired individuals who laid the foundations of public health medicine in the UK. One such person was Thomas Percival (1740–1804), who worked in Manchester and collected data on the patterns of disease and causes of death towards the end of the 18th century. His important contribution was an essay entitled *Observations on the State of the Population of Manchester and Other Adjacent Places*, based on a survey of Manchester and Salford in 1773 (population 27 246) and comparing this industrial conurbation with surrounding rural towns and villages [1]. Table 2.1 indicates the causes of death and it is interesting to note that old age was second to consumption (tuberculosis). Dropsy was an illness characterised by swelling of the legs and could have been the result of heart failure or kidney disease.

**Table 2.1  Causes of death 1773, Manchester and Salford [1]**

| Diseases | Males | Females | Total |
|---|---|---|---|
| Child-bed | 0 | 2 | 2 |
| Chincough | 0 | 2 | 2 |
| Consumption | 23 | 15 | 38 |
| Diabetes | 1 | 0 | 1 |
| Fever (typhoid) | 12 | 11 | 23 |
| Infants | 7 | 6 | 13 |
| Measles | 0 | 2 | 2 |
| Old age | 11 | 19 | 30 |
| Small pox | 7 | 6 | 13 |
| Dysentery | 1 | 1 | 2 |
| Dropsy | 0 | 3 | 3 |
| Apoplexy | 2 | 1 | 3 |

Percival reported that the population of Manchester and Salford experienced deaths per annum in the order of 1 in 28, similar to 1 in 27.7 in Liverpool. The population fared better in rural locations, many of which were to become industrialised a century later. The death rate per annum in Edale was 1 in 59, in Horwich 1 in 66, in Darwen 1 in 56 and in Hale 1 in 69. Similarly, we find that in Manchester and Salford only 1 in 8 of the population lived beyond their 50th birthday, whereas the corresponding proportion in the rural location of Hale was 1 in 3.5 and in Chinley 1 in 3. In Manchester and Salford 1 out of 2 children died before their 5th birthday but in rural Royton (now a suburb of Oldham) the corresponding number was much lower, at 1 in 7. We therefore have what is perhaps the first accurate recording of the geography of disease.

Defining disease is helped by measurements taken at the bedside or in the laboratory, but an equally important place of measurement has been that of populations based in the community, as a result of the work of individuals such as Thomas Percival. The subject has been reviewed by Ulrich Tröhler, who was born in Bern, Switzerland, and is at present Professor and Chairman of the Department of the History of Medicine at the University of Freiburg, Germany. His fascinating book, *To Improve the Evidence of Medicine* [2], describes the work of individuals such as Percival, and Tröhler emphasises the exceptional contribution of Scotland and its physicians. We shall see later the importance of the accurate recording of disease but on a national basis, which is fundamental to international comparisons.

The great physician William Heberden made similar observations concerning deaths in London, published in 1801 [3]. He was particularly concerned with the changing patterns of disease during the 18th century. Such observations of change can provide important clues regarding cause, as we shall see during later chapters of this book. Some of Heberden's observations are shown in Table 2.2 and it can be seen that consumption (tuberculosis) showed the greatest and most significant increase.

**Table 2.2 Deaths in 10-year periods in the 18th century [3]**

|  | Beginning | Middle | End |
|---|---|---|---|
| Abortive and still-born | 600 | 570 | 750 |
| Colic, flux, gripes, etc. | 1100 | 135 | 20 |
| Consumption | 3000 | 4000 | 5000 |
| Dropsy | 850 | 900 | 900 |
| Evil | 70 | 15 | 8 |
| Fever | 3000 | 3000 | 2000 |
| Gout | 26 | 40 | 66 |
| Lunatic | 27 | 75 | 70 |
| Palsy, apoplexy, etc. | 157 | 280 | 300 |
| Rickets | 380 | 11 | 1 |
| Small pox | 1600 | 2000 | 2000 |

It must be remembered that both Percival and Heberden collected their data at a time of immense social change. The Bridgewater Canal, built by the pioneer canal engineer James Brindley in 1759, allowed coal to be floated from the Duke of Bridgewater's mines in Worsley, lying to the north-west of Manchester, to the centre of the city at Castlefield, close to the former Roman fortress and an area that has recently been redeveloped and restored. The construction of the Bridgewater Canal was part of the infrastructure that allowed the development of a city such as Manchester. The canal supplied fuel for its industry and for its rapidly growing population. George Stephenson's Liverpool and Manchester Railway was opened in 1830 to allow this process to develop even further. Similar industrialisation was happening in London and other cities, but whether the population growth and industrialisation of cities such as Manchester in the early part of the 19th century should be considered a good thing is a matter of opinion. It created a pattern of development and urban growth that has been replicated world-wide and it is a process that continues to the present day, most obviously in China.

The process of industrialisation and the concentration of its workforce in new big cities had several important social effects. Science and education, which developed in the age of enlightenment and which stimulated the process of industrialisation, also played an essential part in the development and organisation of health care. The very process of concentrating the population, at a time when industrialisation was taking place and medicine was developing in its wake, meant that the pattern of illness could, for the first time, be recorded by individuals such as Percival and Heberden. The health profile of the rural populations in earlier times had not been recorded in a structured way.

The information that Percival provides is that, in 1773, 1 child in 9 died from smallpox and the other major cause of death was measles, this being the cause of death in 1 in 52 children. Both are microbial diseases.

I use the word 'microbial' to describe diseases that are caused by a micro-organism, for example a cellular organism, a bacterium or a virus, no matter how the disease is spread. Infectious diseases are those that spread rapidly from one person to another, usually by droplet infection through the respiratory tract. The common cold and measles are examples of these. Contagious diseases are also communicable from one person to another, but through the process of direct contact, that is touching. Examples would be certain skin diseases, including smallpox. Water-borne diseases are those resulting from contamination of the water supply. Food poisonings are to the result of microbial contamination of food. Micro-organisms can be passed from one person to another by sexual activity. Transmission can also be by the transfusion of blood or blood products. Finally, micro-organisms can be transmitted from other animals, such as malaria from the mosquito and avian flu from birds. The opportunities for micro-organisms to cause disease are immense and continuous. I believe that more diseases than generally recognised are caused by micro-organisms, including possibly coronary heart disease, and this will be dealt with later in the book.

The number of deaths from measles decreased during the 19th and 20th centuries, even though the disease itself remained common. Measles became virtually eradicated in the UK in the late 20th century, when immunisation was introduced, but it is important to realise that the numbers of deaths attributed to measles and similar diseases were declining well before the introduction of immunisation. We will look at this in the next chapter.

Cholera became a significant cause of death in the 19th century, arriving in Europe in a series of pandemics, probably introduced with the increased volume of shipping from the Far East, where the disease was endemic. The first pandemic of cholera was in 1817 and the second reached the UK in 1831. Cholera is a water-borne infection caused by a bacterium called *Vibrio cholera*. It is still an important disease and cause of death at a world-wide scale and it is effectively the result of the concentration of populations. More directly it is the result of contamination of the water supply by faecal excrement, and it indicates that, when large numbers of people live together in small geographical locations, organisational and engineering processes must be developed to separate domestic effluent from the water supply.

Although cholera had been identified as a specific disease early in the 19th century, its cause was unknown and indeed, at that time, microbiology had not developed. The existence of micro-organisms was unknown. It was not even appreciated that cholera was a result of contaminated water supplies until an inspired physician, Dr John Snow, made the deduction. He must be regarded as one of the fathers of epidemiology, the study of the patterns of disease. Epidemiology demonstrates the clues that allow us to form hypotheses or theories regarding how a disease might occur and what the cause might be. Epidemiological investigations will form a very major part of this book.

John Snow was a physician working in London at the time of an outbreak of cholera in 1854. He investigated the local geography of the disease by drawing a map and on it identifying the houses of those who developed the disease. He noted quite clearly a clustering effect, that the disease had a distinct geographical pattern and that the cluster had the common and central feature of a water pump in Broad Street. His observation led him to suggest, in a forcible way, that the water coming from the pump in Broad Street and being consumed by the local population was contaminated by something that caused the disease of cholera. At that time, the Divinity was usually invoked as the causation of disease, in retribution for some form of communal sin, and so Snow's hypothesis fell on stony ground, ignored by those in authority over the community. However, Snow was a man of conviction; he took things into his own hands, by removing and hiding the handle of the water pump in Broad Street so that the pump could not be used. This understandably caused an outcry from the population, who consequently had to walk a considerable distance to obtain water. Snow became very unpopular but, after only a few days, no new cases of cholera were reported; the epidemic had come to an abrupt end. Snow was proved correct, not only in his action in making the Broad Street pump unusable, but also in his assertion that cholera was a water-borne disease.

Typhoid (previously simply called 'fever', a less specific term) was another disease that assumed epidemic proportions and was responsible for large numbers of deaths in 19th century England, most notoriously, in 1861, that of Prince Albert, husband of Queen Victoria. The disease was again ultimately recognised as being microbial but the bacterium, *Salmonella typhi*, was not identified until later.

Typhoid was such a serious problem that each city community throughout the UK developed a fever hospital. It usually had two wards, one for typhoid and enteric (diarrhoea) infections and the other for measles and acute respiratory infections. With the improvement of public health, these hospitals generally closed down or were transferred to other functions in the mid-20th century.

Rheumatic fever was not fully established as a single disease process in the 19th century but it was becoming increasingly clear that a sore throat, what we now call a streptococcal throat or tonsillitis, could be followed by acute arthritis or joint pains and then progressive damage to the valves of the heart, leading to disability and death from heart failure. In 1827, Richard Bright, a London physician, published *Reports of Medical Cases*, in which he defined the recognised illness of dropsy (an accumulation of fluid in the tissues, especially the legs) as being a manifestation of kidney disease, characterised by large amounts of protein in the urine (which therefore coagulated on boiling) and shrivelled kidneys at autopsy. However, it was not appreciated that what came to be called Bright's disease had the same cause as rheumatic fever, namely a streptococcal sore throat. We now know that Bright's disease is the result of an immune-mediated process and, with a greater level of understanding, it now carries the pathology-based name of glomerulonephritis. It can have acute, subacute and chronic forms, and end-stage renal failure can develop within a matter of weeks, months or sometimes years after the initial disease.

To understand the nature of present-day diseases, it very important to appreciate that both rheumatic heart disease and glomerulonephritis can have a long latent interval between the onset of the disease process and later clinical manifestations, a characteristic often seen in conditions caused by micro-organisms. As rheumatic fever and Bright's disease became more clearly defined during the 20th century, the incidence reduced considerably, for reasons that are not really obvious.

Syphilis was a very major disease during the 19th century, but initially there was no conceptual unification of a disease that had many features and differed from one person to another. The late stages of the disease were very well described and had three major forms. The first was the presence of tumours or gummas (gummata) occurring in a variety of parts of the body, including the skin. These could be locally destructive. The second major feature was that of cardiovascular disease, with the development of aneurysms (dilatations) of the aorta, the main artery leading from the heart.

These aneurysms could burst, with a rapidly fatal result. Alternatively, the aortic valve of the heart could become damaged, with poor function leading to the gradual development of heart failure, ultimately fatal. The third form involved the nervous system, with two major patterns. General paralysis of the insane (GPI) was a rapidly progressive dementing disease that would affect the sufferers during middle age rather than later life. The other was tabes dorsalis, a disease of the peripheral nerves and spinal cord, resulting in unsteadiness and neurological disability.

At the start of the 21st century, it is easy to underestimate the public health problem of syphilis a century ago, in particular its disabling and neurological manifestations. In fact, the large mental hospitals, or lunatic asylums as they became known, were built in the late 19th century to house the large number of people demented by GPI. The size of these hospitals, frequently with more than 1000 beds, is a reminder of how widespread the disease was at the time.

However, it was not appreciated in the mid-19th century that these late manifestations of syphilis were all part of the same disease and indeed that they might have a common microbial aetiology. As is usually the case, it was an inspired physician (this time Sir Jonathan Hutchinson) who arrived at the hypothesis, many years before the culprit organism *Treponema pallidum* was identified. Further details of syphilis and the lessons to be learned from it follow in Chapter 8.

Another common disabling disease of the 19th century was consumption, what became named as Koch's disease and we now know as tuberculosis. It is particularly well described in the literature that death from consumption was common and that it was associated with a chronic productive cough, wasting of the body and anaemia. It also was noted to cluster in families and was considered to be 'constitutional', that is part of the physical inheritance of the individual. The work of Robert Koch demonstrated that it was the result of a micro-organism, *Mycobacterium tuberculosis*, initially known the tubercle bacillus. The history of tuberculosis is immense and Chapter 11 is devoted to more detail of the importance of it.

But the disease that was feared above all by the population was smallpox. It was not only epidemic and contagious but at best disfiguring and at worst fatal. Isolation of affected people was essential, and by the late 19th century this was in remotely situated municipal hospitals. Immunisation against the disease (variola) was developed during the late 18th century by Edward Jenner (1749–1823), a country practitioner in Gloucestershire, UK. The process was called vaccination because it was based on the related cow-pox vaccinia. Jenner had noted that those working with cows who had developed cow-pox appeared to have protection (what we now call immunity) against smallpox. Isolation policies and vaccination led to the eradication of smallpox in the late 20th century, but a century earlier the disease was still significant.

It important to appreciate that, in the 19th century, the major disease processes leading to death were microbial. There were, of course, other causes of death that must not be forgotten. One of the most important was childbirth and indeed this was a very significant cause of death in young married women; the counterparts in men were industrial accidents and warfare. The major medical breakthrough of the 19th century was the understanding that many diseases were indeed the result of micro-organisms. This may seem obvious now, but it was not a conclusion that was easily reached by the medical profession of years gone by.

# 3

# THE CHANGING PATTERN OF DISEASE IN THE 20TH CENTURY

Industrial development in the late 18th and the 19th centuries was immensely important to public health. It created the infrastructure that allowed the prosperity that finally emerged at the end of the 20th century, delayed by almost a century of European and world war. The triumphs of industrialisation were those of mechanical and social engineering. The end of the 19th century saw the building of huge numbers of houses for working class and new middle class people in the cities. All these houses were provided with piped uncontaminated water, flush toilets, sewage disposal, adequate lighting and ventilation, a supply of gas and ultimately electricity. The transport infrastructure had supplemented the earlier canals with an extensive network of suburban and national railways and a network of roads with street patterns providing a good level of ventilation. City-wide transport was provided by tram services.

Social engineering in England, with an emphasis on education, established the universities of London, Manchester, Birmingham and Leeds to supplement the existing universities of Oxford and Cambridge, and more were to follow. Universal primary and secondary school education was established. Medical care had previously been based on general practice, with a rudimentary pre-payment system depending on local initiative. During industrialisation the local authority of each major town developed a hospital (the general hospital) together with a fever hospital, a tuberculosis sanatorium and often, in a particularly remote location, a smallpox hospital. Many towns had also developed, on private initiative, voluntary hospitals (infirmaries) funded by public subscription.

With all these developments in place, the end of the 19th century culminated in what the French recognised as the glorious 20 years, leading into the Edwardian era with rapidly growing prosperity and the Art Nouveau movement of design and building. The hard work and social deprivations of the 19th century were beginning to reap the long-awaited rewards. But, as the economist John Maynard Keynes remarked in 1919: 'That extraordinary episode in the economic progress of man … came to an end in August 1914' [1].

The first 'epidemic' of death of the 20th century erupted in 1914. The massive mortality was, of course, of the young men caught up in a pointless war. The First World War was followed by the second epidemic of death, the major influenza epidemic that is thought to have been responsible for the deaths of just as many people as the war itself.

Great Britain, and Europe in general, therefore staggered into the 1920s in a much weaker state than they had entered the 20th century. A major social initiative of the Edwardian era in the UK was the Social Security Bill of 1911, introduced by the government led by the Liberal prime minister, David Lloyd George. This created a number of initiatives but perhaps the major one in respect to health was the introduction of social insurance, a progressive form of taxation, meaning that it was related to income. This was a funding stream levied on all working people and it meant that they could receive certain benefits at times of hardship, including specific aspects of health care, sickness pay and a pension. The health care component would pay for general practice care, enabling all of the population to have a general practitioner who would be paid from government funds, using social insurance contributions, on the basis of a capitation fee paid to the doctor. It meant that not only would the poor receive the care of a doctor but also that doctors would receive an income irrespective of the prosperity of the local community that they would serve.

The initial proposal of the Social Insurance Bill went further, to provide a social insurance funding stream for hospital care, but this was ultimately withdrawn from the Act because of very strong opposition from the consultants of the country through the British Medical Association. In retrospect this can be seen to have been a very major misjudgement, leading to later nationalisation of the hospitals.

The First World War necessitated the diversion of industrial production and construction into warfare and munitions, and resulted in a major loss of manpower. As a result, throughout the 1920s and 1930s, the country was pushed back into relative poverty. The economic and social progress made at the turn of the century was reversed and was not to recover for more than half a century.

Because of political paralysis, health improvement would still depend upon enlightened individuals rather than the government. One of these was Dr Macaulay, who was responsible for the vision that created a network of high-quality municipal hospitals throughout Middlesex. This could have become a national blueprint for delivery of hospital care in the UK but in fact failed to do so. The reason for this was that the country was once again plunged into war in 1939, with the war effort requiring almost the totality of industrial production, the male and increasingly female workforce and, perhaps most importantly of all, the attention of the government.

There are few benefits from war, but both the First and Second World Wars did provide a major impetus for the development of surgical techniques and surgical training. Wars in the 19th and 20th centuries have provided important opportunities for the development of surgical practice and its organisation. Penicillin was also introduced during the Second World War.

The development of surgery was based on two major foundations. The first was the introduction of anaesthetic gases. The second was the recognition of micro-organisms as a cause of disease and, in particular, as the cause of suppurating wound infections (discharging pus). We owe this advance in understanding to the chemist Louis Pasteur, working in Paris, France, who first identified bacteria. Joseph (later Lord) Lister, an Edinburgh surgeon, realised the importance of Pasteur's work in respect to wound infections, and he challenged the previous idea that oxygen in the atmosphere was the cause of pus. Lister's work was helped by his father's occupation, refining the achromatic lens, which enabled good-quality microscopes and the routine identification of bacteria to be developed. Lister's important next step, after his initial work in 1865, was the introduction of antisepsis with chemical disinfectants, carbolic and phenolic acids, which destroyed bacteria. It was, however, a considerable time before his methods of asepsis and antisepsis were widely applied.

The economic problems of the inter-war years created a major funding crisis for the voluntary hospitals of the UK, which were facing bankruptcy even at the turn of the century. Expenditure was greater than income, and the infirmaries were surviving on their financial reserves; clinical activity was increasing ahead of fund-raising, still a characteristic of health services as we move into the 21st century. The crisis of funding of the infirmaries precipitated the creation of the National Health Service (NHS) in 1948. It was quite clear that the population was entitled to expect a better hospital service than the one that was rapidly deteriorating even before the Second World War began.

Despite everything, mortality rates from specific diseases were falling during the first half of the 20th century, probably for reasons of public health engineering inherited from the late 19th century. It can be seen from Figure 3.1 that the most important improvements in mortality were achieved before 1930. It can also be seen that these were not really the result of medical interventions, which, other than improvements in hygiene, had little to offer at that time. The steep fall in mortality had flattened out by the time the NHS was created in 1948.

**Figure 3.1 Standardised mortality ratio, England and Wales [2].**
(base year 1950–52 = 100)

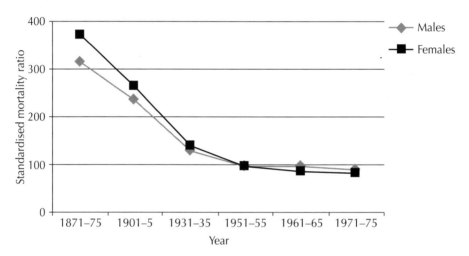

I introduce here the term 'standardised mortality ratio' (SMR) and we will meet this on many occasions. It is a way by which the death rates of different groups of people are compared. In this example it compares one time with another, but it can also compare one location with another. One group is assigned a standard of 100 and the other is a proportion relative to that. In Figure 3.1, the death rate of 1950–52 is assigned 100 and the other years are expressed relative to it. In 1871–75, the mortality rate was three to four times higher.

The improvements in health and survival were given a major boost by the introduction of penicillin during the Second World War and then, in about 1950, the introduction of streptomycin, which would provide a treatment opportunity for tuberculosis, still a significant cause of death. However, as shown in Figure 3.2, the number of people dying from tuberculosis had fallen dramatically before the introduction of specific medical interventions. Immunisation was achieved with an attenuated (low virulence mutation) strain of *Mycobacterium tuberculosis* called Bacillus Calmette–Guerin (BCG), named after the researchers who developed it in 1923 at the Pasteur Institute in Lille, France, and introduced widely in the 1950s. Having a relatively low pathogenicity, it produces an immune response without causing significant disease, the objective of all immunisation procedures.

**Figure 3.2 Deaths from tuberculosis expressed as standardised mortality ratio [2].**
(base year 1950–52 = 100)

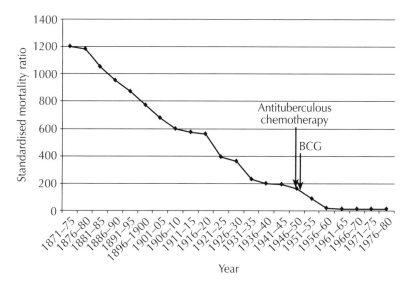

Figure 3.3 shows that the number of children dying from whooping cough (pertussis) had similarly fallen before immunisation became available in 1956.

**Figure 3.3  Deaths from whooping cough expressed as annual death rate per million aged under 15 years.**

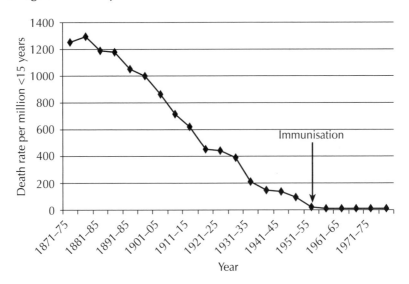

Perhaps, however, the most important health crisis of the mid-20th century occurred on 4 December 1952, the start of the Great London Smog. During the following 5 days a combination of a winter anticyclone and a dramatic increase in atmospheric pollution from coal-fired factories and domestic coal fires led to 4075 more deaths than usual for that time of the year.

The government had to respond to this major crisis as public health was a major responsibility. A bill was rapidly passed through parliament, and the Clean Air Act of 1956 was arguably the most important piece of social engineering of the 20th century. The immediate response was for domestic homes to burn smokeless fuel, thereby reducing particulate emissions into the atmosphere. Factories increasingly turned to oil-fired power generation or electricity from the National Grid. Houses increasingly became heated by oil or gas, and railways changed to diesel oil and electricity.

The last 40 years of the 20th century saw a remarkable reduction in deaths from a wide range of diseases that were identified as being the result of micro-organisms. Syphilis, in all its manifestations, was controlled by penicillin together with a well-organised public health campaign against sexually transmitted disease, with the tracing and treatment of sexual contacts.

But the 20th century saw the emergence of a new disease, publicly known as heart attack but technically called myocardial infarction. It seemed to peak soon after the mid-20th century and then decline for reasons that were not entirely obvious, and we will look into this in more detail later.

The final years of the 20th century saw the emergence of another new disease, at an international scale. This initially started as a series of uncommon clinical phenomena creating a new pattern or syndrome, in other words a new disease entity. It soon became clear, with sophisticated public health monitoring, that the manifestations were mainly low pathogenicity infections that were occurring in people with seriously suppressed immune mechanisms. The disease was AIDS, acquired immune deficiency syndrome, and it was identified as being caused by a transmissible micro-organism, human immunodeficiency virus (HIV). The effects of this virus on certain populations in the world have been devastating, at a time when, in other ways, health has been better than could ever have been imagined.

The opinion of many people is that, with the exception of AIDS, the latter half of the 20th century has seen the conquest of infectious disease in Europe and North America, and that we are now dealing with diseases that are considered to be degenerative. This assessment is wrong; micro-organisms are probably the cause of many diseases that are thought to be the result of something else. To understand such a conclusion requires an understanding of the causation of disease in general and the recognition of the huge potential danger to humans from microbial infection.

# 4

# THE CAUSATION OF DISEASE AND INDIVIDUAL SUSCEPTIBILITY

The cause of disease has different meanings to different people. As far as individuals are concerned, the cause is identified as a life event of that individual. For example, when I developed life-threatening pneumonia at the age of 7 years, my mother was quite convinced that it was the result of snow inside my wellington boots. Many people will have different stories but all will have what is generally called a life event as the explanation for the disease and thus the rational cause. These are specific factors that are applicable only to individuals, as opposed to the general features that are applicable to all.

However, we should not dismiss such stories out of hand. We may, in our scientific society, talk about pneumonia being to the result of the bacterium *Pneumococcus,* otherwise known as *Streptococcus pneumoniae,* and this is the general factor that is present in all people with lobar pneumonia. But then we must ask ourselves what it is about an individual person who develops pneumonia compared other people in the household that do not. This is where the life events do have some importance and where the concept of causation becomes rather blurred.

In reality, most diseases and accidents have a complex causal trail and indeed can be regarded as being multifactorial. Our scientific philosophy identifies causation in physical or biological terms and looks for a common occurrence affecting a number of different people with a given condition. If we look at lobar pneumonia, we can determine that the common finding is the bacterium *Pneumococcus* and we can recognise that, even though snow in wellington boots might have been important for one individual, it was not a common theme across the experience of a large number of people suffering from the disease.

Undergraduate clinical medicine is based very much on the physical and biological sciences. Anatomy, the study of the structure of the body, leads on to pathology, which is the study of the disturbed structure of the body and the identification of specific disease processes, of which pneumonia would be one. Knowledge of biochemistry and its counterpart pathophysiology provides an exciting new glimpse into the fundamental chemical mechanisms of disease, and these can be pursued by research in the laboratory.

However, epidemiology is something different, the breadth of which I never really appreciated whilst an undergraduate. The studies of anatomy, pathology and the clinical specialties look at individual people, whereas epidemiology looks at populations, something that was beyond my vision at a time when my perspective was only the laboratory, the ward or the outpatient clinic. It was only after I had completed my postgraduate medical examinations that, in 1974, whilst browsing a medical bookshop, I came across a small book entitled *Causal Thinking in the Health Sciences* [1]. Its author was Mervyn Susser, who was at the time Professor of Epidemiology in New York, USA, but had been a senior lecturer in the Department of Social and Preventative Medicine at the University of Manchester, UK, when I was an undergraduate. It was a book that changed my way of thinking as I realised the importance of the cause of a disease in general being different from what appeared to be the cause of the illness in an individual person. It also introduced me to the concept of the ways in which two variables might be associated, and the importance of not jumping to a conclusion about the nature of a cause–effect relationship.

But more of this later. For now, it is clear that, when an individual develops a disease, it is because of an interaction between the universal or general cause of that disease and the specific attributes of the individual. By this I mean that the susceptibility to disease will vary between one person and another. So we can see that:

$$\text{cause} + \text{susceptibility} \longrightarrow \text{disease}$$

There is also the issue of a precipitating event. Why should a disease that had been developing slowly over a number of years suddenly produce a serious illness? An example is a heart attack. We will see in later chapters that this is the result of a disease process that starts quite early in life but, after a long latent period, the clinical manifestations suddenly emerge, usually as an illness called myocardial infarction. There might be certain precipitating events for myocardial infarction, and it is a matter of opinion regarding whether these can be considered causative. A sudden emotional upset or sudden strenuous exertion can precipitate myocardial infarction. This is the well-recognised 'acute excited state' appearing to cause sudden death, and this is often the legal conclusion, ignoring the underlying established medical illness that might have been previously unrecognised [2].

An unusual example was described by George Davey Smith, Professor of Clinical Epidemiology, and his colleagues at the University of Bristol, UK [3]. The national football team of England was defeated by that of Argentina in the World Cup by a penalty shoot-out on 30 June 1998. On that day and during the following 2 days, the number of patients between the ages of 15 and 64 years who were admitted to hospital in England on account of acute myocardial infarction increased by 25%. There was no excess of admissions for other diagnoses and there was no excess for admission for myocardial infarction on the day of the other England matches. The only event that seemed to be responsible for this increase was the football match itself. We cannot really regard watching the football match as the cause of myocardial infarction, but this example illustrates the importance of the precipitating event, the acute excited state, the specific factor as opposed to the general factor.

The science of epidemiology has made great contributions to the understanding of disease and thus the pattern of clinical medicine during the past 150 years. It has been based on the tradition of John Snow, the doctor who removed the handle of the Broad Street pump to prevent the spread of cholera. Snow looked at individual episodes of illness and grouped them in terms of time, place and person. Although this relatively simple approach is well suited to acute infectious disease, it is also applicable to chronic disease, the cause of which is not immediately obvious.

The important Framingham study was set up in 1948 to investigate heart disease and try to determine its cause. The study is based on the population of Framingham, a small town in Massachusetts, USA, to look in detail at individual citizens and to identify characteristics that are associated with disease. These characteristics can only be called risk indicators or risk factors and cannot be regarded as causes at this stage. It has been suggested that the major risk indicators that have been identified provide less than 25% of what might be called the understanding of the causation of coronary heart disease [4].

To help appreciate the significance of risk factors, it has been necessary for epidemiologists to continue the tradition of John Snow and intervene.

If the risk factor is removed, does that reduce the incidence of the disease? To progress in this direction, it has been necessary for epidemiologists to work with clinicians, to obtain a better understanding and make useful interventions to improve the natural history of disease [5]. Sometimes these are what might be called lifestyle interventions but there are also interventions regarding medications. Of course, many risk factors might be applicable to the population but not necessarily to individuals.

It is sometimes necessary to influence the lifestyle of many people in order to help the few within that group. For example, not everyone who stops smoking will benefit, as we know only too well that some people who smoke can live healthily for many years and die as a result of old age. Similarly, immunisation is a process given to virtually all children knowing that only a few will benefit. It is in this way, however, that the health of populations can be improved.

We must be cautious in our interpretation of risk factors and, if two variables are associated, for example a lifestyle factor (A) and a health measure (B), we must consider the ways in which they might interact. The major models are shown in Figure 4.1

**Figure 4.1 Models of the interaction between lifestyle factors (A) and measures of health (B).**

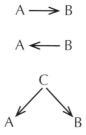

The lifestyle factor that has the strongest association with a variety of indicators of good health is that of eating a family meal sitting around a table when a child. It is difficult to conceive of a direct relationship between the two, and the first model does not appear to be applicable. This is an example in which we must invoke a factor C, something that we do not understand, that can be highly complex but it results in both the lifestyle factor and the health advantage. It could be genetic, environmental or behavioural, as we will see in the next chapter.

# 5
# POSSIBLE CAUSES OF DISEASE

It is important to think in the broadest possible terms of the ways in which diseases can be caused, and it is equally important to separate the cause from mechanisms of production of the disease state, the pathology:

$$cause \longrightarrow mechanism \longrightarrow disease/pathology$$

In the most general terms, a disease is caused by either an incident that occurs before birth or an external event that occurs afterwards.

Genetic disorders occur at the moment of conception. Sometimes genetic abnormalities are the inevitable result of genes acquired from either parent. These most frequently result in disorders of metabolism that can be expressed in a disease pattern shortly after birth or later in development. They are generally classified as dominant, recessive or sex-linked, depending on the precise details of genetic location or action.

Genes are inherited from the parents, each parent supplying one of a pair genes. If the gene from one parent is abnormal and the other normal, this is called the heterozygous state. If the two genes from the two parents are similarly abnormal, this is called the homozygous state.

Congenital spherocytosis is an inherited disorder in which the red blood cells are spherical rather than doughnut shaped. It makes them more fragile, and we will see the effects of this later when we meet the importance of the spleen. It is a dominant genetic disorder; when one gene encoding the disease is present, the disease occurs, even though the paired gene acquired from the other parent might be normal.

The expression of a recessive genetic disorder requires both of a pair of genes, one from each parent, to be abnormal, as one normal gene would enable the metabolic pathway of the offspring to function and therefore no disease would arise. The presence of one abnormal recessive gene results in the carrier state, usually, but not always, without disease expression.

Haemophilia is a sex-linked disease because the gene necessary for the production of blood-clotting factor 8 is carried on the X chromosome. A male child has only one X chromosome and so, if it contains the abnormal gene, then disease will result; a female offspring has two X chromosomes and so, if one is abnormal, the other will enable factor 8 production. Haemophilia will occur in a female only if both X chromosomes carry the abnormal gene, an extremely rare occurrence requiring the mother to be a carrier and the father to have haemophilia.

Mutations can occur as a result of an abnormal gene being created in the reproductive cells of a parent, without it being present in the cells of the body of the parent. Such a disorder, for example achondroplasia, will occur in only one offspring and not in other siblings. It must be a dominant gene for just one of a pair of genes to result in disease; it will then be passed on to the next generation, but statistically only to half of the children if the gene from the other parent is normal. Mutations producing recessive genes will go unnoticed until two such recessive genes are paired.

Sometimes a recessive gene will produce some expression of disease if only one gene is abnormal, the heterozygous state, but much more severe disease will be present if both of the pair of genes are abnormal, the homozygous state. Examples of this are sickle cell disease and familial hypercholesterolaemia. The heterozygous state is many times more common than the homozygous state.

Genetic disease can occur as the result of an apparent accident of the restructuring of genetic material during conception, remembering that a set of chromosomes from the mother contained in the ovum must link with a similar set of chromosomes from the father transmitted in the fertilising spermatozoon. Occasionally during this process part of a chromosome comprising a number of genes might translocate, that is move, from one chromosome to another, a process called genetic scrambling. In the animal world this can produce a new species that can no longer breed with members of the parent species because the chromosomes no longer match. In theory, genetic misadventure can lead to an evolutionary advantage, but this is not usually the case. In the human the most well-known example of genetic scrambling is Down's syndrome, the result of either genetic translocation or, alternatively, trisomy, in which the embryo receives a duplicate of a single chromosome from one parent, thus making a total complement of three rather than two of chromosome 21.

There are, however, a number of diseases apparent at birth that are not determined by genetic disorders but are accidents of development. Examples are club foot and hare lip/cleft palate. Although these can be viewed as accidents, there might be external factors and, for example, the risk of hare lip/cleft palate (craniofacial deformity) is increased considerably by phenytoin taken by the mother for the treatment of epilepsy. These are congenital disorders, not the result of genetic factors.

During birth and thereafter, several other causes of disease can be encountered. Trauma (injury) is quite clearly understood and indeed trauma is a major risk during the process of birth and during childhood. It is the major cause of death of young men. It might be the result of freak accidents but there may be certain factors increasing their susceptibility to accidents. A well-known factor is young men aged between 17 and 25 driving a motorcycle or motorcar. Alcohol further increases susceptibility to death from trauma without itself being the cause of death. From these examples, the interaction between the individual and the environment is becoming obvious. Maternal death during childbirth, particularly in times before useful medical intervention, can be regarded as an additional form of trauma, with a significant susceptibility factor obviously being female sex. Other factors include first pregnancy, especially after the age of 30 years, small stature and childhood rickets causing pelvic deformity.

Deficiency states are also well recognised. We require a variety of nutrients to maintain good health and without them disability and death can occur. Deficiency of oxygen in certain situations and deficiency of water are the most extreme and obvious examples. Deficiencies of protein, vitamins and trace elements can cause specific disease types and death. Vitamins are complex chemical compounds essential for life that the body is unable to synthesise, not having the necessary genetic programming. These substances must therefore be provided in the diet.

The most important early research of vitamins was based on observations of scurvy affecting sailors on long sea voyages, undertaken by the Scottish physician James Lind in 1753 [1]. He was the surgeon on board the *Salisbury* and he successfully treated 12 sailors who had succumbed to scurvy. He wrote [1]:

*On 20th May 1747 I took 12 patients in the scurvy on board the Salisbury at sea. Their cases were as similar as I could have them. They all in general had putrid gums, the spot and lassitude, with weakness of their knees.*

He compared six treatments, cider, elixir vitriol, vinegar, sea water, a laxative and citrus fruit. Only the last was effective, leading to 'the most sudden and good effects'. This led much later to the identification of vitamin C (chemically ascorbic acid), and the identification of several other vitamins was to follow. Deficiencies of trace elements, dietary proteins and calories were also identified. Such discoveries were accepted slowly and with considerable scepticism, as is usually the case with the introduction of new ideas. It was not until 1794, more than 40 years after the work of James Lind, that the British navy introduced lime juice for the prevention of scurvy among sailors.

We are often told to increase something in our diet because it is good for us, often without a very good research base and without any suggestion that we might have a deficiency of it. A surplus does not usually lead to an advantage. Too much of something can be dangerous, and we are now coming to an area of disease that is generally called poisoning or perhaps toxicity. Too much alcohol can cause cirrhosis of the liver, a variety of brain syndromes and neuromuscular disorders. Too much paracetamol can cause death from liver failure within a few days. Lead poisoning became very well described in the 19th and 20th centuries and can still occur today in countries without legislation to control lead use. Too much food in general can cause obesity, with a variety of disabilities resulting from it.

We are told that too much cholesterol causes heart attacks, but the research base of this will be looked at critically in later chapters. A message of this book is that, contrary to conventional wisdom, coronary heart disease is not because of cholesterol poisoning and cholesterol is not toxic. However, it is a suggestion that must be taken seriously as most people believe it to be true.

Infections have been major causes of disease and death historically, and we are in an environment in which living organisms are a continuing danger to us. These can be viruses, small bacteria that can live only within cells, larger more well-known bacteria, single-cell organisms including fungi, and multicellular organisms such as worms. A newly recognised infection agent is the prion, the existence and disease potential of which has led science to review what is meant by a life form. These forms of infestation act mainly internally and are obviously somewhat different from the very obvious threats from life forms such as large carnivorous or poisonous animals.

That is actually the totality of causes of disease. Some would argue that psychological factors can cause disease, but my feeling is that psychological factors will influence the development of the illness rather than the development of the disease itself. Behavioural factors, which are closely linked to psychology, can have a major influence on susceptibility to disease, most obviously trauma, but again they are not what I would view as the cause.

Whatever we think of the cause of a disease, we must consider the possibilities under the above categories. We often find that by a process of exclusion we are looking at infection as a possible cause, even though the micro-organism concerned might not have been identified.

# 6
# RESISTANCE TO INFECTION

Wherever there is water in a liquid state, life forms will exist. This will happen at temperatures above 100 degrees Celsius, in deep-water geothermal vents, and below 0 degrees Celsius, beneath thick ice. It is natural for many life forms to co-exist and live in harmony with each other; the presence of one life form might be of apparent disadvantage to another but necessary for the overall balance of nature.

Symbiosis is a situation in which two or more life forms co-exist in a balanced way, with neither being particularly disadvantaged and in a relationship of mutual gain. In a human being, the skin is occupied by millions of bacteria per square centimetre and they appear to be neutral, not causing disease. In addition, there are tiny creatures called mites that find a comfortable warm home in the human skin and an ample supply of food in the dead cells that we shed from our skin every day. The benefit is that the mites actually clean the skin and prevent sweat pores from being clogged by old, desquamated skin. The symbiosis works well.

Also in the human being, we have a large intestine in which is found a large number of bacteria of many strains, that function in a highly complex fashion and appear to make a significant contribution to health, in particular to bowel health. In fact, most faecal excrement is the biomass created by these bacteria. They feed on food residue and synthesise short-chain fatty acids that are an advantage to the human and indeed an important form of nutrition in other animal species. The disturbance of this colonic microflora by, for example, antibiotic therapy can have very significant detrimental effects and is one cause of what is generally called irritable bowel syndrome, and even more serious illnesses.

A parasite, on the other hand, is a life form that lives off another life form. The host becomes disadvantaged; the parasite ultimately causes physical incapacity (disease state) and death. Regarding microbial disease, we are dealing with parasites on and in the human body.

The relationship between micro-organism and human host is not always as clear-cut as described above. An organism may live off another in what might be thought of as a symbiotic relationship and then, one day, that relationship changes to that of a parasite on a host. The change is often related to the circumstance of the host rather than the parasite.

We can carry within our bodies organisms of serious pathological potential, and perhaps the most striking is the bacterium *Meningococcus*, or *Neisseria meningitidis*. It can be carried in the nose of a human being for prolonged periods of time to no detriment, until one day the host develops meningococcal meningitis or septicaemia and, if untreated, death occurs within a matter of hours. What causes the sudden change in the relationship between *Meningococcus* and the human host is a mystery. It is obvious, therefore, that the human being must be equipped biologically and socially to resist parasitic infection, and there are a number of protective mechanisms.

The human skin is very delicate compared with that of other animals, which might be protected by much thicker skin (pachyderms), dense hair cover, feathers or scales. It is necessary for a human being to adopt behavioural forms of protection, including clothing, combing, washing and drying. However, the skin is a route through which parasites might, and indeed do, enter the body.

The gastrointestinal tract is also an important route of parasitic infection, and the main protection is the production of hydrochloric acid by the stomach. Hydrochloric acid has the function of sterilising food and water, and thus the upper gastrointestinal tract, but this protective function can create problems and hydrochloric acid can become a disadvantage. It has been known for some time that people whose stomachs no longer produce acid are more prone to the development of cholera. More recently, it has been noted that people who take prolonged acid suppression therapy are also slightly more prone to intestinal infections, for example *Clostridium difficile* enteritis [1]. Once again, it is necessary for a human being to develop social and behavioural controls to prevent infection via the intestinal tract. These are the careful selection and organisation of a water supply, together with the selection and cooking of food and the washing of hands before eating.

The third major portal of entry for parasites is through the respiratory tract, and it is perhaps through this route that we are most vulnerable. We inhale air through the nose and mouth approximately once every three seconds, and this is under limited control. We cannot easily select or prepare the air that we breathe, and the only behavioural ways of controlling the inhalation of parasites is to avoid other people known to have infection or to use a barrier mask. Infections of the respiratory tract are very common.

Resistance to infection can also be part of our genetic inheritance. There are rare inherited disorders of immunity that affect unfortunate individuals but, because they are rare, they do not affect the health of the general public. There are also genetically determined differences in the susceptibility to infection and disease in general in different populations in different locations. For example, white European people going to Africa have a much higher susceptibility to malaria infection than the indigenous black population, although the indigenous advantage does have a price to pay.

Resistance against malaria can be provided by a type of haemoglobin that is inherited. When there is no malaria in a country, we anticipate a 'normal' adult haemoglobin type, such as is found within the vast majority of the population of the UK. However, what we in the UK regard as 'abnormal' haemoglobin and identify as a disease state can be protective against malaria. Such diseases are sickle-cell disease and thalassaemia. Although these haemoglobin types put individuals at a disadvantage when they are in the UK, they have an advantage in areas where malaria is common. This is the clearest instance in which genes can be identified as being protective against external disease. However, the science of genetics must still be regarded as new and many other examples are likely to be identified in the future. Later in this book we will see the occasions in which familial hypercholesterolaemia can be an advantage or a disadvantage.

The Australian Aborigines, like the indigenous Pima people in North America, now frequently exhibit extreme obesity, diabetes and a short life expectancy. It is considered that much of this is related to the large amounts of food that are now available to them as a result of their contact with a highly productive food industry. Although the gene itself has not been identified, it is felt that they have what is called a 'thrifty gene', which means that they are able to survive with a minimum of food because of an inherited metabolic effect that probably reduces the amount of heat production following food ingestion. In reality, most of our food goes into heat production and other metabolic processes, and the balance goes into fat deposition. The ability to survive in times of scarce food availability will obviously be an enormous evolutionary advantage in times of famine, but not in the USA and Australia at the dawn of the 21st century when food is abundant.

Further insight into the genetics of resistance to infection has emerged from studies of the major blood groups [2]. People with blood group O appear to be protected against viruses that correspondingly more commonly infect people with blood groups A, B and AB. If viruses were the only form of infecting micro-organisms, only group O people would survive in the long term. However, bacterial infections appear to be more common in people with blood group O and so a balance is achieved. An association between blood groups and disease has long been known but it has not been understood. Further study of micro-organisms acting at a molecular level is likely to shed more light on this subject.

The human being, like other animals and plants, has evolved subtle processes to supplement physical barriers to infection. The body has a system of learning to recognise foreign proteins and to develop the ability to neutralise them; this process is immunity. There are two forms of immunity. The first is humoral immunity, which involves circulating antibodies, called immunoglobulins, of classes IgA, IgG, IgM and IgE. The second is a cellular form of immunity, and the two have different embryonic origins.

The infection of a body by a parasite such as a virus will cause the immune cells of the body to synthesise complex proteins called antibodies, which damage (neutralise) the infecting organism and allow other body defence mechanisms to kill it. It may well be that the virus infection can invade the body much more quickly than the antibody response can act, and the infection might thus be overwhelming and fatal. However, if the individual survives this initial infection, the antibody response has been learned and this means that re-infection at some time in the future will be dealt with promptly and without the development of a significant disease. Most antibodies of the classifications IgG and IgM are found circulating in blood. Those of class IgA are secreted into body fluids, particularly in the respiratory tract, to provide a defence before infection can move into the body in general.

The other form of immunity, cellular immunity, is not as easily measured or as easily understood. Antibodies can be transferred from one individual to another, in a process called passive immunisation, but cellular immunity cannot be transferred in this way.

The immune suppression that occurs in AIDS is mainly impairment of cellular immunity, as a result of damage to lymphocytes by the AIDS virus. It is not possible to replace this immunity by external forms, and the treatment of patients with AIDS depends on the active treatment of a given infection together with suppression of the AIDS virus itself.

It is also known that newly born babies are particularly vulnerable to infection because their immune systems have not fully developed. However, their immunity is helped by IgG antibodies, which transfer across the placenta but disappear within a few weeks of birth, and also by IgA antibodies, which are acquired from the mother's milk.

The identification of immunity has been very important to our understanding of protection against infection. However, there is clearly more to resistance to infection than is at present understood. For example, it is well known that malnutrition (under-nutrition) makes individuals much more prone to infection, and this is thought to be an important reason for the re-emergence of tuberculosis in populations impoverished by war and famine. The precise relationship between nutrition and immunity is unclear, other than the suggestion, in the broadest possible terms, that adequate nutrition is necessary for normal cellular processes, including those in the immune system.

Although vitamin D is most widely known for its function in the maturation of bone, in recent years it has been recognised as having an important role in the immune mechanisms of the body. Insufficiency of vitamin D, mainly the result of inadequate exposure to the sun, produces its own form of acquired immunodeficiency. We will be exploring this in subsequent chapters.

# PART 2

# INFECTIONS AND THE ENVIRONMENT

# 7
# THE SEASONALITY OF ILLNESS

I t is obvious to most of us that we tend to be healthier in the summer than in the winter. This is particularly true with respiratory infections, colds and coughs, which are more common in the winter, and also a variety of non-specific viral infections that generally go under the name of 'flu'. People suffering from bronchitis tend to be worse in the wintertime, and generally there are more visits to the family doctor and more emergency admissions to hospital. There are more days lost from work because of illness during the winter than the summer, and more days are lost from school. There are certain illnesses more likely to occur in the summer. The most obvious is sunburn, but food poisoning is also more common in the summer, because of the ability of bacteria to proliferate on food that is not kept cool.

The major burden of illness occurs during the winter and, although limb fractures because of slipping on ice and road traffic accidents resulting from darkness are fairly obvious, it is difficult to explain why other diseases are more common during the winter months. Data published by the UK Office of National Statistics in 2000 show clearly that there is a seasonal variation of deaths, higher in the winter than in the summer [1], as shown in Figure 7.1.

**Figure 7.1 Deaths, by months of occurrence, in 2000, England and Wales [1].**

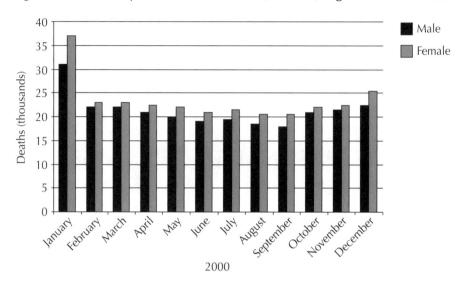

The seasonality of disease has been known for many years; a pattern of more deaths in the winter than in the summer has been observed in the UK since about 1840. The excess winter deaths have been reported in a number of countries, mainly in Europe but also in other, warmer countries, as outlined in Table 7.1. For the purpose of this study, the excess winter death index is shown for the months December to March, relative to the months of September to November and April to June [2].

**Table 7.1 Mean excess winter death index, 1976–84 [2]**

| Country | Number of deaths | Country | Number of deaths |
|---|---|---|---|
| England and Wales | 21 | Austria | 11 |
| Scotland | 20 | Bulgaria | 19 |
| Northern Ireland | 18 | Germany (east) | 10 |
| Irish Republic | 24 | Czechoslovakia | 9 |
| Denmark | 9 | Canada | 7 |
| Finland | 8 | USA | 9 |
| Norway | 9 | Israel | 26 |
| Sweden | 10 | Japan | 17 |
| Belgium | 11 | Australia | 20 |
| France | 11 | New Zealand | 25 |
| Germany (west) | 8 | | |
| Italy | 19 | | |
| Netherlands | 9 | | |
| Portugal | 26 | | |
| Spain | 19 | | |
| Switzerland | 10 | | |

Michael Curwen, author of this study [2] and medical statistician at the Office of Population Censuses and Surveys of the UK, was open-minded about the explanation of this phenomenon and he rightly felt that his role was simply to make valid observations. Robert Scragg, reporting from Adelaide, Australia, had earlier identified a similar seasonality in Queensland [3]. He noted excess winter deaths from cardiovascular and respiratory diseases and, because of the location of Queensland on the edge of the tropics, he felt that temperature could not be the explanation. He proposed that the important factor is the seasonal variation of ultraviolet light at ground level, a suggestion of great significance to which very little attention has been paid.

A further study by Curwen looked at the seasonal variation of mortality between the years 1949 and 1990; he reported a diminution in the variation between the summer and winter during this period of time. This has also been reported by Drs Crawford, McCann and Stout from the Department of Geriatric Medicine at Queen's University, Belfast, UK. Their study looked at the period 1979–98 and showed a seasonal variation of deaths from myocardial infarction, with an excess in the winter, together with a diminution of that variation during the period of the study [4]. The reason for the decline in seasonal variation is likely to be related to the cause of the seasonal variation overall.

It is generally considered that the higher incidence of disease in the winter is because of the colder temperatures, hence older people in the UK are given a winter heating allowance through government policy. But we are warm-blooded mammals and isothermic, that is our body temperature remains constant; our hands and feet might be cold in the winter but not the inner parts of our bodies. We inhale colder air in winter, and so it might be thought that our nasal passages can become cold and thus more susceptible to infection, but they have a very rich supply of blood vessels (hence the fairly frequent occurrence of nose bleeds) and there is no evidence that the nasal passages are hypothermic during cold spells.

A study from the University of Lund, Sweden, of 259 municipalities, has demonstrated a high mortality rate from myocardial infarction in the cold parts of Sweden [5]. However, it could not be concluded that cold itself was the cause of increased morbidity and mortality in the winter months and it was suggested that the reason is a different but unknown factor. In a subset of 37 municipalities, there was no association between serum cholesterol and coronary mortality but there was a significant association between serum cholesterol and coldness. We will be dealing with these important issues later.

A major challenge to the temperature hypothesis comes from a comparison between Ontario, Canada, and the UK. Anderson and Lerache [6] found that, while the seasonal variation of temperature is greater in Ontario, the seasonal variation in coronary heart disease mortality is greater in England and Wales, which are significantly warmer countries. It is perfectly clear from this observation that temperature variation cannot be the cause of the variation in coronary heart disease mortality.

Further support for this view comes from a study comparing the seasonality of deaths in the Grampian region of northern Scotland and Kuwait in the Middle East [7]. The populations of both experience an increase in mortality during the winter months, and this is from all causes, respiratory disease and coronary heart disease, as can be seen in Figures 7.2–4. The seasonal changes are remarkably similar in both places and it is perhaps surprising that death from respiratory disease shows a greater winter peak in Kuwait. Please note that the data for Kuwait are from the years 1981–84 and 1986–88, and for Grampian from the years 1974–88. Averages are shown.

**Figure 7.2  Relative mortality from all causes by month [7].**

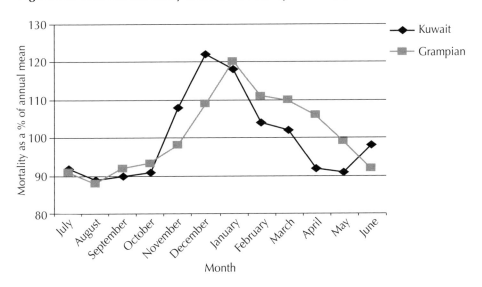

**Figure 7.3  Relative mortality from respiratory disease by month [7].**

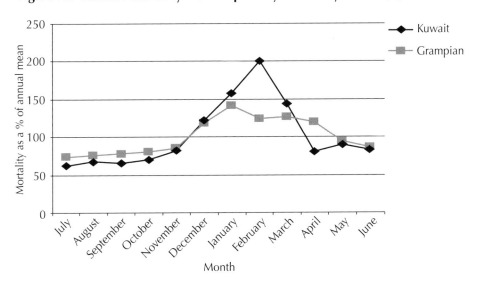

**Figure 7.4 Relative mortality from coronary heart disease by month [7].**

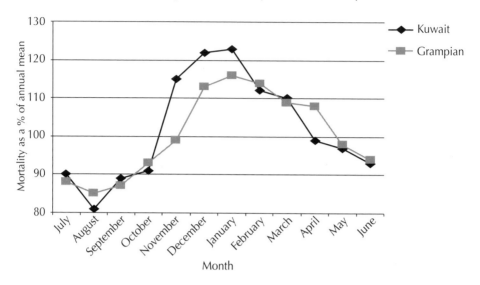

Figure 7.5 shows the seasonal temperature variation in Kuwait and the Grampian region of Scotland. The minimum temperature in Kuwait is about the same as the maximum temperature in Grampian and so it would appear that temperature itself would be unlikely to provide an explanation of the annual variation of mortality.

**Figure 7.5 Average maximum daily temperature [7].**

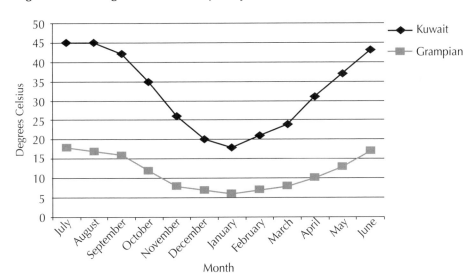

Most winter illnesses appear to be respiratory; we talk about winter colds, we expect to have influenza in the winter and pneumonia is more common. We can see that the seasonal changes of respiratory disease and coronary heart disease are very similar and it has been suggested that winter respiratory illness might be the cause of the winter increase in coronary heart disease. This introduces the idea that coronary heart disease might perhaps be caused by a micro-organism, an interesting theme that will be developed in later chapters.

However, it also begs the question why respiratory infections might be more common in the winter. There is a popular feeling that the increased incidence of respiratory infections during winter months is because the micro-organisms 'wake up'. This defies all biological reason in that activity is proportional to temperature, usually reaching a peak at the human body temperature of 37 degrees Celsius, especially important in non-mammalian and more simple creatures that have no control over internal temperature.

Biological plausibility must indicate that the increased incidence of disease in the winter months is the result of increased susceptibility of the human host, in other words reduced resistance to infection. We have already seen that resistance to infection is mainly immunological, and so there is a suspicion that immunity of the human being living in temperate zones is lower in the winter than in summer. There is every reason to suspect that warmth is necessary for the activity of parasites. When the temperature of hibernating mammals or amphibians drops, there is no indication that they are more likely to develop microbial diseases during the cold season; the parasitic organisms require the higher normal body temperature to become active.

If cold is not the reason for the increased burden of illness during the winter, we must look for another explanation. The reason for the lower temperature in the winter is a reduction of sunlight exposure, and it is obvious, but rarely stated, that a reduction of sunlight exposure of the population during the winter might be the reason for the peak of illness and mortality. This suggestion was made by Wong and colleagues [8], who reported in the *British Medical Journal* that the population of Hong Kong also has a seasonal variation of mortality, with a peak of deaths from coronary heart disease during the winter. In Hong Kong there is a variation of mean temperature between 15 and 30 degrees Celsius throughout the year. Wong and colleagues suggested that variation in sunlight could well be important in determining the seasonal variation of mortality rate and would correlate with temperature.

We know that sunlight exposure has an effect on human metabolism; it is necessary for the production of vitamin D. One of the functions of vitamin D is the development of immunity.

We have seen that there is a phenomenon of winter mortality from all causes, and specifically from coronary heart disease and respiratory disease. Against this background, a study of the seasonality of clinical presentation of tuberculosis was undertaken, using the National Notification System for Tuberculosis in England and Wales [9]. In this particular study, the pattern was based on 57 313 tuberculosis notifications between 1983 and 1992. It looked at deaths from pneumonia, confirming peaks in the winter and a low incidence in the summer, but the pattern for tuberculosis showed exactly the opposite: the notifications were low during the winter months and rose from April onwards, diminishing again in October. This might at first sight appear to a paradox but, whereas pneumonia is an acute illness with a short time scale of development, tuberculosis is a more chronic illness with a long time scale. The authors felt that the observation fitted in with tuberculosis being a disease that is activated by vitamin D deficiency. Following a winter of impaired sunlight exposure and depletion of the vitamin D reserves of the body, the disease would activate and become clinically obvious during the early summer months, before vitamin D levels were restored.

The same observation has been made recently in India [10]. The study was made possible by the development of tuberculosis control programmes that have been developed across India since 1998, allowing, for the first time, the collection of population-based data using standard registers, essential for good-quality epidemiological research. The study covered locations with a total population of 115 million people and, during the 5-year study period, there were 11 101 cases of tuberculosis. The study concentrated on three districts, and the incidence of tuberculosis was highest in the most northern, Hamipur. The incidence was lowest in Pathanamthitta, the most southern location. This indicates a geographical gradient, with increasing incidence of disease with distance from the equator, a phenomenon that we will be looking at in more detail in later chapters. We can see this geographical gradient in Figure 7.6, which also indicates a seasonal variation. The new cases of tuberculosis are reported by quarter, and the peaks of incidence occur mainly in quarter 2, April–June.

**Figure 7.6 Tuberculosis in India [10].**

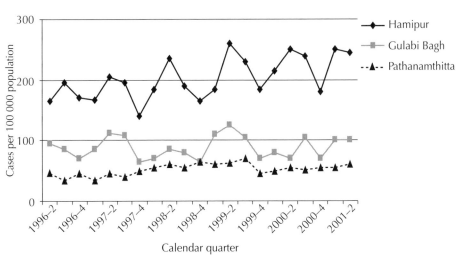

As in England and Wales, the incidence of clinical presentation of tuberculosis is maximal in the early summer, conforming to the view that biological activation of the disease starts in the late winter, when vitamin D reserves are depleted. We can also see that the amplitude of the seasonal variation is greatest in the most northern location, where the seasonal change of sunlight exposure is greatest. This study strongly supports the idea to be developed, namely that lack of sunlight and consequent insufficiency of vitamin D increases susceptibility to infections, in this case to tuberculosis.

We can see that it is not only respiratory infections and deaths that are more common in the winter but there is an increased risk of myocardial infarction and death from coronary heart disease. There is a greater risk of stroke during winter months, and blood pressure tends to be higher in the winter. The Medical Research Council of the UK undertook a trial of treatment of mild hypertension and, for this purpose, it recruited 17 000 men and women with slightly elevated blood pressure, diastolic between 90 and 109 mm Hg. Recruitment was a continuous process, and one of the interesting observations of the study was a seasonal variation of blood pressure. The average blood pressure was clearly higher in the winter than the summer [11], an observation that had previously been made by Professor Geoffrey Rose in 1961, based on a much smaller number of observations.

A similar observation was made by a long-term study of 96 people, aged between 65 and 74 years, from a general practice register in Cambridge, UK. They were visited at home every 2 months and blood pressure was recorded on each occasion. It can be seen in Figure 7.7 how many of the 96 people had a given range of blood pressure. The blood pressure range shifted to a higher level in the winter months compared with the summer [12]. The data shown display systolic blood pressure; the same phenomenon was observed in diastolic blood pressure.

There is also some evidence that vitamin D has an effect on control of blood pressure, and it has been suggested that the unexplained greater elevation of blood pressure during the winter is because of reduced levels of vitamin D [13]. It has been observed that exposure to ultraviolet light (UVB) has an effect in reducing blood pressure [14] and this has been advanced as a theory regarding how sunlight might help cardiovascular morbidity. It has also been proposed as the reason for the increased susceptibility to hypertension of dark-skinned populations living at a great distance from the equator, Afro-Caribbeans in the USA and south Asian Indians in the UK. This will also be dealt with in more detail later.

**Figure 7.7 Distribution of systolic blood pressure by season [12].**

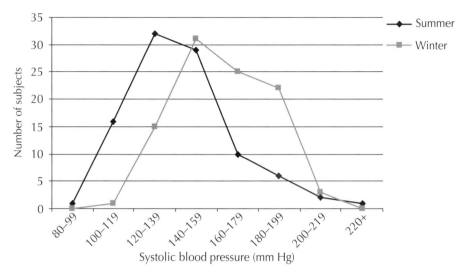

A recent review of the seasonality of death rates appeared in the *Health Service Journal*, written by John Appleby, chief economist at the King's Fund in London, UK [15]. His data indicate that the excess of deaths in the winter is much greater among elderly people, that is people with an age greater than 75 years, as shown in Figure 7.8.

**Figure 7.8 Excess winter mortality by age group (UK) [15].**

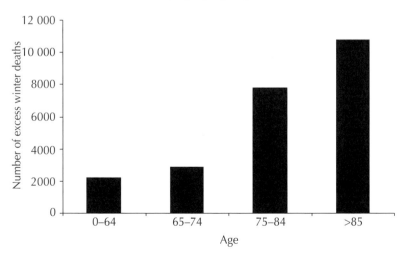

The greater winter mortality among elderly people could be a manifestation of the well-recognised vitamin D deficiency among this age group, resulting mainly from their reduced mobility and thus a reduced outdoor exposure to the sun [16]. Vitamin D deficiency also contributes to muscle weakness, and so there develops a spiral of reduced mobility, being housebound and vitamin D reserves becoming even lower.

Vitamin D deficiency in older people is extremely important and is usually not recognised. Although it can create poor bone quality, as we will see later, it is the muscle weakness that is perhaps of greater importance but not appreciated. It is the muscle weakness that will lead to falls, and fractures as a further result. Clinical trials may not show a conclusive effect, and so in recent years there has been a move to meta-analysis, the pooling of the results of a number of trials. A meta-analysis combining the results of five clinical trials demonstrated that vitamin D supplements reduce the frequency of falls in elderly people, and this obviously indicates that the elderly people must have been deficient of vitamin D in the first place [17]. We can thus see that falls and the winter excess of deaths in older people are likely to be mediated by vitamin D deficiency, because of inadequate exposure to the sun.

Appleby also demonstrated that the excess winter mortality has fallen substantially during the latter half of the 20th century (Figure 7.9). This is a pattern that we will see in later chapters and it could be the result of reduced winter air pollution.

**Figure 7.9 Trend in excess winter mortality [15].**

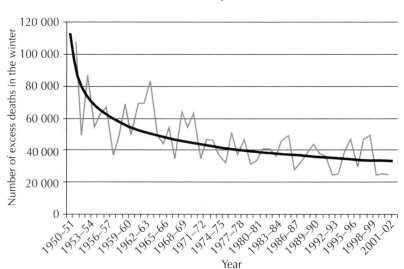

A study in Scotland, England and Wales looked at children and young people up to the age of 14 years developing diabetes. The study was of a total of 4665 people and the month of birth was the particular subject of investigation; the result was that the majority had been born during the summer months [18]. A previous suggestion that stimulated the study was that the development of diabetes might be based on intra-uterine, or gestational, factors. Birth during the summer, with a risk of subsequent development of diabetes higher than expected, indicates that gestation during the winter months is a disadvantage. During this time the important transfer of vitamin D from mother to the developing foetus is suboptimal because of reduced synthesis of vitamin D by the mother. We will be looking at vitamin D and diabetes in later chapters, and also maternal factors influencing health later in life.

While touching on the subject of pregnancy, it is interesting to note the study by a team from Liverpool and Chester, UK, as reported to the British Fertility Society Conference in 2004. The observation was that *in-vitro* fertilisation (IVF) was more likely to be successful in the summer months, and that ovulation occurred more readily during months with more daylight. The rate of successful pregnancy was higher after summer treatment, based on the study of 3000 IVF cycles carried out between 1997 and 2001; 20% of treatments resulted in successful pregnancy in the summer months, compared with 16% in the winter months [19].

This is another example of how sunlight has a favourable influence on human health but, once again, it would be interesting to identify the intermediary mechanism. In this case, the researchers suggested that it could be melatonin, a hormone that varies during light and darkness, but its physiological mechanisms are not clear. Vitamin D was not suggested in this study, whereas it is a hormone that is known to increase with sunlight exposure and which has well-established and widespread physiological actions.

The other condition that is receiving increased prominence in recent years is seasonal affective disorder (SAD), a depressive type of illness that is more common in the winter. It is generally thought to be psychological, the result of being miserable during shorter days with darkness and poor weather, but there is a fundamental difference between unhappiness and depression. If SAD does exist as a disease entity, and there is compelling evidence that this is the case, then it might be pathophysiological rather than psychological, and part of the larger pattern of increased morbidity (illness) in the winter. It has been suggested that the well-recognised increased mental illness of the winter months might be the cause of the increased incidence of coronary heart disease that occurs at the same time [20]. The weakness of this argument is that it presupposes that psychological factors are directly causal of coronary heart disease, and it also fails to appreciate the wider burden of illness excess during the winter. The winter burden of mental illness would appear to be a response to the climatological changes that influence other illnesses.

The seasonal variations of the blood-clotting agents fibrinogen and factor 7 show increased levels in the winter and the suggestion is that this is an acute phase response, probably the result of respiratory infections that are more likely to occur in the winter [21]. The increased incidence of myocardial infarction during the winter is unlikely to be a direct result of increased blood clotting tendency, as the disease is much more complex than that. It might be more closely related to respiratory infection.

Thrombosis in the veins is thought to be a rather more simple process of blood clotting and, unlike myocardial infarction, it occurs in people with thrombophilia, a genetically determined pre-disposition to excessive blood clotting. The clinical expressions of this are deep vein thrombosis (DVT) and pulmonary embolus (PE). There have been many reports indicating an increased risk of fatal PE during the winter. A report from Nice, France, confirms this and shows an increased incidence of DVT during the winter months. This is thought to be an expression of increased fibrinogen and blood-clotting factor 7 concentration [22].

It is clear that the seasonal variation of excess winter mortality and morbidity shows a consistent pattern that is international. Because it is a phenomenon of many nations and many diseases, we must look at a general climatological or geographical explanation and it is no use trying to find the explanation by looking at just one disease or just one location. It is the suggestion of this book that the phenomenon of excess winter deaths is an expression of vitamin D insufficiency and consequently a suppression of immunity.

# 8

# HEPATITIS, TUBERCULOSIS AND SYPHILIS

Following the inspiration of John Snow (see Chapter 2), scientific thinking was directed to consider that certain illnesses might be the result of transmissible agents rather than divine interference. The pattern of disease was important in identifying these and, even in the present day, diseases can be accepted as having a microbial cause before the identification of the micro-organism, for example 'virus negative viral hepatitis'. It is important to follow the patterns of thinking that have led up to the recognition that a disease is caused by a micro-organism, irrespective of its identification. Hepatitis, tuberculosis and syphilis provide very important examples of this.

The pattern of illness that came to be identified as indicating a microbial cause was that of acute (sudden) onset followed by either rapid death or fairly rapid recovery, with no evidence of chemical poisoning that might create the same pattern. The clinical symptoms could be either respiratory, with nasal congestion or cough, of a gastrointestinal nature, with vomiting, diarrhoea or jaundice, or of a neurological nature, with headache. There could simply be a fever and sometimes a rash.

Over the years, specific clinical syndromes have been identified and hepatitis is a good example. A syndrome is a grouping of symptoms, signs or investigation results that constitute a recognisable pattern. Infectious hepatitis was known and characterised by non-specific pyrexia (fever) and feeling unwell, followed by the development of jaundice over a period of a few days and then gradual resolution; this is its syndrome. It tended to occur in epidemics, with a latent period of about 3 weeks between exposure of an affected individual and the appearance of the illness. Serum hepatitis was similar but the previous history was of exposure to blood products or possibly contaminated needles.

Bacteria had been identified by microscopy but there was a failure to identify a bacterium related to hepatitis. It became clear that transmissible diseases such as hepatitis were not caused by bacteria but something much smaller, something that could pass through a filter. They were called viruses but could only been identified with the advent of electron microscopy. The term viral hepatitis was applied to the disease and it was by accident that the causative virus was recognised in the late 1960s. It was first identified by antibody tests in a blood transfusion laboratory, and it was initially called the Australia antigen without realising that it was related to hepatitis. Electron microscopy of the blood of patients with viral hepatitis who were Australia antigen positive showed it to be teeming with virus particles. This observation had previously been disregarded, in keeping with Thomas Kuhn's comment that people see what is determined by their previous visual–conceptual experience [1].

Later still it came as some surprise to realise that there were several viruses that cause hepatitis. Infectious hepatitis became known as hepatitis A and serum hepatitis (Australia antigen positive) became known as hepatitis B, one of the most common infections in the world. Hepatitis C is also very common, usually without an obvious illness onset but a history of transfusion of blood or blood products, for example concentrates of clotting factor 8 in the treatment of haemophilia. More hepatitis viruses have since been identified, and the diagnosis of virus-negative viral hepatitis indicates that more are at present undiscovered.

The important thing to note about the story of hepatitis is that the condition was accepted as being caused by a virus many decades before the causative viruses were identified. It was the pattern of an acute illness with a history of exposure to the disease or the occurrence of an epidemic that provided the characteristic model of a microbial disease. Even today, if an individual experiences an acute pyrexial illness with generalised non-specific symptoms, he or she will usually say 'I have a virus' without there being any laboratory evidence available to support this assertion. The diagnosis is made on the pattern of illness, the syndrome, rather than identification of its cause.

The story is rather different for tuberculosis, because it is a chronic illness that will run its course over many years. It did not seem to have a beginning and, for many sufferers, it never really had an end, it just became part of life, but for many the end was death. It was very common and so there was no easy identification of one person catching it from another. It would cluster within families who lived in the same household, and this gave the impression it was constitutional, meaning an ill-defined form of inheritance. Family clustering always raises the problem of whether the important factor is genetic or perhaps environmental, and I shall return to this theme later. It is particularly important regarding coronary heart disease.

I have already mentioned that it was Robert Koch who felt that tuberculosis, or consumption as it was known, might be the result of a transmissible agent. Koch instinctively and correctly realised that tuberculosis was caused by a micro-organism, challenging the paradigm of the day that it was constitutional. The fact that he could not identify the organism did not deter him from his quest for its expected identification.

Bacteria in general are identified microscopically by the use of various staining techniques. The Gram stain shows that certain bacteria, mainly *Streptococcus* and *Staphylococcus*, take up a blue pigment that allows them to be identified from the surrounding tissues, counter-stained in red. Other bacteria, called Gram negative, do not take up the blue Gram stain but can be stained red. Koch was disappointed to find no evidence of bacteria when he examined microscopically the sputum produced by sufferers of tuberculosis. Eventually the Ziel–Nielson stain was produced. It is taken up by the tubercle bacillus (*Mycobacterium tuberculosis*, the cause of tuberculosis) and retained only by this organism after washing the specimen with acid and alcohol, thus leading to the microscopic identification of the cause of tuberculosis.

Soon after the development of microscopic techniques to identify bacteria, it was realised that they grow easily on culture media and that the growing colonies are composed of the bacteria themselves. The culture of bacteria in colonies played an important role in the identification of bacterial illness. Koch had a further disappointment when it was discovered that bacteria such as staphylococci and streptococci will grow in culture within 24 hours, but this could not be achieved with sputum cultures from sufferers of tuberculosis. Once again, his persistence was rewarded and, after experimenting with a variety of culture media, he finally induced colonies to grow, but not reliably until after 6 weeks of incubation.

However, Koch felt that more rigorous testing was needed before he was satisfied that he had identified the cause of tuberculosis. He therefore injected the cultured bacteria into guinea-pigs, and found that they developed the disease, as demonstrated when the animals were killed and their internal organs examined microscopically. Not only that, but he went on to isolate the bacillus from the animal tissues. He was then satisfied.

Robert Koch recognised and demonstrated the causative micro-organism of a chronic disease that was not obviously microbial at the time. He therefore opened the eyes of the medical profession, and the scientific world at large, to the breadth of opportunity in identifying a new dimension of the causation of disease.

A similar process took place with syphilis, which had appeared in Europe in 1493. The acute clinical onset in an individual is characterised by a genital sore, obvious in men but frequently hidden internally in women. It was quite clear that this 'primary chancre' was the immediate result of sexual activity with a stranger or with the partner of a stranger. The primary manifestation was followed a few days later by a rash that was frequently profound when syphilis first appeared in Europe but gradually became less so. It has been postulated that this change and moderation of features was because of an improved resistance of the population of Europe, perhaps through the development of what has been called herd immunity, but it has also been postulated as being because of a mutation of the organism into a less virulent form. This is a general principle: if the incidence of a microbial disease changes over a period of time, is this the result of a change in the micro-organism (mutation) or a change in the resistance or susceptibility of the population?

The cause of the appearance of syphilis in Europe was unclear but was said by some to be to the result of the conjunction of the planets Saturn and Jupiter that occurred at 6.04 p.m. on 25 November 1484, as reviewed by Deborah Hayden in her book Pox [2]. However, most people felt that the cause, rather than being divine intervention or otherwise celestial in origin, was the return of the first voyage of Christopher Columbus from the New World. Dietary theories were also expounded, that the disease might be because of the introduction of the potato, but it became quite clear that sexual contact was the major precipitating event that initiated the disease. It is interesting to note that the Italian physician, philosopher and polymath Girolamo Fracastoro (1478–1553) postulated in 1530 that tiny invisible living things might be the cause of the disease. This was the first expression of germ theory.

The late features of syphilis appear after a long latent period of several years and are not obviously part of the same condition; the association was not even considered until almost 400 years after the introduction of the disease into Europe. In 1875 Francis Welsh, a British Army Surgeon, studied the records of 53 men who had died from ruptured aortic aneurysm (it could not be treated surgically at that time) and noted that two-thirds had a documented history of syphilis. He felt that this frequency was greater than would be expected among the general population and he wondered, quite correctly, whether syphilis might be the cause of the aortic aneurysm. It was not until 1905 that the German zoologist Fritz Schaudinn and dermatologist Eric Hoffmann first observed, in autopsy specimens of aorta, the causative spirochete bacterium that later became classified as *Treponema pallidum*.

The common neurological disorders of the 18th and 19th centuries were tabes dorsalis (TD) and general paralysis of the insane (GPI). They did not have a known cause and were not linked to syphilis until 1879, when the French dermatologist Alfred Fournier (1879–1944) proposed that syphilis was the cause of GPI, and in 1886, the cause of TD. Previously they, like tuberculosis, had been thought to be constitutional (what we would now term familial or possibly genetic), as there was a strong familial tendency. The late effects of syphilis in its various forms could be present in more than half of family members, predominantly caused by non-sexual transmission in the secondary infective stage by common use of cups and face-cloths, etc.

Within living memory, we have taken for granted that tuberculosis and syphilis are caused by infections and it is not easy to put ourselves in the position of those clinical scientists of the late 19th century to whom this was by no means obvious and to whom the concept of infection had not been taught. It is difficult for us to imagine the depth of thought and the persistent hard work of people such as Robert Koch, Alfred Fournier and others to provide sound foundations that enabled the advances that were made in clinical medicine in the 20th century. But even with our present-day knowledge and research opportunities, we are still sometimes slow or resistant to recognise that a disease, of which the cause is not clear, might be caused by a micro-organism.

# 9
# PEPTIC ULCER: A MICROBIAL DISEASE

The message from Chapter 4 is that the simple association between a bacterium and a disease does not automatically imply causation. This process requires much more vision and much more work. Peptic ulcer provides a good model for how thinking has developed concerning the cause of disease, and it is worthwhile considering the history of this.

It had been noticed for several years that, when the lining of the human stomach was examined by microscopy, curved bacteria could be seen on its surface; the first observations were made early in the 20th century. However, it had been noted by then that bacteria can be found everywhere, and so these observed micro-organisms in the stomach were regarded as commensals, that is organisms that live on or in the body without doing any harm. They were regarded as irrelevant to any disease process; after all peptic ulcer, by far the most common disease of the stomach, was obviously constitutional or perhaps dietary. It took the Australian microbiologist Robin Warren, and his physician colleague Barry Marshall, working at the University of Perth, western Australia, to think what was effectively the unthinkable, and to ask themselves in the early 1980s 'Could this micro-organism be the cause of peptic ulcer?', leading to a series of publications providing supporting evidence [1].

Peptic ulcer had always been an interesting disease of great clinical relevance because of its ability to cause severe dyspeptic symptoms, vomiting, haemorrhage and perforation. The ultimate treatment, removal of most of the stomach, made it very much a surgical disease. Throughout the 20th century, there was felt to be a declining incidence of ulceration of the stomach itself, with an increasing incidence of ulceration of the duodenum, the first part of the small intestine, 12 fingerbreadths (12 cm) in length. There was a tendency to divide peptic ulcer conceptually into two groups, gastric ulcer and duodenal ulcer, without really knowing where to place the ulcers clustered around the pylorus.

The first written description of peptic ulcer was by William Brinton (1823–67), physician at the Royal Free Hospital London, UK, in a monograph published in 1857 [2], in which he reported the result of 7000 autopsies performed by himself and others. He observed that ulcers occurred predominantly in middle-aged and elderly people, with twice the frequency in women compared with men, and that gastric ulcer was much more common than duodenal ulcer.

A study of acute perforated ulcers in Glasgow and the west of Scotland looked at the trends during the first half of the 20th century, between 1924 and 1943 [3], and this was followed by a second study, of the years 1944–53 [4]. The number of perforations per annum increased from about 200 to 700 during this time but despite this, and probably because of surgical advances developed during the Second World War, the number of deaths remained constant and therefore the mortality rate decreased.

The incidence of both forms of peptic ulcer declined during the 20th century, the incidence of gastric ulcer declining first. Perforation of duodenal ulcer was much more common than perforation of gastric ulcer, by a factor of 20, and, for both types of ulcer, perforation was much more common in men than in women, as shown in Table 9.1.

**Table 9.1  Perforated peptic ulcer in the west of Scotland, 1924–53 [4]**

|                | Male | Female | Totals |
|----------------|------|--------|--------|
| Gastric ulcer  | 248  | 71     | 319    |
| Duodenal ulcer | 5175 | 378    | 5553   |
| Totals         | 5423 | 449    |        |

It is interesting to note that R. A. Jamieson, a surgeon in Glasgow, UK, looked at the seasonality of perforation of peptic ulcer and observed a summer dip (and therefore a corresponding winter peak) of deaths from this cause, shown in Figure 9.1. This is another example of the seasonality of disease, and the role of vitamin D needs to be considered.

**Figure 9.1  Deaths from perforated peptic ulcer in the west of Scotland, 1924–53 [4].**

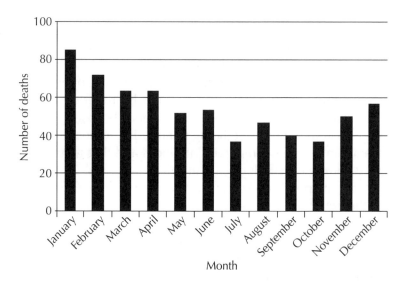

*Adapted with permission from the British Medical Journal Publishing Group.*

It became quite clear during the first half of the 20th century that acid secretion by the stomach was of great importance in the development of peptic ulcer, as it was observed that people whose stomach did not produce acid (achlorhydria) did not develop ulceration at all. But there was much more to it than acid, as some people who produced a great deal of acid showed no features of gastric or duodenal ulcer and some people producing just a normal amount of acid might develop an ulcer.

A general model of understanding is that the body produces, within the stomach, an amount and concentration of hydrochloric acid that is critical and potentially dangerous. Although it has the undoubted advantage of sterilising food, and thus protecting the intestinal tract from infection, there is inevitably a potential problem of acid-related damage. The stomach is able to cope with this by special defence mechanisms, which have never been entirely understood but a major part of which is the layer of mucus secreted by the stomach to protect itself against acid damage. We therefore have a balance between acid causing potential damage and defence mechanisms located within the stomach. This model is generally refined to suggest that in duodenal ulcer the acid production is generally increased and in gastric ulcer the defence mechanisms are reduced.

The recognition of hydrochloric acid produced by the stomach as the major factor leading to duodenal ulcer led to surgical and medical treatments. But acid could only be a mechanism and it was necessary to develop ideas of causation. During the inter-war years of the 20th century, it was felt that nutrition was of fundamental importance and that gastric ulcer in particular had faulty diet as its cause. This idea was probably based on the observation that peptic ulcer was more common in what were then called 'the lower social orders' but what we would now regard as the lower income group or the socio-economically deprived.

Sir Arthur Hurst (1879–1944), physician at Guy's Hospital, London, UK, and the father of British gastroenterology, wrote in 1920 [5]:

*The patient must be made to realize the danger he runs of an ulcer developing unless he eats slowly and chews his food very thoroughly. He should take nothing which is chemically irritating to the stomach, such as alcohol, vinegar, unripe fruit, mustard, pepper, chutney, and curry.*

Gastric diets were devised and persisted through the 1960s, even though Richard Doll (later Sir Richard Doll) and his colleagues at the Middlesex Hospital in London, UK, demonstrated, in 1956, a lack of effectiveness of a variety of dietary treatments for peptic ulcer [6]. The general population accepts very readily dietary explanations of stomach disorders and disease in general. Food is something that can be seen and it obviously has a physical relationship with the stomach. Even today, people feel by instinct that stomach problems must be caused by faulty food, even though there is no evidence to support this as a general concept. Anecdotes by individuals that a certain food causes indigestion might be important for that individual but cannot be applied to the population in general. Furthermore, it has been shown quite clearly, in the era of fibre-optic endoscopy, that most people with dyspepsia (indigestion) do not have an ulcer and also that most people with a peptic ulcer identified as a consequence of bleeding have never experienced dyspepsia.

A new line of thinking had developed at the end of the 19th century, with the influential French neurologist, Jean-Martin Charcot, and his pupils Josef Breuer and Sigmund Freud, at the Saltpêtière Hospital, Paris, France, who developed the concept of the psychological cause of illness. They and their followers proposed that a disordered mind would cause a disordered body and thus disease. From this base, the concept of psychosomatic disease developed progressively throughout the 20th century and was applied to the causation of duodenal ulcer, among many other conditions.

It was thought that there was a social dimension to peptic ulcer. In the early 20th century epidemiology had not developed as a science, but nevertheless there was an impression that gastric ulcer was a disease of poor people who were not eating properly; they were thus their own victims. 'Victim blaming' developed very much as a concept during the 20th century and persists today, leading into a more general 'lifestylism', that illness and disease are the result of the ways in which we live our lives. Lifestyle change then becomes a treatment, and this has been described clearly by Faith Fitzgerald, an outstanding 'clinician–educator' at the University of California School of Medicine, Davis, USA [7]:

> Certain failures of self-care have become, in a sense, crimes against society, because society has to pay for their consequences. And society now looks to health care providers for the education and direction to eliminate behaviour that leads to disease.

It became clear that professional people were suffering from peptic ulcer that was identified more as the duodenal ulcer variant. I must emphasise that the diagnostic methods that we know today had not been developed. I and countless other medical students were taught that the distinction between gastric and duodenal ulcer was the delay between eating and the development of pain, immediate pain indicating gastric ulcer and pain about an hour after eating indicating duodenal ulcer. This was later shown to be of no discriminatory value, but only after the introduction of diagnostic gastroscopy.

To explore the social dimension further, and with much greater accuracy, an important review was undertaken by Michael Langman, Professor of Therapeutics at the University of Nottingham, UK. He confirmed that, throughout the 20th century, peptic ulcer, in both the UK and the USA, has been a disease mainly of the poor, with the exception of duodenal ulcer being more common in the wealthier classes in the UK in the early part of the century [8]. His findings can be seen in Table 9.2.

**Table 9.2 Ulcer mortality in England and Wales and the USA, in men of differing social classes (expressed as standardised mortality ratio) [8]**

| | Social class | I | I and II | II | III | IV | V |
|---|---|---|---|---|---|---|---|
| | Site | | | | | | |
| *England and Wales* | | | | | | | |
| Early 20th century | Gastric | | 86 | | 86 | 105 | 123 |
| | Duodenal | | 133 | | 92 | 92 | 82 |
| Late 20th century | Gastric | 46 | | 58 | 94 | 106 | 109 |
| | Duodenal | 70 | | 84 | 113 | 102 | 136 |
| *USA* | | | | | | | |
| Late 20th century | Gastric | 54 | | 74 | 94 | 113 | 159 |
| | Duodenal | 70 | | 84 | 113 | 102 | 136 |

Although it was acceptable to criticise the lifestyle of the poor, it was not quite so acceptable to criticise the lifestyle of those who were succeeding in the national economy and who were the social equals of doctors. It became fashionable to talk of over-work together with more general concepts such as stress, responsibility and pressure as the cause of duodenal ulcer. It was even suggested that if an executive had not developed a duodenal ulcer then he was probably not working hard enough or earning his money. We were therefore led into 'work-blaming' for the middle classes rather than 'victim-blaming' for the working classes and this was actually very convenient. An executive who developed a duodenal ulcer was rewarded by less work and less responsibility. As we shall see, the same principles were applied to victims of heart attacks in the latter half of the 20th century.

At this time, when the science of epidemiology had not been developed adequately, many ideas were based on anecdotes and very restricted experience of medical practitioners. Indeed the clinical experience of Sigmund Freud was extremely restricted, but he was a good and influential writer, at a time when ideas of causation of disease were lacking, what Kuhn calls the 'pre-paradigm era'. If people required an explanation for a disease the cause of which was unknown, a plausible psychological cause could readily be introduced and accepted, especially if presented by a grave-looking man with a beard who wrote and spoke very well. Psychology was based on anecdotes and theories, what Karl Popper would call 'the pseudo-science of untested and untestable hypotheses'. Scientific rigour was not applied until quite late in the 20th century.

It was against this background that Barry Marshall and Robin Warren took the immense intellectual step of suggesting that peptic ulcer might be caused by an infection. They had identified and cultured the spiral organism long known to exist in the stomach; it has been fully identified and is now called *Helicobacter pylori*.

Marshall and Warren were working at a time when fibre-optic gastroscopy was widely used, leading to a much more accurate diagnosis of peptic ulceration than had been the case. Whereas the diagnosis was previously based on clinical judgement and shadow pictures of barium X-rays, fibre-optic gastroscopy allowed direct inspection of the inside of the stomach and duodenum with high-quality images; furthermore, biopsy specimens were readily available. Marshall and Warren were able to develop a strong scientific background for their work, leading to the observation that *Helicobacter pylori* was present in 90% of patients suffering from duodenal ulcer and 70% of patients suffering from gastric ulcer. Their judgement was to recognise *Helicobacter pylori* as perhaps not the only cause of peptic ulcer but certainly the major cause.

But, before reaching this conclusion, they had to identify more than a strong association between *Helicobacter pylori* and peptic ulcer. They had to demonstrate that, after isolation, the organism was capable of causing the disease in susceptible animal models.

When investigating tuberculosis, Robert Koch was able to transmit the disease to guinea-pigs, creating an animal model that was of immense value to his work. But animal models are not always available and a given micro-organism might cause a severe disease in one animal species but not in another. This was the case regarding syphilis and hepatitis. Transmission studies, the basis of the demonstration of infection and necessary to improve understanding of the causation of disease, could not be applied to laboratory animals, as none was susceptible. The studies were therefore undertaken on human subjects without their knowledge, usually prisoners or residents of institutions for sufferers of mental handicap.

Such research processes that were undertaken in the 19th and early 20th centuries are totally unacceptable in the present time, in which we acknowledge ethical considerations and respect for human beings irrespective of their ethnicity and any misfortune at birth or afterwards. Barry Marshall therefore undertook the experiment on himself, ingesting a culture of *Helicobacter pylori*, and it made him very ill. This was a sample size of only one but, as an experiment, it could not be extended. Despite his qualities and commitment as a researcher, no doubt Marshall would not have undertaken the experiment on himself if, firstly, the infection had potentially fatal results and, secondly, the treatment possibilities had not been very high.

Marshall and Warren needed to add plausibility to the case that peptic ulcer might be caused by *Helicobacter pylori*. The first step was to identify the organism in association with the disease. The second step was to demonstrate that infection with the organism would lead to the disease, but the opportunity for this as an experiment was very much restricted. The third step was to see if eradication of the organism with appropriate medications would bring about cure of disease. These are principles that we will also consider regarding other diseases, for example coronary heart disease and Crohn's disease. Eradication of *Helicobacter pylori* was demonstrated to be effective when antibiotics, combined with bismuth agents or acid suppression therapy, were found to cure gastric and duodenal ulcers in the long term, but only a high proportion and not all.

The work of Marshall and Warren fell on a surprisingly receptive medical audience, perhaps because of the charisma of the researchers and their presence at a number of well-attended international conferences. It was also because, in the pre-paradigm era, there was no plausible competing hypothesis; during the course of the 20th century the dietary and psychological theories had been found to be implausible. A great deal of work had been undertaken on gastric acid physiology and the large research infrastructures within hospitals, universities and the pharmaceutical industry were looking for additional research opportunities, which Marshall and Warren clearly provided.

The *Helicobacter pylori* story became popular very rapidly, helped by the advertising campaigns of the pharmaceutical companies who were to provide the eradication regimes. In fact, the acceptance of the theory was taken to an over-extreme position by the United States National Institute of Health, which identified *Helicobacter pylori* as being 'a grade one carcinogen'. It had been suggested that stomach cancer might be caused by *Helicobacter pylori* because there were studies showing an association [9]. However, this is by no means a definite cause–effect relationship and conclusions cannot be drawn on the basis of this observation alone. It had been clearly demonstrated previously that people who suffer from duodenal ulcer, more definitely associated with the organism, have a low incidence of stomach cancer and therefore appear to be protected.

Another gastric bacterium has been identified, formerly called *Gastrospirillum hominus* and now *Helicobacter heilmannii* [10]. Its clinical importance is uncertain and its identification is not part of standard clinical practice.

The story of peptic ulcer tells us that a disease for which the cause was unclear but which was thought to be dietary or psychological suddenly, and against all expectation, turned out to have a micro-organism as its cause. The inspirational work of Marshall and Warren with *Helicobacter pylori* (for which they were awarded the Nobel Prize for Medicine in 2005) is comparable with that of Koch with *Mycobacterium tuberculosis*. Proof has been based on the association of the organism with the disease together with the benefits of eradication. The concept of proof in the *Helicobacter pylori*/peptic ulcer story was much less rigorous than applied by Robert Koch but this is a subject that will be discussed more fully in a later chapter. It is to be hoped that at the present time medical science might be more receptive to suggestions that chronic diseases of unknown cause might be caused by micro-organisms, but I am by no means certain that this is the case.

The decline of peptic ulcer during the 20th century can in part be the result of the introduction of powerful and safe medications to inhibit acid secretion by the stomach, but it is clear that the decline pre-dated the introduction of medication. The decline was similar to that of other microbial diseases that we have seen, and has probably been the result of improved resistance of the population against infections and perhaps reduced exposure of the population to the micro-organism as a result of improved sanitation. The seasonality of perforation suggests that vitamin D might provide a protective role.

Peptic ulcer brings us again to the geography of disease. Perforation of duodenal ulcer in men has been shown to be twice as frequent in the north of England than in the south (adjusted for population size and age) and four times as frequent in Scotland. There is also the social dimension: peptic ulcer in men is twice as common in socio-economic group V (unskilled) as in group I (professional). We will meet more of these issues in later chapters and also the associations between peptic ulcer and other diseases, with further suggestions of a protective role of vitamin D.

We have seen in the examples of tuberculosis, syphilis and peptic ulcer, that familial constitutional disease is more likely to be environmental than genetic, and that there are strong relationships between the micro-organism, the human host and the environment. Looking at tuberculosis in more detail will enable us to learn much more.

# 10
# TUBERCULOSIS AND SOUTH ASIAN ETHNICITY

W e have seen that the incidence of tuberculosis in the UK decreased substantially during the 20th century, but the pattern seemed to change and it appeared that the condition was not being eradicated in the way that might have been expected. During the second half of the 20th century it became clear that immigrants to the UK from south Asia have a high incidence of tuberculosis. Although this is sometimes in the pulmonary form, with cough and chest X-ray abnormalities, it can also be in other parts of the body, such as lymph nodes, brain, spinal cord and intestine. The presentation is often non-specific, with fever, malaise and weight loss. When a disease is in an inaccessible part of the body, such as internal lymph nodes, the diagnosis is often based on the clinical pattern rather than identification of the causative organism concerned.

Tuberculosis is a major disease in sub-Saharan Africa at present because of the epidemic of AIDS, this condition reducing immune competence and therefore the defences of the body against the disease. Tuberculosis is an important disease in Asia for reasons that we will investigate later, but its incidence in immigrants from south Asia into the UK is very much increased compared with what would be expected in their countries of origin. It is clear that the occurrence of tuberculosis is dependent on impaired immunity of individuals.

There is no doubt that the burden of tuberculosis within the UK is unevenly distributed, with a particularly high incidence among those whose origin is the Indian subcontinent. In a survey of all tuberculosis notifications for a 6-month period in England and Wales in 1978–79, a total of 3732, it was noted that 35% were from patients whose origin was India, Pakistan or Bangladesh, almost 10 times greater than their proportion of the population [1]. It is thought that the risk of an immigrant from south Asia developing tuberculosis in the UK is 30–40 times that of the indigenous population.

This presents a very serious problem to those who have come to this country from south Asia. It might be anticipated that the peak incidence of disease would be on arrival in this country, the immigrants having brought the disease with them. It might also be expected that there would be a steady decline in the incidence as the population became adapted to living in the UK, with its greater wealth. Those initially having disease would be treated and the ethnic group would then enjoy the decline of tuberculosis, as in the indigenous population defined in Figure 3.2. This, however, turned out not to be the case, as determined by a survey conducted in Wandsworth, south London [2].

The initial study included 620 patients from south India who were diagnosed between 1973 and 1988 as having active tuberculosis. The peak incidence of diagnosis was found to be at about 5 years after immigration, indicating that the disease was not present as such on arrival in the UK but developed subsequently. A further study by the same group from St George's Hospital Medical School, UK, indicated that as many as two-thirds of the cases were notified more than 5 years after arrival in the UK [3]. Clearly living in the UK was not a good thing with respect to tuberculosis, and it appeared that there must be an environmental factor responsible.

Because the background population of the UK at the end of the 20th century had a low incidence of tuberculosis, it was considered unlikely that those entering this country from south Asia would acquire (catch) the organism after arrival. It was felt to be much more likely that the observed high incidence of the disease was explained by activation of latent disease after arrival in the UK, as a result of encountering a new susceptibility factor found in the UK. It is well established that tuberculosis can be dormant or latent and emerge many years later as an active disease, usually at times of suppression of immunity, such as with AIDS. Could the south Asian immigrants have developed some form of immunodeficiency after moving to the UK?

Further evidence came from an analysis of the subgroups of those from south Asia who developed tuberculosis. The immigrant population is, in fact, diverse and by no means homogeneous, comprising people of different religions and different cultural traditions. We are talking about people coming from a total population of 1.5 billion. The analysis was broken down initially according to two major religions, Islam and Hinduism [3]. The results are summarised in Table 10.1.

Of those south Asians diagnosed in Wandsworth as having tuberculosis, the Hindus had a significantly greater risk than Muslims, the overall Hindu:Muslim ratio being 4.5:1. The incidence was highest of all in those Hindus who were lactovegetarians and who would eat no form of animal products, including fish and eggs.

It was concluded that the susceptibility factor to tuberculosis lay somehow in south Asian ethnicity, whatever the religious or cultural subgroup. However, the observations from this study led the researchers to suspect that meat and other animal products offered significant protection. The south Asian Muslims consumed a moderate amount of meat but still had an increased susceptibility compared with the background local population. It was also felt that the rather lesser amount of meat but the consumption of fish and eggs by the Hindu population would offer minimal protection, but there would be no dietary protection for the lactovegetarians, who had an 8.5-fold risk compared with regular meat and fish eaters from the same ethnic group.

**Table 10.1  Risk of developing tuberculosis among ethnic groups in Wandsworth [3]**

| Group | Risk |
| --- | --- |
| Hindu:Muslim | 4.5:1 |
| Vegetarian:meat/fish | 4.3:1 |
| Lactovegetarian:meat/fish | 8.5:1 |

It was not possible to draw an absolute conclusion from these studies as they were observational and not experimental. Observational studies can only produce hypotheses that might be tested, and subsequent experiments might be undertaken at some stage in the future. There were four main observations regarding tuberculosis among the south Asian immigrants: it was more common than in the indigenous population; it usually occurred after 5 or more years in the UK; it was more common in vegetarians; and meat and fish appeared to be protective.

The explanation and hypothesis presented by the study group is that, when south Asian immigrants arrive in England, their sunlight exposure diminishes suddenly and substantially. Vitamin D synthesis in the skin reduces as a result of this, and body stores of vitamin D, mainly in the liver, are gradually mobilised for metabolic use until they are exhausted. The hypothesis goes on to suggest that vitamin D derived from sunlight provides significant protection against tuberculosis for all the ethnic groups whilst they are in their original south Asian country, usually India or Pakistan. The increased distance of the UK from the equator, the increase in cloud cover and perhaps a more indoor life because of the cold atmosphere, will lead to less sunlight exposure and vitamin D synthesis. This will be exacerbated by their skin pigmentation, dress and behaviour. During the 5 years following immigration, vitamin D stores are gradually used up and not replenished. It is at this stage that tuberculosis will activate.

These studies suggest that insufficient sunlight and vitamin D are likely to be the cause of the increased susceptibility of the south Asian population of the UK to tuberculosis. A further study investigated the role of vitamin D, looking at Gujarati Asians in west London; it found that the incidence of tuberculosis is three times higher in those with the lowest blood levels of vitamin D [4].

The studies described are particularly important because they lead us to identify that disease can occur because of a susceptibility factor rather than an altered exposure to the cause itself, in this case a micro-organism. Furthermore, they identify a powerful environmental factor, namely sunlight, that has a modulating effect on a microbial disease. We see an interaction between genetic factors (skin pigmentation), behavioural factors (dress and cultural sun avoidance) and the environmental factor sunlight. This can be summarised as in Figure 10.1.

**Figure 10.1 Model of the protective effect of vitamin D on tuberculosis and the influence of ethnic factors**

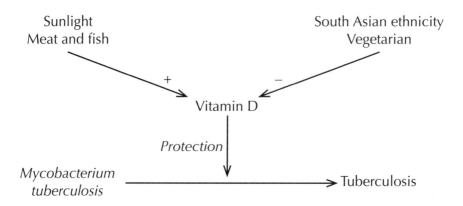

The logical extension of this hypothesis is to conduct an experiment to determine whether either artificial sunlight or vitamin D supplementation protects against the development of tuberculosis following immigration into this country. It would need to be randomised so that only half of those investigated received the hypothetical protection and the other half did not. To my knowledge, such an experiment has not yet been conducted. It is interesting to note that, whereas tuberculosis in south Asians is treated using standard microbicidal therapy, no attention is given to vitamin D insufficiency, either by vitamin D supplement or heliotherapy (treatment by the sun).

Whereas acquired immunodeficiency resulting from vitamin D deficiency is the cause of the high incidence of tuberculosis in people born of south Asian ethnicity, the incidence of tuberculosis in the UK is now much higher in black Africans born in Africa [5]. This is because of another form of immunodeficiency, AIDS. Once again we see the importance of the susceptibility factor rather than just the causative micro-organism. We need to explore in more detail the nature of tuberculosis and also the biology of vitamin D to help us understand this important health issue.

# 11
# LESSONS FROM TUBERCULOSIS: A MULTIFACTORIAL DISEASE

Tuberculosis represents the battle that is a perpetual process involving an interaction between infection and the body. A dead body undergoes the process of putrefaction under the influence of micro-organisms that are then totally uninhibited, and it is the intrinsic vitality of life, virulence, that keeps micro-organisms at bay to prevent deterioration of the body, in other words to prevent disease. The weaker the life force, the more liable the body is to infection and deterioration. The life force, the vitality, of the body is clearly of immense importance and its nature must be understood. There are several factors involved, and tuberculosis can be regarded in many ways as a multifactorial disease because there are certain aspects of life that make the condition more likely to develop and therefore may be seen as causative.

Malnutrition, usually meaning under-nutrition, has been and still is associated with tuberculosis. This was the case in western Europe in the 19th and early 20th centuries and is observed in many poor countries of the world. It is not just malnutrition itself but also poverty that has been closely linked with tuberculosis; it has been assumed that the major mechanism by which poverty and tuberculosis are linked is malnutrition.

Poverty has often been linked with industrial cities, with the hungry poor dying in unheated homes (such as Mimi in *La Bohème*), but it can also be applied to rural communities with little wealth. It is mainly city dwelling that has been identified as a risk factor for tuberculosis, with treatment historically being provided in sanatoriums built in rural environments.

Tuberculosis tends to run in families but, whereas this was originally thought to imply an inherited or constitutional causation, scientific thought in the 20th century has considered the familial clustering to be the result of close proximity and exposure to a transmissible environmental factor. There would be common susceptibility rather than genetic inheritance. However, none of the risk factors for tuberculosis could be considered to be the cause; it was always possible for people developing tuberculosis to have none of the risk factors (family history, low socio-economic status, living in cities, faulty nutrition), even though this might be exceptional. In times before the identification of the tubercle bacillus as the cause of tuberculosis, environmental, family and social factors were seen to be of the greatest importance.

If a disease is multifactorial, then there must be the suggestion that removing any of the factors will lead to a reduction of incidence of the disease, and that appears to have been the case with tuberculosis. We have seen that, during the 20th century in the UK, the number of deaths caused by tuberculosis decreased quite dramatically, and this was before the development of effective microbicidal chemotherapy and before the development of BCG immunisation. The reason for the decline in tuberculosis is by no means clear but it is assumed to be because of the modification of various social susceptibility factors, mainly environmental and in particular the relief of poverty with an improvement of nutrition and housing.

The decline of tuberculosis can be regarded as because of either a mutation of the organism leading to a lower level of pathogenicity, or an increased resistance of the human host. The general impression is that the latter view is correct, and this becomes clear if we look at the big picture: it was not just tuberculosis, but the incidence of several other microbial diseases (including peptic ulcer) declined at the same time. It would be a great coincidence if several micro-organisms had simultaneously undergone a mutation to lower virulence; it is much more likely that the change has been within the human host.

We can therefore build up a model of a cause of tuberculosis, with a series of susceptibility factors that make the disease more likely to occur. These factors are under-nutrition, poor socio-economic status, living in cities, having the disease in the family, Asian ethnicity and more recently, suffering from AIDS. The model is:

$$\text{cause} + \text{susceptibility} \longrightarrow \text{disease}$$

This is an important model that we will return to later. It is from the study and example of tuberculosis that this very important model can be developed, but it is applicable to a number of other conditions. In many diseases the susceptibility factors are called risk factors, whether they are on the causal pathway or whether they indicate something that is not easily measured. Remember that having a meal as a child sitting at a table with the family is the most powerful predictor of good health in adult life, but we do not regard eating a meal in front of the television as causing disease. The example of tuberculosis illustrates that the causation of a disease is not always simple and that there is usually an interplay of genetic, social, behavioural and climatic factors.

# 12
# GLASGOW: A MICROCOSM OF THE INDUSTRIAL SOCIETY

Glasgow must be viewed as one of the greatest cities of the world, having made immense contributions not only to industrial production but also to art, education and commerce during the past two centuries. Glasgow was a small and unimportant place before the industrial era, Edinburgh being the major centre of government and tradition of Scotland. However, Glasgow embraced the industrial revolution, with the development of heavy industry based on education and learning. The population of Glasgow grew from 77 000 in 1801 to 740 000 in 1901. The industry for which Glasgow became best known was ship-building on the River Clyde, but this in itself required an enormous industrial infrastructure of steel, railways, coal and also the craftsmanship that went into the finished products. It is quite remarkable to think that towards the end of the 19th century almost 20% of all the ships in the world had been built in the shipyards of the Clyde, which employed at their height 38 000 workers.

The wealth generated by this industry produced what, at the time, were high-quality tenement houses for the population. This housing fell into disrepair in the mid-20th century, and most of it was demolished in the 1960s to be replaced by housing that many people now regard as inferior. Glasgow had developed a strong architectural tradition, with high-quality buildings designed by such architectural geniuses as Alexander 'Greek' Thomson and Charles Rennie Mackintosh. Unfortunately, many architectural gems were replaced during building programmes in the late

20th century, and some of the new buildings detracted from, rather than enhanced, the greatness of the city. The industrial production also led to the creation of personal fortunes, witness the vast art collection of Sir William Burrell that can be seen in Glasgow today.

But industrial and wealth production in Glasgow and elsewhere came at a considerable price, and that price was the health of its population. As Charles Dickens expressed on visiting the industrial cities of the north of England during the mid-19th century, 'May God forgive us for what we are doing'. As well as being arguably the industrial capital of the world, Glasgow became the tuberculosis capital of the world, with an exceptionally high incidence of the disease among its citizens. Once again, we have a high density of population, with large families living in cramped surroundings, so that the transmission of an infective agent would be common-place. In addition to the susceptibility factors of close contact and over-crowding, there is a distinct possibility that sunlight deprivation was an important and key factor. The 19th century was a time of a major movement of the British population from rural work that was, of course, outdoors in a clean atmosphere, to industrial work of long hours, indoors, sometimes underground and in a city in which the atmosphere was becoming steadily more polluted, with little sunlight penetration to ground level.

Glasgow also became the rickets capital of the world. Rickets is a developmental disease of the growing bones of children, leading to stunting of growth and deformity. It is caused by a deficiency of vitamin D, which will be the subject of a later chapter; it is usually the result of sunshine deprivation, particularly in people living in cities. Even today, children of south Asian immigrants living in Glasgow have a greater incidence of rickets than those living in Bradford or Coventry [1].

Accurate comparative data are not readily available but, during the 20th century, Glasgow appeared to become the peptic ulcer capital of the world. This was certainly the perception of people who were aware of research into peptic ulcer. It could be that the reputation was based on the learning and research of such outstanding individuals as Professor C. F. W. Illingworth and R. A. Jamieson of the vey influential Department of Surgery of Glasgow University, UK, whose work from the mid-20th century we have seen. It is likely that the detailed investigation by the researchers was stimulated by the high prevalence of the disease in Glasgow.

Glasgow can also be viewed as the myocardial infarction capital of the world, with an extremely high incidence almost equalled only by Northern Ireland and Finland. Statistics released by the British Heart Foundation in March 2001 indicated that Glasgow was top of the world league for heart attacks (coronary events) in women, at 265 per 100 000 women aged 34–65 years, taken from data collected in 1999 from 35 different locations [2].

We have up-to-date data on the health of the population of Glasgow. As reported in *The Guardian* on 10 March 2004, the UK average life expectancy for men is 77 years. In the Shettleston district of Glasgow, the average life expectancy for men is 63.9 years, and in Springburn 66.6 years. These two locations in Glasgow are described as the UK's most socially deprived, and so we see the interaction between place of residence and social geography. Is the health record of Glasgow explained purely by its social order or is there still something special about Glasgow?

A further disease for which Glasgow has considerable notoriety is dental decay, and it is generally felt that the dental health of the population of Glasgow is perhaps the worst in the world. It was said for many years that the standard 21st birthday present for a citizen of Glasgow was a set of dentures. Things have improved since then, but we must not leave Glasgow without acknowledging this characteristic.

It is possible to look at each of these diseases as unrelated entities, but Glasgow provides us with the opportunity to observe the clustering of diseases in the same population group. Is it mere coincidence that one population has had particularly high incidences of tuberculosis, rickets, peptic ulcer, coronary heart disease and dental caries? This is unlikely, and we must look at the possibility of such associations being more than chance. It is difficult, however, to conceive that all these diseases have the same cause, and we are more likely to be looking at a common susceptibility to disease. Is there something about Glasgow that leads to a particularly common susceptibility to these various and common diseases? The examples of tuberculosis and rickets suggest that a key factor might be vitamin D deficiency as a result of poor sunlight penetration, because of the high latitude, low altitude, atmospheric pollution and housing characteristics. This is something that we must explore further as it might be relevant to other diseases.

Comparative data between cities and between populations is important but it is also vital that the data are collected in a reliable and accurate way. I touched upon Northern Ireland, and in particular its capital city Belfast, perhaps the equal of Glasgow regarding coronary heart disease. In the British Heart Foundation report mentioned above, Belfast was the runner-up to Glasgow regarding heart attack rates in women, with 180 per 100 000 [2]. We must visit Belfast and look in more detail at the health characteristics of that city, just a short distance from Glasgow and sharing many of its social and historic features.

# 13
# BELFAST AND TOULOUSE

The ill-health of the population of Glasgow became legendary, but there has been considerable concern regarding the comparative health of people living in a wider area of north-west Europe, in particular the north-western parts of the British Isles, and those living in the Mediterranean countries. Until recently only speculation was possible, most of which was based on lifestyle features, either diet or stress. A further puzzle was the apparent decline of coronary heart disease in the latter half of the 20th century, the details of which we will see later. The search for more evidence led to a study initiated within the UK by Hugh Tunstall-Pedoe, Professor of Epidemiology at the University of Dundee, and co-ordinated by WHO [1]. This is the international MONICA project, 'multinational monitoring of trends and determinants in cardiovascular disease'. Alun Evans, Professor of Epidemiology and Public Health at Queen's University, Belfast, developed MONICA in Belfast and also a similar project, the PRIME study, 'prospective epidemiological study of myocardial infarction' [2].

Although these studies have been concerned with coronary heart disease, they have provided very interesting additional information. Rather than the broad approach of comparisons between countries, the studies have targeted in detail two particular cities, Belfast and Toulouse, which have certain similarities and, in that respect, comparability, but are located in different parts of Europe.

Belfast is situated on the north-east coast of Ireland, at the head of a large sea loch that provides shelter and makes it eminently suitable for shipping. It developed as a sea port and a ship-building city before the days of steam, and it became the location, until very recently, of the world's largest rope works. Despite the paucity of coal reserves in Ireland, Belfast embraced the industrial revolution, importing coal mainly from the coast of Cumbria across the Irish Sea. It became a major ship-building city, the home of Harland and Wolfe, from whose shipyard *Titanic* was launched in 1911.

Belfast has a history very similar to that of Glasgow. Its population has been highly productive, creating a vast industrial output with the very minimum of natural resources other than its manpower. Both Belfast and Glasgow lie close to the sea and are at sea level. They lie on a similar latitude, Belfast 54°36′ North and Glasgow 55°52′ North. It is interesting to observe that latitude 55° North passes through Alaska, Hudson Bay and Siberia. Both Belfast and Glasgow lie further north than any part of China. They are quite close to the Arctic and, as we shall see later, they are under the influence of a cold Arctic air stream. They are habitable with comfort only because of the warming influence of the Gulf stream.

Toulouse lies in the south of France and is also an industrial city, one of the most important in France. It is not on the coast and its single main industry is aircraft production. Toulouse lies about 820 miles (1300 km) to the south of Belfast and Glasgow, on latitude 43°38′ North.

The MONICA study provides accurate data concerning the mortality patterns of Belfast and Toulouse. It is a prospective study and the investigators had agreed descriptive terms in advance. The overall death rate for men aged between 45 and 64 years is much higher in Belfast compared with Toulouse, as shown in Table 13.1. This confirms earlier impressions and reinforces public health concerns. For men in the age-group 45–54 years, the death rates per 100 000 are 638 in Belfast and 459 in Toulouse. This is worrying, but for the age group 55–64 years the deaths rates are 2112 in Belfast and 1197 in Toulouse, an excess mortality rate of 76% in Belfast [2]. This is dramatic and must cause great concern for those with responsibility for public health.

**Table 13.1 Age-specific mortality data from Belfast and Toulouse [2]**

| Cause | Belfast | Rate/100 000 Toulouse | Ratio |
|---|---|---|---|
| | | **Men aged 45–54 years** | |
| All causes | 638 | 459 | 1.4: 1 |
| Coronary heart disease | 237 | 56 | 4.2: 1 |
| Stroke | 32 | 24 | 1.3: 1 |
| Other cardiovascular disease | 30 | 22 | 1.4: 1 |
| Cancer | 188 | 159 | 1.2: 1 |
| | | **Men aged 55–64 years** | |
| All causes | 2112 | 1197 | 1.8: 1 |
| Coronary heart disease | 761 | 175 | 4.3: 1 |
| Stroke | 130 | 61 | 2.1: 1 |
| Other cardiovascular disease | 130 | 92 | 1.4: 1 |
| Cancer | 694 | 195 | 1.3: 1 |

*Adapted from the QJM, with permission from the Oxford University Press.*

If the overall death rate is higher in Belfast, then the specific diseases responsible for this need to be identified. The main one is coronary heart disease, the death rate for men being more than four times greater in Belfast than in Toulouse in both age groups. Other cardiovascular diseases, mainly stroke and peripheral vascular disease, also show a higher rate in Belfast than Toulouse, the death rate for men aged 55–64 years from stroke being twice as high. It is also worth noting at this point that death rates from cancer are also higher in Belfast than Toulouse, by a factor of 20–30%.

We will consider these specific diseases in later chapters, and the geography of cancer towards the end of the book. At present we must acknowledge the disturbing information identified by the MONICA study. Belfast and Toulouse were chosen for detailed study, but we have already seen that Glasgow has an even worse health record than Belfast. We will be looking at various other locations in the UK and Europe. We will also be looking at possible explanations for the remarkable susceptibility of the population of Belfast to early death from a range of diseases. The important thing to note at present is that the excess mortality in Belfast is not the result of a single disease but several diseases. Their association might provide a clue to cause, and that will be the subject of the next chapter.

# 14

# ASSOCIATION AS A CLUE TO CAUSATION

An important part of the process of clinical medicine and the clinical management of individual patients is identifying patterns. A patient may have just one or two features of illness, which is therefore straightforward. For example, a productive cough and fever of a few days duration would indicate a high probability of acute tracheobronchitis or perhaps pneumonia. Another patient might have a number of different features of illness and a more complex clinical presentation. When the association becomes more frequent than would be expected by chance, the collection of features, the combination of symptoms, the various aspects of disease process or abnormal blood tests, will make up a pattern that is called a syndrome.

The identification of a syndrome is an important intellectual resting place in the understanding of disease. A syndrome often carries the name of the physician who first identified the pattern. For example, the great French physician and neurologist Jean-Martin Charcot (1825–93) identified two triads, syndromes of three features. The first was the association of fever, jaundice and pain in the right upper quadrant of the abdomen, which later was recognised as cholangitis. The second was the association of dysarthria, ataxia and nystagmus (slurring of speech, unsteadiness and tremor of the eyes), later becoming recognised as characteristic features of multiple sclerosis. It is important to note that such syndromes were not defined statistically but based only on clinical impression, by a physician with great experience.

A syndrome is thus a pattern of illness that is recognised and has an identity leading to understanding, perhaps of causation, and ultimately treatment. The syndromes bearing the eponym of Charcot were based on simple clinical features, for example fever, rather than what might be called complete disease processes. The medical world has been able to accept these but has found it more uncomfortable when it comes to the grouping of defined diseases, although some people appreciate that this must be done. As expressed by Ronald La Porte, Professor of Epidemiology at the University of Pittsburgh, USA [1]:

*We need to examine and model the evolution of patterns of disease. We need to break away from our orientation towards single disease and begin to focus on the big picture.*

An example is Saint's Triad, first defined in print by the Johannesburg radiologist Dr C. J. B. Muller in 1948, but he attributed it to his former colleague Professor C. F. M. Saint, who was Professor of Surgery in Cape Town, South Africa [2]. The triad is the association of hiatus hernia, gallstones and diverticular disease of the colon. Each of the three is recognised as being a disease in its own right, and this brings us back to the concept of disease. Saint and Muller recognised that they were associated more often than would be expected by chance. Each of the three can be defined in terms of pathology, that is a structural abnormality, but none is understood regarding causation or even pathogenesis, the mechanism by which the structural abnormality is produced. Saint and Muller made no attempt to propose a common cause in this continuing pre-paradigm phase: their common purpose was to draw clinical attention to the association so that patients could be diagnosed more readily.

Denis Burkitt (1911–93) worked after the Second World War in the Colonial Medical Service as a government surgeon in Africa (1946–62). He became interested in the pattern of disease and thereby became well-known as an epidemiologist. His main claim to fame is the identification of what became known as Burkitt's lymphoma, which presents clinically as a large facial swelling. He noted that its geographical location was defined by altitude limits, and this led to the identification of its cause, the Epstein–Barr virus, transmitted by mosquitoes within a specific habitat. This conclusion is of major importance because it is an example of cancer caused by a micro-organism; we will see more examples later. An outstanding clinical review of Mphatso, a child suffering from Burkitt's lymphoma, appeared in the Christmas 2006 edition of *The Lancet*, as the Wakely Prize Essay [3].

As part of his more general surgical work in Africa, Burkitt noted that he saw the three conditions making up Saint's Triad extremely rarely, whereas he had seen them commonly in the UK when he undertook his medical education and surgical training. Thinking in terms of 'association is a clue to causation', he felt that there must be a common cause. As they were all gastrointestinal diseases, he thought that they might be the result of faulty nutrition. In 1969 he proposed that the refinement of flour in the UK and the western world was the common cause, a simple proposal that was readily received at the time, when dietary theories were thought to be plausible [4]. His ideas still influence treatment.

A further important example of the association of diseases being a clue to causation is the observation that led to the understanding of syphilis, in the way described earlier. We have seen that Francis Welsh and Alfred Fournier, working independently, noted that a variety of well-defined diseases, GPI, TD, gummas (tumours composed of inflammatory tissue) and thoracic aortic aneurysms, were likely to be associated more commonly than would have expected by chance. This was all brought together shortly afterwards by Sir Jonathan Hutchinson (1828–1913), surgeon at the London Hospital and President of the Royal College of Surgeons, UK. This was in the days before formal statistical analysis, but the clinical impressions were based on extensive clinical experience and proved to be correct. Welsh used data collected from the well-recorded deaths of soldiers, and was able to identify the association between syphilis and death from ruptured aortic aneurysm. He would not have been able to do this for the general population as the data were not available. Welsh, Fournier and Hutchinson assembled these defined illnesses effectively into a syndrome, grouping them into a single disease entity (syphilis) that allowed identification of the cause, *Treponema pallidum*, and ultimately lead to specific treatment with penicillin.

The clinical doctor delivering patient care will frequently, in daily practice, identify a syndrome affecting an individual. Of equal importance, or in the long term of even greater importance, is the public health dimension of looking at the association of disease patterns within communities and populations, creating a population syndrome that provides an opportunity for the identification of a common cause or susceptibility, and the opportunity for preventative intervention.

We have seen the historic clustering of disease in the population of Glasgow, tuberculosis, rickets, peptic ulcer, coronary heart disease and dental decay, and we might be led to the most simple conclusion that they all have the same cause. This was true for the triads of Charcot and the identification of the late manifestations of syphilis. But our increasing knowledge of pathology and understanding of causation should warn us to be cautious and not jump to conclusions. We must remain wary of the views of Burkitt and others, who insisted that there must be a common dietary cause for the cluster of what Burkitt called the diseases of western civilisation. We must also be open to the fact that a number of apparently specific diseases might share a common cause. An alternative view of the association of diseases that I would like to propose is that it does not necessarily mean a single cause but a common susceptibility factor, a very different thing.

I have used the words 'cause' and 'causation', which are different. A cause is an entity, something that can be seen or measured; causation is a process leading to the development of a disease. Disease can arise from the interaction of the cause with susceptibility factors, and the term pathogenesis is also used to define this process.

The association of tuberculosis and rickets suggests that sunshine and vitamin D provide the link. The susceptibility of the population of Glasgow to both diseases was because of the environmental factor of atmospheric pollution and industrial working practices. In a similar way, because of rather different environmental factors, the south Asian immigrants into the UK have developed a high incidence of vitamin D deficiency and also susceptibility to tuberculosis.

We need, then, to look at the association of diseases that appear to lead to the poor health and reduced lifespan of the population of Belfast compared with that of Toulouse. Rather than a common cause, could the association be that of a common susceptibility factor? Could it be a geographical and climatic factor, a lower exposure to the sun of the population of Belfast? This is the theme that will be developed in later chapters but, in the meantime, we need to look at vitamin D in more detail, starting with its discovery.

# PART 3

# VITAMIN D

# 15
# RICKETS AND THE DISCOVERY
# OF VITAMIN D

Rickets is a disorder of growing bone and is thus seen as an active disease in children, but the resultant deformities can persist into adult life. The equivalent active disease in adults is osteomalacia, meaning soft bones.

Bone formation starts as the production of a fibrous substance called osteoid, which is laid down in a structural pattern called matrix. Under the influence of vitamin D, specialised cells called osteoblasts then convert this matrix into mature bone with the addition of a calcium-containing compound, a process called ossification. When vitamin D is deficient the ossification fails, leaving bone that is not rigid, and so it can bend and deform during growth and weight-bearing. The characteristic deformity is bow-legs. Vitamin D deficiency occurring during adult life produces bones that can fracture through an osteoid seam that has not ossified. This is possible because bone is always in the process of reconstruction and new osteoid is constantly being laid down to be formed into new bone.

Although rickets is usually caused by deficiency of vitamin D, it can also occur because of rare metabolic disorders that lead to a lack of activity of vitamin D within the body. This resistance to vitamin D is because of a genetic abnormality of what are called vitamin D receptors (VDRs) that are found within cells. This is a general principle: all hormones, chemical messengers, require a receptor in the target cells, and it is the receptor that drives the metabolic action. The receptor is a complex molecule within the cell; it turns on specific cell functions, but only after it has been activated by a hormone. Vitamin D, like other hormones, acts as an all-important key to 'unlock' the dormant receptor. VDRs are, of course, found in osteoblasts, but they are also found in a surprisingly large number of cells, normal cells and some tumour cells. When VDRs are abnormal, vitamin D is ineffective because it cannot turn on the defective receptor. VDRs are inherited and, as we will see later, the inheritance can result in an abnormal receptor.

It was in the new industrial cities of the UK, and particularly in Glasgow, that the emergence of rickets was first observed. A child with rickets (a rickety or rachitic child) is recognised by growth retardation and general sickliness with failure to thrive. The first specific features of rickets relate to the epiphyses of bones, the growing plates close to the ends of long bones, which become characteristically swollen just above the wrists, forming the rickety (or rachitic) bracelet. The epiphyses also expand close to the junctions of the ribs with the sternum, leading to the appearance of the rickety (rachitic) rosary. It is when a child starts to walk that the bones of the legs bear weight and bend, creating the deformities characteristic of rickets that will survive into adult life, even if the deficiency of vitamin D is corrected.

There had to be an explanation, there must be a cause, for this new disease of rickets. It had not been seen in the old coastal fishing communities that were characteristic of pre-industrial Scotland, and it was correctly felt that the movement of the population from one environment to another must hold the key. The answer was probably provided by the observation that a folk medicine, fish oils, was protective against illness when given to infants and was found to be protective against rickets. Organic chemistry had not developed at the end of the 19th century; fish oils were simply noted to contain a substance essential for child development, and it was later classified as vitamin D. It was subsequently identified as a steroid compound, called calciferol because of its physiological effect on bone formation.

The same clinical problem was encountered in Austria but the deduction of its cause led to a different conclusion. Industrialisation had occurred in most European countries at a slightly later time than in the UK, but once again rickets was observed in children living in the new industrial cities. It had not been seen previously in the typical farming communities of Austria and, as in Scotland, a change of environment was felt to hold the key. But lack of fish or indeed any dietary change did not seem to be important in central Europe. It was observed that sick and rickety children improved when they were moved back to a farming village or high location: sunshine, or lack of it, appeared to be the answer. It was suggested that, under the influence of the sun, the skin was producing a substance that was necessary for bone development. This chemical messenger, hormone, was subsequently called cholecalciferol. It was later shown to have identical actions as the vitamin D obtained from fish oils.

Vitamin D thus has two sources, the sun and diet, and the relative importance of the two depends on location, season and individual attributes. We have seen that, in south Asians living in the UK, sunlight is generally inadequate and therefore diet is critically important. Research from Australia has demonstrated that the contribution of dietary vitamin D is insignificant in the summer but in the winter it is of some importance, but inadequate as a total replacement for sunshine [1]. Fortunately, being fat soluble, vitamin D can be stored in the liver and the fat cells of the body during the summer months of sunshine for use during the winter.

Although it became clear that sunlight deficiency was responsible for the development of rickets, it was subsequently noted that rickets could occur in severely malnourished children who had had adequate sunlight exposure, mainly in Africa. In these circumstances a very severe deficiency of calcium can give rise to rickets, even when vitamin D supplies are adequate.

Children with rickets had also been recognised as being sickly, that is to have a more generalised disorder, with frequent respiratory illnesses in particular. This could possibly be because of chest deformities resulting from rickets but could also arise from a more direct effect of vitamin D, which is now known to be necessary for the development of immunological protection against infection. Children with physical and learning disabilities have been more prone to rickets and vitamin D deficiency. This is probably because of an almost exclusively indoor existence, especially in the days of institutional residence, with lack of outdoor exposure to sunlight. Deficiency of vitamin D, with reduced immunocompetence, could be a reason why people with physical and mental disabilities tend to have a shortened lifespan.

A particularly important survey of rickets in Glasgow was undertaken in 1918 by Dr Margaret Ferguson, working for the Medical Research Council, UK [2]. The paper, sponsored by the new National Insurance of the UK, is fascinating in that it was at a time when the cause of rickets was not clear. Although fish oils were known to be helpful for reasons that were unknown, Ferguson was obviously struggling to make sense of the substantial and important data that had been assembled. She looked at the various social and economic factors, identifying social deprivation and poverty as being the major risk indicators of rickets. It was clear that poverty was characterised by poor diet and a lack of fresh air and exercise.

Ferguson brought to attention a clear, close relationship between lack of fresh air and rickets, but was unable to separate the importance of dietary factors, as in Glasgow poor diet was always very closely related to lack of fresh air. As we understand now, there is an additive effect of dietary deficiency of vitamin D when associated with sunlight deprivation.

The publication was probably distributed quite widely, as it came to the attention of Dr H. S. Hutchison, who had been posted to the Nasik district of the Bombay presidency in India [3]. He observed that children of the poor were generally free of rickets, despite a very inadequate diet with, in particular, virtually no meat or animal products, but they did have plenty of fresh air. He noted that, whereas the children of the poor in Glasgow had an inadequate diet, sunlight deprivation and lack of fresh air, leading to rickets, the children of the poor in India had an inadequate diet, plenty of fresh air and no rickets. This led him to the conclusion that fresh air (what we now know to be sunlight exposure) was the major factor in prevention of rickets.

Hutchison and his assistant S. J. Shah also investigated the wealthier population of India, and discovered rickets to be quite common among their children. They conducted a comprehensive house-to-house survey of the district, identifying disease patterns and also dietary patterns. Whereas the poor (called class II in this study) had very little animal protein intake, the wealthier (class I) had a significant amount of animal products and, even if they were vegetarian, they would take butter and ghee. As part of the house-to-house survey they found that 13.7% of children of class I Hindu families had rickets and 10.2% of class I Muslim families, compared with 0.3% of class II Hindu children and 2.7% of class II Muslim children. This is shown very clearly in Figure 15.1. Hutchinson and Shah also noted that the women and their children of the poorer classes were of much finer physique than those of wealthy families.

**Figure 15.1  Prevalence of rickets in Indian children [3].**

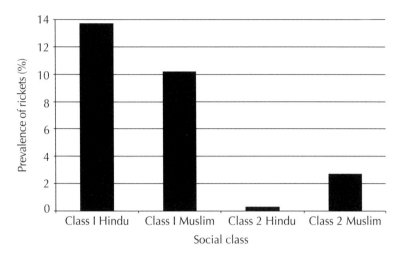

*Adapted from the* Quarterly Journal of Medicine *with permission from the Oxford University Press.*

The conclusion was that the high incidence of rickets in the well-to-do class was because the women were superfluous to industrial and agricultural production needs and therefore were able to practice purdah, remaining indoors for virtually all of their married life. Women of the poorer families had to work out in the fields and purdah was a luxury that they could not enjoy. Hutchinson and Shah felt that the slightly higher incidence of rickets in the poor Muslim families compared with the Hindu families was because even the poor Muslim women did practice a certain aspect of purdah and remained indoors much of the time. The lifestyles of the populations concerned were described very well in the paper by Hutchison and Shah, published in 1920. It is also interesting that they reported that the Brahmin women, who were vegetarian and practiced purdah, were well nourished but 'phthisis' (tuberculosis) and anaemia were rampant among them. Here was a strong suggestion of rickets and tuberculosis being closely associated, and both resulting from sunlight deprivation.

Rickets is still seen in the UK today. The epidemiology has not been clearly defined but, certainly in the northern industrial towns, rickets is quite commonly seen in babies born to mothers from south Asia. It was in Glasgow in 1962 that the first observations were made that rickets and osteomalacia were much more common in the Asian ethnic population than in the white population [4]. The impression is that rickets does not occur commonly in India and Pakistan at the present time but it is the result of immigration to a more northern latitude, associated in particular with social aspects of sun avoidance, an indoor life pattern and a great deal of skin covered by clothing, We can remember Leila living in Kabul, which is at latitude 34°34′ North. Karachi (Pakistan) lies on latitude 24°7′ and Delhi (northern India) on latitude 28°39′; Glasgow lies on latitude 55°52′, almost 2000 miles (3300 km) to the north.

Evidence of osteomalacia can be found in a high proportion of the south Asian ethnic population in the UK at the present time. While it may not reach overt clinical disease, it can certainly be found very commonly if it is looked for carefully. How south Asian people living in the UK become deficient in vitamin D is slightly controversial; the main area of controversy is skin pigmentation. Research suggests that south Asian people have the same capacity as white-skinned people to synthesise vitamin D but social factors are of great importance. It is felt that, within the UK, south Asian people tend to be congregated in inner city areas, where opportunities for sun exposure are reduced, and that they are culturally disinclined to expose themselves to the sun. Because the skin tends to go darker with sun exposure, girls in particular may try to avoid the sun. Muslim women minimise exposure of the skin out of doors and may have a tradition of fully covering themselves when outside the house. In contrast, observation in the parks and cities of northern Europe during the summer suggests that the fair-skinned indigenous population has a genetic characteristic that impels them to remove their clothes when the sun shines; if so, obviously a protective gene for people living at that latitude.

The differential rates of rickets between children born to Muslim and Hindu mothers has not been identified, as far as I am aware, but the south Asian immigrant populations in the northern industrial towns tend to be predominantly Muslim. Although Muslim women may receive more vitamin D from meat compared with their Hindu counterparts, they tend to have a greater skin cover as part of the Muslim dress code. As we will see later, such populations have serious health problems in later life and it is the main theme of this book that such ill health is determined by the susceptibility factor of vitamin D insufficiency, which can often be traced back to infancy and indeed to the mother before conception.

Vitamin D deficiency has been reported in Israel, a country with a great deal of sunshine. It has been found among young ultra-orthodox (Haredi) women and is considered to be because of their dress habit, long-sleeved dresses, high necklines, opaque stockings, hats and other headgear worn for reasons of modesty and tradition [5]. In a paper describing these findings, Professor Yosef Weisman of the University of Tel Aviv, Israel, commented that about 40% of Haredi women would not be able to synthesise adequate amounts of vitamin D because of the high level of skin cover. Figure 15.2 shows the results of this study and also the beneficial effects of vitamin D supplements. Vitamin D insufficiency is defined as a low blood level of calcidiol (25-hydroxy vitamin D) and deficiency is when this is associated with biochemical features of osteomalacia.

**Figure 15.2  Vitamin D insufficiency in Jewish mothers in Israel [5].**

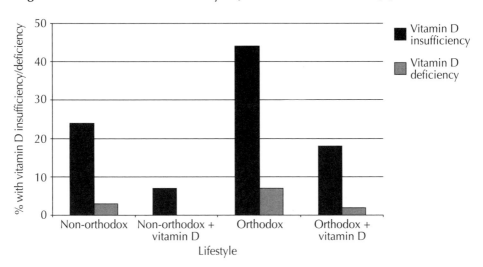

*Adapted with permission from the* Journal of the Israel Medical Association.

Vitamin D deficiency in adults can occur because of other diseases, in particular intestinal disease with impaired absorption of vitamin D from the food, kidney disease and, occasionally, liver disease, for reasons that will be seen later. However, the most common cause of vitamin D deficiency in adult life is inadequate sunlight exposure together with inadequate dietary sources of vitamin D. It can be seen in the indigenous white population of this country, when it might be called privatational osteomalacia because it is encountered mainly among elderly people, who are housebound by necessity, and the reclusive, who are housebound by choice.

A study undertaken in the Johns Hopkins University School of Medicine, Baltimore, USA, investigated the vitamin D status of elderly people who were housebound [6]. It included 64 residents of nursing homes and 121 people living at home. The predominant disease processes in these people were cardiovascular diseases, including coronary heart disease, stroke and peripheral vascular disease. There was also a control group of 128 subjects who were healthy, mobile elderly people. The average vitamin D level from the control group was 68.4 pg/mL; in the sun-deprived group it was significantly lower, at 53 pg/mL (both measuring 1-25 vitamin D, calcitriol).

There are different interpretations of the association between vitamin D deficiency and being housebound. The most obvious is that being confined to the home diminishes sunlight exposure and diminishes vitamin D levels in the blood. However, although this is perfectly reasonable, plausible and almost certainly true, there is no doubt that vitamin D deficiency can interfere with mobility and so there could be a vicious circle of continually reducing mobility with vitamin D depletion causing osteomalacia. It is interesting to note that the major disabilities of those who are housebound are cardiovascular disease, and we shall see later that there is a strong association between vitamin D deficiency and cardiovascular disease.

A study from Japan has indicated that vitamin D deficiency is common in people with Parkinson's disease [7]. The average blood level of vitamin D (measured as 1-25 vitamin D, calcitriol) in a control group was 49.6 pg/mL; in those with Parkinson's disease it was 26.8 pg/mL in one group and 30.2 in another group. We once again have an association that needs interpretation. The authors of the study felt that the low vitamin D level was the result of restricted movement, mainly indoor living, as a result of the Parkinson's disease, and therefore low vitamin D synthesis in the skin. This seems to be a sensible interpretation and is another example of how vitamin D deficiency can occur in disabled people, resulting in further ill health, disability and reduced life expectancy. Another interpretation might be that vitamin D deficiency predisposes to Parkinson's disease. Although it cannot be eliminated as a possibility, it is not an explanation that is plausible at the present time, and so the first interpretation would appear to be more acceptable.

Rickets has emerged in the USA recently, but has been reported only in black children [8]. It is suggested that the cause is a combination of skin pigmentation together with behavioural features, such as the children being indoors all day, fear of outdoor crime, parents at work, concerns about exposure to atmospheric pollution, and fear of the sun causing skin cancer (heliophobia).

Another effect of vitamin D deficiency in infancy is poor development of teeth, with the delayed appearance of primary dentition but, more importantly, poor enamel formation on permanent teeth. It is interesting to remember that Glasgow has been noted for both rickets and poor dentition of young adults. We will return to dental health later, but for now we need to understand more about the biology of vitamin D.

# 16
# THE BIOLOGY OF VITAMIN D

The main thesis of this book is that sunlight is protective and that insufficiency of it increases susceptibility to disease. We must look at the mechanisms by which sunlight interacts with the human body to produce vitamin D, and this is going to necessitate a biochemical review with some technical detail.

Sunlight can act favourably on the human body through vitamin D synthesis and also by two indirect mechanisms. Air temperature is one of these. We associate absence of sunlight with the cold of winter, but air temperature is also determined by air movement, cloud cover, distance from the oceans, sea temperature, latitude and altitude. The other intermediary between sunlight and the human body is food, agricultural production being very dependent on sunlight. These factors will be discussed in later chapters but for now I would like to concentrate on the direct effect of sunlight, the production of vitamin D.

The metabolic interaction between sunlight and the body results in the synthesis and probable degradation of vitamin D within the skin, an organ that is metabolically active rather than just a waterproof coating to the body. Research has shown that vitamin D is in fact a group of related chemical compounds with different levels of biological activity. It is important to understand the formation of vitamin D because it is very closely related to the formation of cholesterol, a subject that we will meet in a later chapter. The subject may appear to be very complicated but the basic outline is as follows, and is shown in Figure 16.1.

**Figure 16.1 The metabolic pathway of the various forms of vitamin D.**

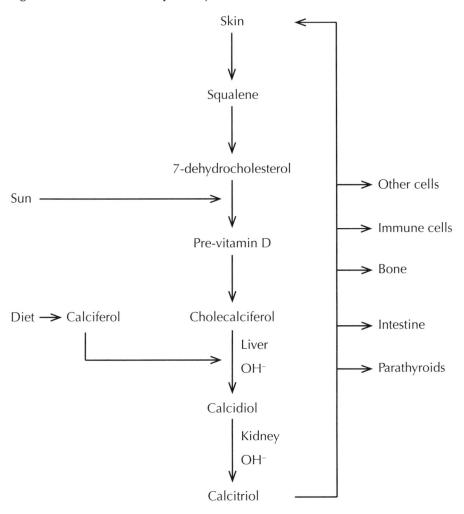

*Adapted with permission from* Annals of Clinical Biochemistry.

The metabolic pathway is within the cells of the skin and the compounds concerned are shown in Figure 16.2. Our starting point is the synthesis of a long-chain unsaturated hydrocarbon called squalene, one of the omega-3 fatty acids. Squalene was first discovered in shark liver by Dr Mitsamaru Tsujimoto of the Imperial Industrial Laboratory, Tokyo, Japan in 1916 [1]. Through further enzyme activity, the squalene molecule becomes folded to create a basic sterol nucleus, which has four joined rings. The specific molecule created at this stage is the important 7-dehydrocholesterol.

The next stage in the production of vitamin D requires input of energy from the specific ultraviolet wavelengths of sunlight, UVB 290–315 nm. As a result of the energy of this irradiation, the sterol ring structure is split to form pre-vitamin D; the site of the split can be seen in the structure of pre-vitamin D in Figure 16.2. This molecule instantly undergoes a change of shape, with partial unfolding, to create the first vitamin D compound, cholecalciferol (Figure 16.2). It can be seen that this has a similar structure to calciferol (ergocalciferol), which is derived from fish oils. It is important to note that this process is one of physical chemistry and not biochemistry. It can occur in creatures that live in the sea close to the surface and it can occur *in vitro*.

It will be seen later that, whereas in the presence of sunlight vitamin D is synthesised in the form of cholecalciferol, in the absence of sunlight the metabolic process from 7-dehydrocholesterol maintains a complete sterol ring structure. It is directed into the synthesis of the closely related and more well-known compound cholesterol, the major animal sterol.

Vitamin D as found in food, in particular fish oil, has the name of calciferol, which is also known as ergocalciferol and it is absorbed from the small intestine, then passing through the portal vein to the liver. Within the liver an important chemical transformation takes place, with the addition of a hydroxyl (OH) group, to form calcidiol, so-called because the molecule now has two (di-) hydroxyl groups.

**Figure 16.2  Molecular variations of vitamin D.**

Squalene

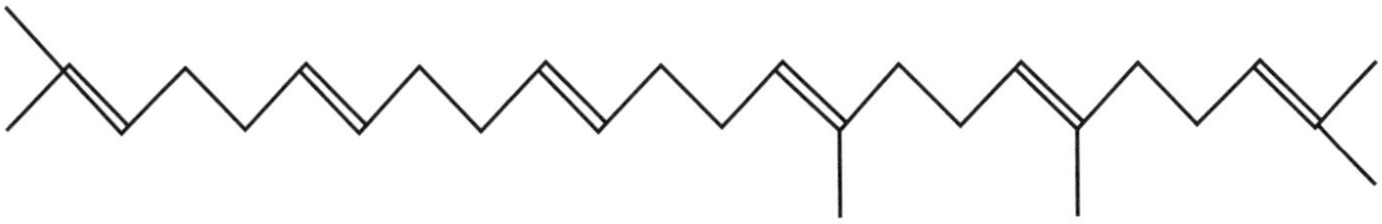

7-dehydrocholesterol

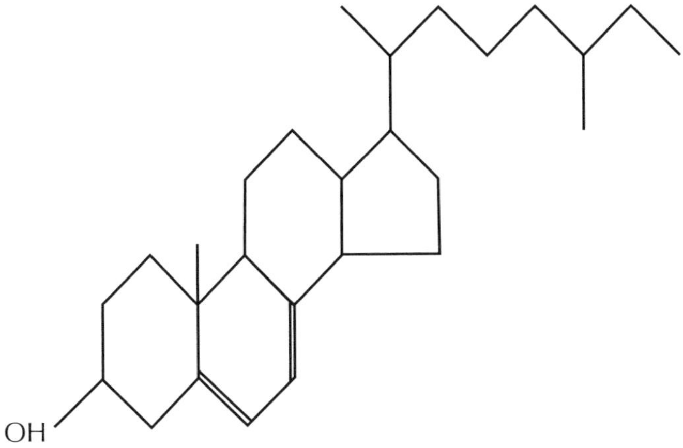

OH

Pre-vitamin D

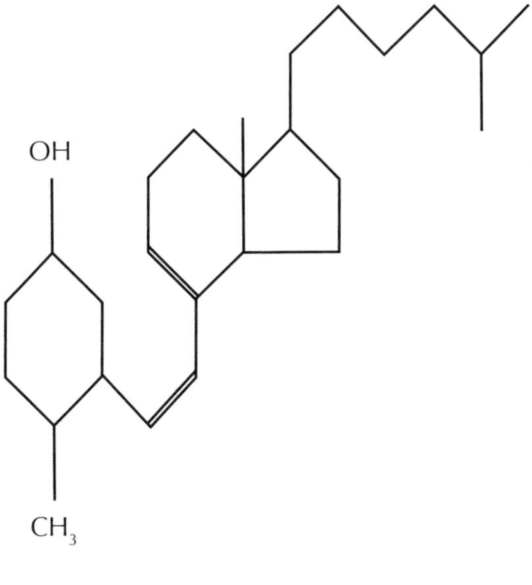

OH

CH₃

Cholecalciferol

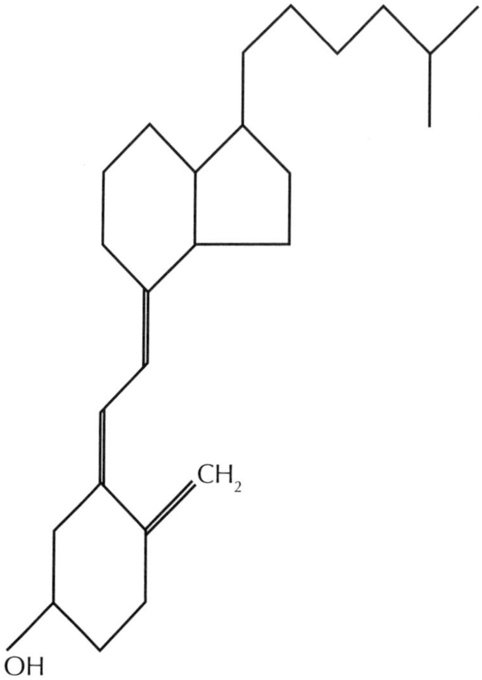

Calciferol (ergocalciferol)

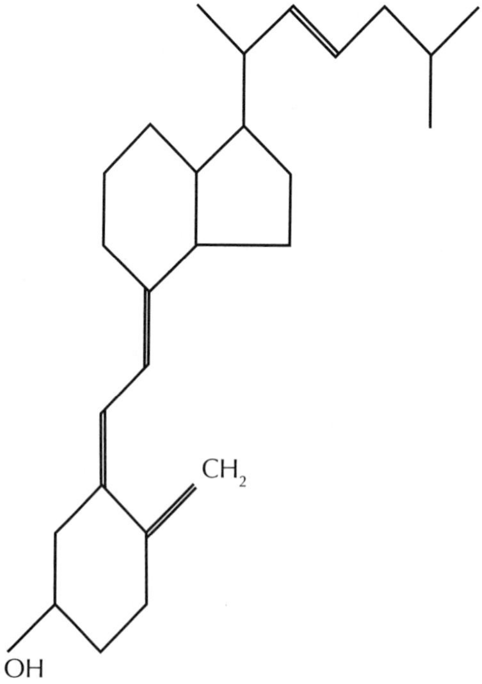

Calcidiol, 25-hydroxycholecalfierol, 25-hydroxyvitamin D, 25(OH)D

Calcitriol, 1,25-hydroxycholecalfierol, 1,25-hydroxyvitamin D, 1,25(OH)2D

There is a convention of numbering the corner carbon atoms of the sterol ring structure. Calciferol and cholecalciferol have a hydroxyl group at position 3 and this can be seen in Figure 16.2. Calcidiol has an additional hydroxyl group at position 25. Calcidiol is sometimes called 25-hydroxyvitamin D, 25-hydroxycholecalciferol or, more simply, 25(OH)D. Calcidiol is the more simple name that I will be using.

Calcidiol leaves the liver and enters the general circulation, but as it passes through the kidney it is altered by the addition of a further hydroxyl group, to form calcitriol. This third hydroxyl group is placed at position 1 and so calcitriol is also called 1,25-hydroxyvitamin D, 1,25-hydroxycholecalciferol or, more simply, 1,25(OH)2D. Calcitriol is again the simple name; it is the most metabolically active form of vitamin D within the body.

Cholecalciferol, like calciferol, is metabolically weak. In exactly the same way, its biological activity is enhanced by two stages of hydroxylation, the first in the liver, to calcidiol, and the second in the kidney, to calcitriol. There is an implication from this that the effects of vitamin D deficiency can be seen in liver disease and kidney disease, but these are rare circumstances and of no further concern at present.

Calciferol is strictly speaking vitamin D, an essential chemical that is obtained from the diet. It is a pro-hormone in that it is converted into calcidiol and then calcitriol to produce its biological effects. The synthesis of cholecalciferol in the skin is usually much more important than calciferol in the diet, but I will use the term vitamin D to include both.

The amount of calcidiol in the blood is a measure of vitamin D derived from either diet or sunlight. The normal range does not have a meaning in a population with overall poor exposure to sunlight. It is measured as either nanogrammes per millilitre (ng/mL) or as nanomols per litre (nmol/L), an obvious source of confusion. What can be said is that the optimal blood level of vitamin D as calcidiol is in the range of 30–40 ng/mL (80–100 nmol/L). Bone disease would be expected with a level less than 10 ng/mL. Insufficiency of vitamin D without bone disease but with significantly detrimental effects on immunity would be expected in the range of 10–20 ng/mL.

The amount of calcitriol in the blood depends on the metabolic conversion of calcidiol, mainly within the kidney. It is about 1000 times more active than calcidiol and it is measured in the blood as picogrammes per millilitre, the normal range in the UK being between 20 and 50 pg/mL.

Because calcitriol is so highly active, the amount of it must be controlled very carefully; not only must it be produced but it must also be inactivated. This is achieved mainly by the enzyme 24-hydroxylase, which adds an additional hydroxyl (OH) group, thereby changing the molecule into a form that has only one-hundredth of the activity of calcitriol [2]. Further inactivation of vitamin D compounds is thought to take place from sunlight energy during circulation through the skin, producing a number of photo-metabolites with no known biological activity.

It is important to point out at this stage that it is possible to receive an excessive dose of vitamin D through medication error, creating a condition called hypervitaminosis D. However, because calcitriol and other vitamin D compounds are inactivated by the action of sunlight on the skin, hypervitaminosis D cannot occur by natural means. It is not possible to develop an excess of vitamin D from sunlight exposure [3].

Calcitriol circulates in the blood and has a number of well-recognised biological activities. First, it promotes the absorption of calcium from the small intestine. Second, in the presence of adequate dietary calcium, it promotes bone formation, and its absence results in rickets and osteomalacia. Another action of vitamin D, and the action that is most important to this book, is the stimulation of immunity. It may also bind to VDRs within other cells and influence their metabolism. Table 16.1 lists the cells in which VDRs have been detected, and it can be seen that it includes some cancer cells [4]. We will see this in more detail towards the end of the book.

**Table 16.1 Tissue distribution of Vitamin D Receptors (VDRs) [4]**

| Normal | Malignant |
|---|---|
| Intestine | Breast cancer |
| Bone | Melanoma |
| Kidney | Colon cancer |
| Skin | Osteosarcoma |
| Lymphocytes | Medullary cancer of the thyroid |
| Monocytes | Myeloid leukaemia |
| Parathyroid | Lymphocytic leukaemia |
| Testis | Pancreas cancer |
| Ovary | Transitional cell cancer of the bladder |
| Placenta | Cervical cancer |
| Pituitary | |
| Pancreas | |
| Thyroid | |
| Colon | |

*Adapted with permission from* Annals of Clinical Biochemistry.

VDRs are complex proteins that are found within certain cells. They are genetically determined and are created within the cells by the process of transcription, that is synthesis from a template provided by RNA. VDRs are synthesised within the cells in an inactive form; they require the incorporation of calcitriol before they become active and stimulate intracellular metabolic processes.

It is suggested that melanin pigment produced within the skin in response to exposure to sunlight has a moderating effect on vitamin D synthesis. Similarly, it is felt that the natural skin pigmentation is at least in part responsible for the high incidence of vitamin D deficiency in south Asian immigrants in the UK. The relative importance of pigmentation and behavioural factors in south Asians is controversial.One study, from Holick and colleagues in the USA, suggests that south Asian immigrants have the same capacity as the white population to synthesise vitamin D [5]. This suggests that deficiency is likely to be almost entirely the result of cultural behavioural characteristics, these being extensive clothing and a tendency to live an indoor life.

This view is supported by a study from Rochdale in Lancashire, UK, which examined the blood vitamin D levels of south Asians living in this town. The levels were low, as could be predicted, but their family members living in Lahore and Rawalpindi in Pakistan had normal vitamin D levels [6]. The conclusion of this study is that deficiency of vitamin D in Rochdale is the result of behavioural and not biological factors, but this view is not conclusive because the sunlight levels are much lower in Rochdale than in Pakistan.

We have already noted the increased susceptibility of people to tuberculosis when they do not have adequate exposure to sunshine because of environmental factors, especially if there is also a diet low in vitamin D. Rickets and osteomalacia can occur, rarely, when vitamin D is present as calcitriol in adequate amounts but does not function because of faulty VDRs in the tissues. This condition, sometimes called vitamin D pseudodeficiency, is the result of abnormalities (mutations) of the gene responsible for the synthesis of VDRs, and the effect is the same as deficiency of vitamin D. It can lead to an increased susceptibility to tuberculosis, and we will meet it again when we look at Crohn's disease.

The process whereby a gene becomes abnormal is called a mutation. When a mutant gene becomes well-established in a population, it is called a polymorphism. There are many 'abnormal' encoding genes and thus a range of polymorphisms of VDRs, with varying levels of metabolic efficiency. With low exposure to the sun, people with very efficient VDRs will be at an advantage compared with those with less efficient VDRs. It is possible that fair-skinned people in north-west Europe have a survival advantage not just because of a lack of skin pigment but also because of natural selection of very efficient VDRs in an area where sunlight intensity is low. This is one way in which the genetic susceptibility to disease is being understood by the new molecular biology; this subject is reviewed well by Wharton and Bishop in a seminar in a recent issue of *The Lancet* [7].

# 17
# TUBERCULOSIS AND THE SUN

I have pointed out that children with rickets have a predisposition to respiratory infection and there appears to be a geographical relationship between rickets and tuberculosis. This is based mainly on the experience of industrial cities in general and Glasgow in particular. We have also noted the susceptibility to tuberculosis of south Asians who move to the UK, and it is therefore useful to explore the experience in the 20th century of the therapeutic use of sunshine in the treatment of tuberculosis. However, it was in Glasgow in 1896 that James Burn Russell (1837–1904), the first full-time and great medical officer of health of that city, remarked in his report *On the Prevention of Tuberculosis* that: 'Sunlight is the only disinfectant which sustains the man while it kills the micro-organism' [1]. The source of this idea lay across the North Sea, in Denmark.

Niels Ryberg Finsen was born in 1860 in the Faeroe Islands, where his father was the governor. He was educated in Reykjavik, Iceland, and obtained a medical degree from the University of Copenhagen, Denmark, in 1891. His initial research looked into observations that sunlight had a detrimental effect on the skin lesions of severe smallpox. He identified ultraviolet light as the damaging part of the spectrum and this led to his use of red light or the 'red room' for the treatment of smallpox.

He realised that sunlight was biologically important and his further research turned to the then common and disfiguring skin disease lupus vulgaris, a manifestation of tuberculosis of the skin. He demonstrated in 1895 that exposure to artificial ultraviolet light would cure this condition, and for this major medical advance Finsen was awarded the Nobel Prize in 1903. His adult life was impaired by ill-health because of constrictive pericarditis (thought to be caused by hydatid disease acquired from sheep droppings in childhood) and this led to his early death at the age of 44 years.

Although tuberculosis of the skin was the subject of Finsen's studies, he suspected that ultraviolet light improved the health of his patients through suppression of internal disease. As tuberculosis is an active disease process, we would expect ultraviolet light to act through a biological rather than a physical process. Immunology as a science had not developed in the early years of the 20th century, but it is now clear that the mechanism by which sunlight heals tuberculosis is the enhancement of immunity by vitamin D.

It had also been noted that tuberculosis was rampant in cities but rare among rural communities and, in particular, with the Austrian experience, almost non-existent in people living at high altitudes in the Alps. The early years of the 20th century therefore saw a new treatment for people suffering from tuberculosis: heliotherapy, treatment by the sun. The Swiss Alps became the centre of this, with the development of high-altitude treatment resorts (Kurort) in locations such as St Moritz (1856 m, 6090 feet, above sea level) and Davos (1560 m, 5118 feet, above sea level). It was realised that the treatment of tuberculosis was based on ultraviolet light and not on temperature, and also that ultraviolet light could not penetrate glass. The hospitals, or sanatoriums as they were called, were built with rooms facing south and each room had a balcony on which the patient would recline on a chair, couch or even bed. The patients were clothed against the cold and the treatment seemed to be effective even when the exposed parts of the skin were limited in the winter to the hands and face. Indeed it is known now that perhaps exposure of only these parts of the body is necessary for some vitamin D production.

Only the wealthy could afford to go to the high-altitude resorts of Switzerland for heliotherapy, but tuberculosis was a major public health problem of the poorer people of Europe in general, and of the UK in particular. We have seen the development of the voluntary infirmaries in the cities of the UK, but they were orientated towards the care of industrial injuries and short-term illness. They did not see the treatment of tuberculosis and other chronic diseases as being their prime responsibility. The municipal authorities had built their own hospitals including, as already mentioned, fever hospitals and smallpox isolation hospitals. In the early 20th century they built sanatoriums that were located out of the cities, usually placed towards the prevailing wind so that the air would be as clean as possible, with the industrial smoke blowing in the opposite direction. They were modelled on the Swiss sanatoriums, with wards facing to the south and with balconies on to which the patients could be wheeled in their beds whenever the sun was shining.

Heliotherapy was an important health care movement in the first half of the 20th century. I have never seen any attempt to evaluate it in terms of patient outcome, but it must be remembered that this was an era before the introduction of the randomised controlled clinical trial. The development of the heliotherapy movement would suggest that it was indeed effective for controlling tuberculosis, rather than necessarily having a long-term curative effect. An extremely interesting and full account of heliotherapy has been written recently by Richard Hobday, also an expert on solar design of buildings [2].

There was also a move to use sunlight as a preventative treatment, and sunshine clinics were often provided as routine to inner-city children, who would sit around an ultraviolet lamp dressed only in knickers and protective goggles. The fashion for this came to an end only in the 1960s.

We therefore see a very close relationship between tuberculosis and insufficient exposure to sunlight. It is quite clear that tuberculosis is caused by the micro-organism *Mycobacterium tuberculosis*, without which the disease cannot occur. I have already established the model:

$$\text{cause} \times \text{susceptibility} = \text{disease}$$

We can now see that, apart from AIDS, insufficiency of sunlight is the major susceptibility factor in determining whether or not a person exposed to *Mycobacterium tuberculosis* develops the clinical illness of tuberculosis.

In the 19th and early 20th centuries, the people most susceptible to tuberculosis were those living well away from the equator in north-west Europe, and especially those living in cities with heavy atmospheric pollution, poverty, cramped living conditions, poor nutrition and indoor life with long hours of indoor work. During the second half of the 20th century, south Asian ethnicity became the most important susceptibility factor. Living at high altitudes in the Alps appeared to be protective, and all these factors are influenced by sunshine.

We are also aware that, in addition to insufficient sunlight exposure, there are other causes of immunodeficiency allowing the development of tuberculosis. The most important factor at the present time is the epidemic of AIDS, mainly in Africa and compounded by the immunodeficiency that appears to be a result of severe malnutrition. Early in the 21st century we find that black African immigrants have the highest incidence of tuberculosis in England and Wales, twice the incidence as those from India, Pakistan and Bangladesh, as reported by the UK Health Protection Agency in November 2006 [3], shown in Figure 17.1.

**Figure 17.1 Tuberculosis in the main ethnic groups in the UK, 2004 [3].**

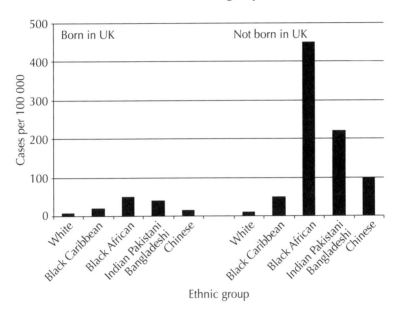

© *Crown Copyright 2006, adapted with permission.*

Another factor identified as a susceptibility factor for tuberculosis is a mutation of the VDR. We have seen that this can lead not only to tuberculosis but also to the development of rickets and osteomalacia in those with adequate sunlight exposure, for example in Nigeria [4].

A study was undertaken in west London, UK, investigating the population of south Asians of Gujarati origin [5]. Many are vegetarian and are known to have a particularly high incidence of tuberculosis. The study included 91 patients with tuberculosis before treatment was started and 116 healthy subjects. The blood level of vitamin D (as calcidiol) was checked and deficiency was found to be associated with active tuberculosis.

Undetectable levels of vitamin D (less than 7 nmol/L) carried the highest risk of tuberculosis. A low level of vitamin D, when combined with certain mutations of the VDR genotype, had the same high risk as undetectable levels. It was concluded that vitamin D insufficiency is likely to be contributing to the high risk of tuberculosis in the Gujarati population. It also indicated that, if there is a relatively mild deficiency of vitamin D, the co-existence of genetic mutations of VDR gives a much higher susceptibility to tuberculosis.

The plausibility of this was enhanced by laboratory observations identifying that vitamin D has a direct effect on immunological processes. In an inspired paper written in 1985, Peter Davies, a physician working in Swansea, UK, and later in the Cardiothoracic Institute in Liverpool, UK, re-introduced the concept of sunlight and vitamin D assisting the body's immunological defence mechanisms in the fight against tuberculosis [6]. Further laboratory investigations have been undertaken and it has been demonstrated that cell-mediated immunity is suppressed in mice that are rendered deficient in vitamin D [7]. Cell-mediated immunity is particularly important in the body's control of tuberculosis. For reasons that I fail to understand, Davies' work has not been absorbed into mainstream medical practice, and south Asian patients with tuberculosis are not normally given vitamin D to supplement the anti-tuberculosis microbicidal therapy (microbicidal meaning that the medications kill the micro-organism; strictly speaking they are not antibiotics because they are entirely synthetic).

It has also been demonstrated that macrophages are important in the body's defence mechanisms against tuberculosis [8]. The word macrophage means 'big eater' and these cells are involved in the inflammatory process, particularly in destroying foreign proteins and cleaning up sites of infection; we will revisit macrophages towards the end of this book. This study also demonstrated that the addition of vitamin D *in vitro* enhances the effects of macrophages.

We have looked at the increased susceptibility of people who have in their environment inadequate exposure to sunshine, especially if there is also little vitamin D in the diet. The strong association between susceptibility to tuberculosis and a mutation of the gene that encodes the VDR is also important. Here lies an important interaction between genetic characteristics and the environment [9].

Therefore it appears that, with an adequate food supply and in the absence of other important diseases, sunshine exposure provides good control of tuberculosis. Improvement of nutrition and increased sunlight exposure of the population of the UK were responsible for the decline in the incidence of the disease during the first half of the 20th century. Important developments were increased leisure time, a shorter working week and the provision of public parks, the lungs of the cities. However, the introduction of the specific antibiotic streptomycin in 1948, supported by the microbicidal compounds para-amino-salicylic acid (PAS) and isoniazid, provided the ultimate treatment and the possibility of definitive long-term cure of tuberculosis in individuals. In fact, the introduction of the antibiotic streptomycin for the treatment of tuberculosis led to the world's first randomised controlled clinical trial.

The trial was conducted by the UK Medical Research Council (MRC) and it compared the outcome of 55 patients with advanced pulmonary tuberculosis given streptomycin treatment with that of 52 similar patients treated with traditional sanatorium therapy. Most of those treated with streptomycin improved and four died, compared with improvement in only 8% of those receiving sanatorium treatment and 14 deaths [10]. However, it became clear that treatment with streptomycin alone (monotherapy) led rapidly to the emergence of strains of the bacillus that were resistant to streptomycin, with re-emergence of disease after completion of the trial.

People have argued about the ethics of the MRC trial on the basis that death could have been foreseen for the untreated and therefore those who died in the untreated group were victims of scientific rigour as much as of the disease itself. What such critics probably did not realise is that the subsequent mortality in the treated group almost equalled that in the untreated group. After 5 years, 35 of the 52 receiving sanatorium care had died, as had 32 of the 55 who had received streptomycin monotherapy. In later trials triple therapy, with a combination of streptomycin, PAS and isoniazid, was shown to have long-term effectiveness. An excellent review of this and other aspects of tuberculosis is provided by Frank Ryan, former physician in Bury, UK, and now successful author, in his book *Tuberculosis: The Greatest Story Never Told* [11].

Tuberculosis is an interesting model that brings out the multifactorial nature of disease, the social and ethnic dimensions, genetics and, in addition, geography and history. It also indicates the important potential of sunshine and vitamin D in the prevention and treatment of disease. It is now time to look at what is generally considered to be the major disease of Europe and North America during the latter half of the 20th century: coronary heart disease.

# PART 4

# CORONARY HEART DISEASE

# 18

# THE EMERGENCE OF CORONARY HEART DISEASE AND ITS DECLINE

It is not easy to recognise a potential new disease until it has developed into a public health problem or achieved a size that might qualify it as an epidemic. This was the case with the emergence of acquired immune deficiency syndrome (AIDS), as it was with coronary heart disease. The first half of the 20th century saw Europe preoccupied with the massive catastrophes of two world wars. However, epidemic water-borne infections had come to a virtual end, infant survival had improved substantially and tuberculosis was on the decline. The epidemic of influenza at the end of the First World War was brief but carried a mortality of millions. Then something new appeared: coronary heart disease.

The origins of coronary heart disease are obscure, probably because there were two other major forms of heart disease in the early 20th century, rheumatic fever and syphilis. With the virtual disappearance of these in Europe and North America in the 1950s, as a result of a combination of personal health factors, public health initiatives and the introduction of penicillin, coronary heart disease became more obvious as the major heart disease of the time.

However, a question remains regarding whether coronary heart disease was common or rare at the start of the 20th century, and opinions are divided concerning this. Was the disease new or just newly recognised? It was not mentioned in the first edition of the first major textbook of medicine, published in 1895 and written by Sir William Osler (1849–1919), Professor of Medicine at McGill University, Montreal, Canada,

119

at Johns Hopkins University, Baltimore, USA, and finally at Oxford University, UK. However, he mentioned angina in the 1912 edition [1]:

*It [angina] is a rare disease in hospitals: a case a month is the average even in the large metropolitan hospitals.*

The expression 'myocardial infarction' was first used by the French physician René Marie in 1896 but it did not come into common use until after a further publication in French literature, by C. Lian in 1921 [2]. These reports were clinical, describing what the authors felt at the time was a new disease. Before this, descriptions of the condition had been provided by pathologists based on autopsy studies. These earlier case reports emphasised the pathological feature of a thrombotic event in the coronary artery, which led to the use of the term coronary thrombosis. This will be discussed in more detail in the next chapter.

The first description of the clinical illness that we now call myocardial infarction was published in 1859 by the Swedish physician J. P. Malmsten and pathologist G. W. J. Von Duben, based on a presentation to the Swedish Medical Society. This has been reviewed in detail relatively recently [3].

The report by Malmsten and Von Duben is of particular importance because they felt that they were describing something new, and that is certainly the way it was received. However, their report was not translated into English and it remained obscure. It was not until 1912 that the condition of myocardial infarction resulting from coronary artery disease was accepted in the USA. In England, this concept was rejected in 1915 by Sir Clifford Allbutt, Professor of Medicine at Cambridge University. Sir James MacKenzie, the father of British cardiology, started his medical research whilst a general practitioner in Burnley, Lancashire. The third edition of his book *Diseases of the Heart* was published in 1913; in it he described the illness of angina but he did not relate it to disease of the coronary arteries [4].

The recognition of coronary heart disease and its incidence increased during the 20th century. The Swedish physician B. W. Johansson and pathologist P. Nicol pointed out that, whereas in 1859 Malmsten and Von Duben identified a single case, in their home city of Malmo in 1978 there were 770 new cases of acute myocardial infarction [3]. This would seem, in the view of most people, an adequate basis for classifying it as an epidemic.

There are, however, dissenters from this view. W. E. Stehbens, from the Department of Pathology, Wellington Medical School, Wellington, New Zealand, expresses this forcibly [5,6]. He criticises the use of the word epidemic, pointing out that, traditionally, the term has been used to indicate an upsurge in mortality associated with a contagious (read 'microbial') disease. He acknowledges, however, that in the latter half of the 20th century the word epidemic was used to describe a sudden increase of mortality of non-infectious disease, and there was great concern about an epidemic of increased mortality from asthma in the 1960s (thought to be to the result of a lack of control of certain medications). Stehbens points out that the increase in the diagnosis of myocardial infarction might not reflect a true increase in the incidence of disease and that, as I have pointed out in earlier chapters, there were no robust data generated before the second half of the 20th century.

Comparing the present to the past must be undertaken with great caution, but we must make some attempts to do so and form a judgement on the basis of the evidence available, whether it is conclusive or not. Stehbens, like others, felt that death from myocardial infarction was the result of an underlying pathology of atherosclerosis, and he expressed the view that atherosclerosis is simply a 'degenerative condition', something that is inevitable in someone who lives long enough. Therefore the great reduction of deaths from conditions such as tuberculosis meant that more people were living long enough to die from degenerative atherosclerosis. The weakness of this view is that he makes an assumption about the nature of atherosclerosis being degenerative or part of the ageing process and thereby ubiquitous. In later chapters, I will indicate that atherosclerosis is in fact a specific disease process and not a result of ageing or degeneration.

During the emergence, real or imaginary, of coronary heart disease, public health and government had other distractions and little attention was given to its cause. The health of the population in general was improving, in particular infant mortality rates.

Controversy about the emergence of an apparently new disease is not confined to coronary heart disease. Neil Painter, surgeon at Manor House Hospital, London, UK, and Denis Burkitt, the British surgeon working in Uganda, who me met in Chapter 14, reporting in 1971 [7] provide early descriptions of diverticulitis and diverticular disease of the colon from the early years of the 20th century, when reports of these conditions were infrequent. The disease had apparently not emerged at the level that was to become obvious later in the century, both as an illness and as a cause of death. In 1920, Sir John Bland-Sutton (1856–1936), surgeon to the Middlesex Hospital, London, UK, and president of the Royal College of Surgeons, England, remarked that [8]:

*Up to the last ten years, acute diverticulitis is recognised with the same certainty as appendicitis and is a newly discovered bane of elders.*

It is interesting to note that diverticular disease of the colon appeared to emerge at the same time as coronary heart disease, as shown in Figure 18.1 using data from Surgeon Commander T. L. Cleave and colleagues in 1969 [9]. Although this could be a coincidence, there must be a suspicion that it could be more than that, and there could be a common cause or a common susceptibility. Painter and Burkitt felt that dietary fibre deficiency was the cause of diverticular disease of the colon, and Cleave and colleagues later suggested that this might also be a major causative factor of coronary heart disease [9]. We will review this later. Painter and Burkitt dismissed the idea that diverticular disease had always been present and only just been recognised, expressing the view that 'clinicians of the last century were just as capable as those of today of recognizing diverticulitis'. The same applies to coronary heart disease.

**Figure 18.1  Crude death rate for diverticular disease [9].**

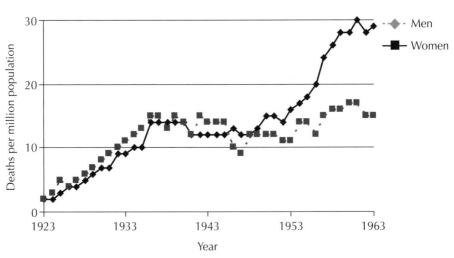

An editorial of the *British Medical Journal* in 1971 indicated that, at that time, the number of deaths from coronary heart disease was increasing, being the cause of death in four out of 10 men and two out of 10 women [10]. It quoted data from the Framingham study, that two-thirds of coronary deaths were unexpected and took place outside the hospital [11]. More than half of the deaths were sudden, occurring within 1 hour of the first onset of the symptoms. Death was more likely to be sudden in younger than in older individuals and more likely in men than in women. Two-thirds of the sudden coronary deaths occurred in people without previous clinical evidence of coronary heart disease. The conclusion was that it was difficult to see how the increasing mortality rate could be reversed by medical interventions, and that only preventative measures could be expected to be effective. The implication was that preventative measures would have to be part of public health arrangements and it was not anticipated that the increase in death would be reversed by factors unknown. However, by the end of the 1970s, it was appreciated that in the UK the increase in deaths from coronary heart disease had reached a plateau in about 1972 and from 1975 appeared to decline [12].

A further editorial in the *British Medical Journal*, written in 1982 by John Hampton, Professor of Cardiovascular Medicine at the University of Nottingham, UK, reported on the falling mortality in coronary heart disease [13]. This was based mainly on data from the USA that indicated a 25% reduction of mortality in the previous decade, and Hampton's review noted that both the incidence of the disease and the fatality rates were falling. Unlike others, Hampton suggested that the trend of reduced mortality rate was apparent before there were any substantial alterations to what were generally thought to be the causative factors, and certainly before the introduction of effective medical interventions.

A contemporary report from New Zealand recorded a 20% reduction in coronary heart disease mortality in the 13 years following 1968 [14]. The data from this study suggested that:

*Factors other than the improved care of myocardial infarction patients are responsible for the decline in coronary heart disease mortality rates in New Zealand.*

The study concluded that improvements of the care of patients in the year following myocardial infarction were not major factors in the decline in coronary heart disease mortality in New Zealand.

The increase in the incidence of coronary heart disease throughout the first half of the 20th century, its peak and its subsequent decline, are shown particularly well in a paper by Jeremiah Stamler from Chicago, USA [15]. His data were obtained from the *US NCHS Monthly Vital Statistics Report* of June 1984 and are shown in Figure 18.2. It can be seen that in the USA deaths from coronary heart disease reached a peak around 1970, and declined by about 30% between 1970 and 1981. It is interesting to note that deaths from stroke declined gradually from 1950 but more rapidly from 1970, the decline being parallel with coronary heart disease deaths.

**Figure 18.2 Trends in coronary heart disease (CHD) and stroke mortality in USA [15].**

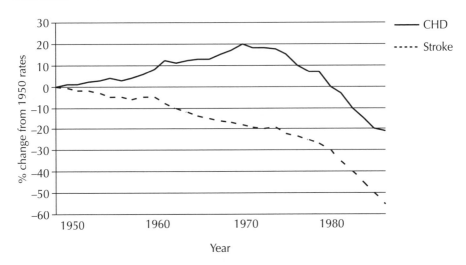

*Adapted with permission from* Cardiology.

A further contribution from Robert Beagleholme, Associate Professor of Epidemiology at the University of Auckland, New Zealand, looked in more detail at possible reasons for the reduction of coronary deaths [16]. His calculation was that in 1981 there were 126 fewer deaths from coronary heart disease in people less than 70 years living in Auckland than would be expected from the 1974 rates. He felt that specific medical interventions probably accounted for 51 (40%) of the 126 fewer deaths. Of these, resuscitation before admission to hospital was responsible for 20 fewer deaths, assuming that successful outcome of resuscitation would be continued following discharge from hospital. Fifteen of the fewer deaths were thought to be to the result of treatment of hypertension, six the coronary care unit treatment and three the use of beta-blocker medications. The impact of coronary heart surgery is difficult to determine with certainty, but it was thought to have been responsible for between seven and 23 of the 126 fewer deaths. Unknown factors were therefore responsible for 60% of the fewer deaths, and it is these unknown factors that are particularly interesting.

The geography of coronary heart disease will be dealt with in later chapters, but for now it is worth noting that the country with one of the highest rates of coronary heart disease in the world has been Finland, and within Finland the region of North Karelia has had the highest mortality rate. This led to a major public health campaign. The peak of mortality in North Karelia was in 1969–70 and thereafter the mortality declined. The published conclusions were that this was the result of the public health campaign [17]. However, one of the major authors of this paper, Jukka Salonen, took a dissenting view, that it was not possible to draw the conclusion that the mortality decline in North Karelia was the result of the public health project. The point is, of course, that there was a public health initiative and there was a reduced incidence of disease, but it was not possible to demonstrate that the association of the two was cause and effect [18].

A study from Melbourne, Australia, looked critically at the improved outcome of coronary heart disease since 1969, this time looking at the long-term outlook of patients who had survived a myocardial infarction rather than looking at the incidence of disease. The report indicated a hospital mortality rate in men of 16.7% in 1969–73 and 8.5% in 1979–83. Of those who survived the initial myocardial infarction, the subsequent mortality 1 year after discharge from hospital declined by an average of 7% per year for both men and women. These changes did not appear to be caused by the severity of disease or the health characteristics of the patients, and it was felt that this change was because of the benefits of medical intervention [19].

Although the reason for the increase in coronary heart disease during the 20th century might possibly have been diagnostic awareness rather than true disease incidence, its decline was in an era of good-quality data collection and could hardly be attributed to lack of medical awareness or apathy, or even an increase in deaths from other causes. The decline was real and dramatic, but of course it was ill-understood and therefore the cause of controversy. There were those who considered that it was the result of medical intervention, others that it was the result of public health initiatives, and others that it was the result of changing environmental factors that could not be recognised. In latter years medical intervention could clearly have made a contribution, but not in the early parts of the decline when the effectiveness of medical intervention was much less than it is today. The appearance of the disease, its increase to epidemic proportions and its decline have all the hallmarks of environmental influences that are not yet clear. The pattern is certainly not that of a genetic disease.

If there was some puzzle regarding the emergence of coronary heart disease, its unexpected decline provoked action in the form of the 1978 Bethesda Conference, held in the National Institutes of Health, Bethesda, Maryland, USA, in an attempt to understand it [20]. The international conference identified the need for more research and, in particular, a more robust effort regarding data collection. This was organised through the World Health Organization (WHO) Cardiovascular Diseases Unit, which recruited different national research groups that would be interested in monitoring cardiovascular disease. This was the start of the MONICA project (multinational monitoring of trends and determinants in cardiovascular disease). It included 38 populations and 21 countries in four continents [21].

An attempt to clarify the relative contributions of medical care and environmental factors was undertaken in the Minnesota Heart Study published in 1998 [22]. This study identified clearly the decline in deaths from coronary heart disease between 1970 and 1990, and looked in detail at deaths classified as caused by myocardial infarction in a population of 2.29 million people from Minneapolis and St Paul, USA. The target population was aged between 30 and 74 years and included 550 719 men and 575 690 women. To try to identify the role of medical intervention, the deaths were separated into those that occurred outside the hospital and those that occurred inside the hospital, assuming the second group to be influenced by medical intervention. The trends in mortality during these 20 years are shown in Figure 18.3 and the decline in mortality is clear, both in hospital and out of hospital. The authors supported the view that the trend of declining mortality from deaths out of hospital reflected the success of primary care preventative methods. This conclusion was not based on evidence but was a self-congratulatory attitude that Voltaire described as 'Doctors taking the credit while nature brings about the cure'.

The authors of the Minnesota Heart Study did not entertain the view that the decline of the epidemic might be the result of factors of which we have no understanding. Mortality rates both in and out of hospital were more or less parallel, indicating that both were under the same influence. Between the years of 1985 and 1990, the decline in deaths for men in hospital was greater than those out of hospital, and the authors seized upon this as evidence of improved medical care. But on the other hand, during the previous years of 1978–85 hospital deaths declined at a slower rate than those out of hospital and this could be interpreted as indicating that hospitals were positively harmful during that period. Combining the 1978–85 and 1985–90 periods effectively produces a straight line of in-hospital deaths parallel with that of out-of-hospital deaths, indicating no effect of hospital stay on the overall health of the public, although clearly it had a significant advantage for certain individuals.

**Figure 18.3 Trends in mortality caused by coronary heart disease (CHD) [22].**

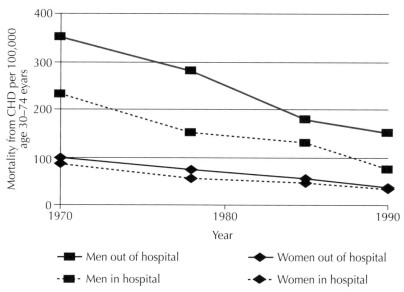

The decline in deaths from coronary heart disease during the past 30 years remains a subject of some controversy, as many doctors take the Minnesota Heart Study view but others feel that it is accepting misdirected responsibility for this phenomenon. It is not only doctors who are claiming to be responsible for the improvement in deaths from heart disease, but also the government. On 25 March 2004, the UK Health Secretary John Reid proclaimed that: 'The NHS is winning the war against coronary heart disease' and that heart services are being improved during the time of the Labour government. This comment introduced the report *Winning the War on Heart Disease* [23]. The report described the decline since 1990, and a prominent graph, shown in Figure 18.4, projected by 2015 the end of the epidemic of coronary heart disease deaths in people below the age of 65 years. The start of the graph in 1990 does not give a full picture of the decline of deaths from coronary heart disease, which started 20 years earlier. The British Heart Foundation has also expressed the view that the organisational changes introduced by the government have had a beneficial effect on fighting heart disease.

**Figure 18.4  Projected decline of coronary heart disease [23].**

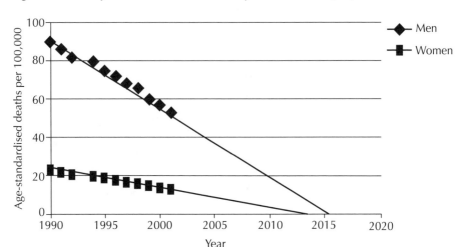

It is important to scrutinise the reasons for the decline in deaths from coronary heart disease, and a further recent attempt has come from the UK. The Department of Public Health at the University of Liverpool has looked at the reasons for the decline in coronary heart disease mortality in England and Wales between 1981 and 2000, noting that the decline in the USA commenced about 10 years earlier than in the UK [24]. The authors observed that, during this period of time, the decline in the USA had been about 62% in men and 45% in women (ages 25–84 years), as seen in Figure 18.5.

The study tried to determine whether this improvement was the result of medical intervention or risk factor reduction, particularly with respect to smoking, cholesterol, hypertension, obesity, diabetes and socio-economic deprivation. The conclusion, based on a rather detailed mathematical model that had been used previously in New Zealand [16], was that 42% of the reduction was the result of medical intervention and the remainder was assumed to be the result of risk factor reduction. The model accounted for 89% of the total mortality decrease in England and Wales (medical intervention plus risk factor reductions) and attributed the remaining 11% to immeasurable factors, suggesting that those factors might be dietary changes and life-style effects.

**Figure 18.5 Age-standardised death rates from coronary heart disease (CHD) [24].**

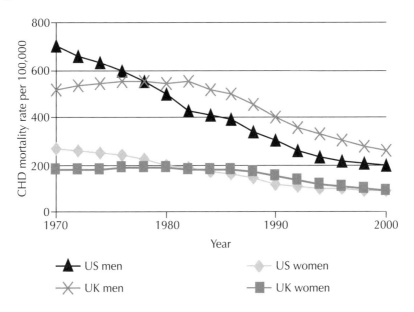

*Adapted from* Circulation *with permission from Lippencott, Williams and Watkins.*

It seems strange that, in both the USA and UK, the decline of coronary heart deaths has been associated with a time of great concern regarding an increasing problem of obesity and over-nutrition in society. These two observations appearing simultaneously suggest that either there is no association between the two or that perhaps over-nutrition has led to the decline in coronary heart disease deaths. It is customary to invoke dietary factors when there is ignorance, and it would have been better had the conclusion of Unal and colleagues from Liverpool [24] ended at 'immeasurable factors' rather than speculating about diet.

It has also been observed that in Northern Ireland, which has about the highest incidence of coronary heart disease in the world, the mortality from myocardial infarction has also declined [25]. This is in keeping with international observations that the epidemic of coronary heart disease reached its peak in the 1960s. The authors of this study, from the Department of Geriatric Medicine at Queens University, Belfast, noted that the seasonal variation of deaths from coronary heart disease remained but that the amplitude of variation throughout the year diminished [25].

The changing incidence of coronary heart disease indicates one thing for certain: it is not the result of a primary genetic disorder, the incidence of which will always be approximately constant. Change gives clues to cause and we will look at these. Before doing so, however, we will consider in more detail the nature of coronary heart disease.

# 19
# THE BIOLOGY OF
# CORONARY HEART DISEASE

We are concerned with a number of clinical expressions of what is considered to be a single disease entity, the cause of which is not clear. The understanding of coronary heart disease is not helped by a significant problem with terminology, and this problem seems to be increasing.

Universally the term coronary heart disease, abbreviated as CHD, is most widely used compared with alternatives, and that is the term that I have used in this book. It tells us three things. Firstly, it tells us that it is a disease entity, and that is a reasonable starting point. It is possible that, when understanding becomes more complete, coronary heart disease could prove to have a number of distinct causes, each with a slightly different clinical expression. Secondly, it tells us that the disease process is centred on the heart. The disease process is, however, considered to be part of a more general disorder of the arteries, called arteriosclerosis (hardening of the arteries) or atherosclerosis (a porridge-like material in the hardened artery wall). Finally, coronary heart disease introduces the word coronary, which has become synonymous with the heart.

Coronary is derived from the word coronet, which means crown. The origin of this is that if the heart is transected horizontally to cut off the atria (or atriums) then the view of the heart from above shows that the ventricles have a 'crown' composed of two arteries that encircle the heart and then send branches over the ventricles to provide the blood supply to the muscle of the ventricles. The two arteries are the right and left coronary arteries. The left starts off with a main stem, dividing into diagonal and a main left coronary branch. The details of the coronary artery circulation can be seen in Figure 19.1.

**Figure 19.1 The coronary artery circulation.**

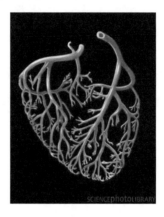

*Source Science Photo Library.*

Occlusion of a coronary artery branch causes infarction, death of the heart muscle supplied with blood by that branch. Sometimes such an occurrence produces no symptoms whatsoever, sometimes it can cause sudden death, but it can also cause chest pain, abnormal rhythm of the heart and failure of the pumping function of the heart.

The final process of occlusion of a coronary artery is a blood clot on the surface of a plaque of existing disease on the internal surface of the artery. The terms coronary artery thrombosis and coronary thrombosis are used to describe this. A person might be said to have had 'a coronary', which is simply an abbreviation but which has led to the word coronary being almost synonymous with heart in lay terminology.

The diagnostic criteria of myocardial infarction must include at least two of the following three features: characteristic chest pain or other characteristic clinical presentation; appropriate electrocardiogram (ECG) changes; a rise in the blood of enzymes released from the dead cells of the heart muscle and, more recently, the appearance in the blood of troponins, also released from the heart muscle cells. A new term has been introduced recently, NSTEMI (non-ST segment elevation myocardial infarction), an acute coronary syndrome in which the above criteria are met but are not adequately rigorous for the institution of thrombolytic therapy, which needs very specific ECG changes of the ST segment elevation of 2 mm or more (Figure 19.2). The terminology almost certainly remains in a state of change, and recent changes of terminology will have an impact on statistical returns of the frequency of the disease. Similarly the introduction of increasingly sensitivity blood tests will increase the number of people diagnosed. This will create further argument about the incidence of the disease, the nature of the epidemic and its decline.

**Figure 19.2 Elements of an ECG.**

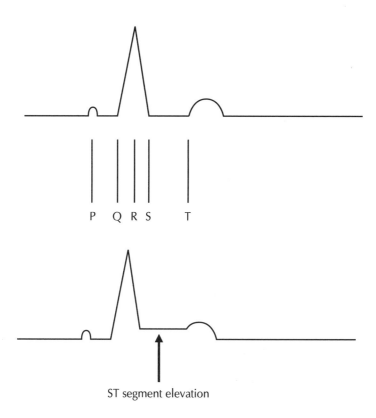

The occlusion of a coronary artery might be gradual, and an incomplete occlusion, say 80%, can cause angina, an intermittent chest pain without death of the corresponding heart muscle. It is the combination of angina and myocardial infarction (coronary artery thrombosis) that is given the all-embracing name of ischaemic heart disease (implying reduced blood supply to the heart muscle) or coronary heart disease.

The thrombotic occlusion described above does not occur in normal arteries but there is an underlying process that gradually and progressively causes a narrowing of the coronary arteries. This process develops over a period of many years and can be diffuse and patchy. It has been suggested that the process starts as fatty streaks in the arterial wall, particularly that of the aorta, as these have been seen at autopsies of young men that died as the result of trauma [1]. Whatever the initial event, the artery ultimately develops within its wall a porridge-like material called atheroma. This can become hard and sometimes calcified, leading to descriptions of atherosclerosis, arteriosclerosis or, more popularly, hardening of the arteries. The porridge-like atheromatous material is known to be rich in cholesterol. The atherosclerotic process is shown in Figure 19.3.

**Figure 19.3 Atherosclerosis of the coronary arteries.**

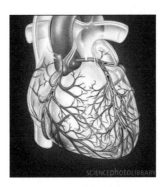

*Source Science Photo Library.*

The process of myocardial infarction is shown in Figure 19.4 and detail of the final thrombotic occlusion is shown in Figure 19.5. The process of coronary angiography is now a widely used diagnostic technology; it can lead to treatment intervention by dilating a narrowed artery with a balloon and introducing a stent (named after an English dentist Charles Stent in 1856 but more correctly called a Wiktor-Stent to include the name of the USA engineer who, in 1984, applied the principle to the repair of arteries).

**Figure 19.4 The process of myocardial infarction.**

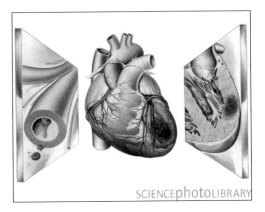

*Source Science Photo Library.*

**Figure 19.5 Blood clot in a coronary artery.**

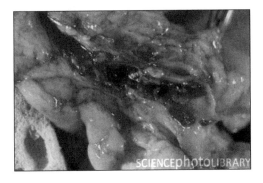

*Source Science Photo Library.*

Early descriptions of the atherosclerotic plaques identified the cholesterol content. It was assumed that the cholesterol enters the arterial wall from the blood stream by a process of diffusion supplemented by elevated blood pressure. This view has persisted to the present time, presenting the idea that the arteries 'fur-up' with cholesterol. The lipid accumulation process was first proposed by the great German pathologist Rudolf Virchow in 1856. Slightly earlier, in 1852, the Czech-born Carl Freiherr von Rokitansky had placed emphasis on the thrombotic nature of the process.

However, the simple physical model of the arteries furring-up with cholesterol does not stand up to scrutiny, as we will see later. The relationship between atherosclerotic plaques and myocardial infarction is not simple. A recent report from Barcelona, Spain, indicated that, although there is a low incidence of myocardial infarction in that locality, autopsy studies show a surprisingly high prevalence of atherosclerotic plaques, one of several paradoxes that we will encounter [2]. The authors comment that the plaques appear to be mainly fibrous or stable. Plaque instability is important and it is this that results in the blood clot that precipitates a myocardial infarction [1]. It is now thought that plaque instability is related to an inflammatory process, something that is far from traditional thought but is of fundamental importance, and we will consider it in detail in later chapters.

The pathological processes leading to coronary heart disease and myocardial infarction are complex, incompletely understood and, for the most part, beyond the purpose of this book. An excellent review was provided recently by Valentin Fuster and colleagues from the Massachusetts General Hospital, Boston, USA, and the Mayo Clinic, Rochester, Minnesota, USA, but it deals with pathological process, the pathogenesis of coronary heart disease, and not its cause [3].

While introducing the role of inflammation in coronary heart disease, I would like to draw special attention to the role of the macrophage cell in the development of atherosclerosis. It was mentioned in the early part of the 20th century but forgotten when coronary heart disease became viewed as degenerative, or perhaps dietary, but the concept has been revived within the past 20 years [4]. It is interesting to remember that vitamin D is essential for effective macrophage function, and we will be looking in detail at the very important relationship between vitamin D and coronary heart disease.

The main point about the biology of coronary heart disease is that the clinical expression may be sudden, unexpected and sometimes fatal, occurring mainly after the age of 70 years. However, it is based on a clinically silent process that develops over many years; during this silent or latent period, the disease is unsuspected and effectively cannot be diagnosed. Fissuring or disruption of an atherosclerotic plaque can take place at any time during the development of the disease, leading to a thrombotic event and possibly a myocardial infarction. In terms of causation, the initiation of the silent atherosclerotic process is the important event and this is not understood.

We must remember syphilis and rheumatic fever: in these conditions there is a long latent interval between the initiation of the disease process and its ultimate clinical expression. We must also remember that the initiating event is an infection and that the clinical diseases are caused by micro-organisms. This is a model that might be applicable to other diseases, perhaps coronary heart disease. We must not forget this when we look at the development of thinking regarding the cause of this common and puzzling condition.

# 20
# THE CAUSATION OF CORONARY HEART DISEASE

Coronary heart disease is a condition that is a major cause of death in what we call the western world and an increasing cause of death in the wider world that is now undergoing industrialisation. Some people feel confident that we understand the disease and can prevent it through various lifestyle initiatives, but others feel that, in terms of causation, we understand very little. If we keep to the rule that the cause is the general factor without which the disease cannot occur, and if we accept that coronary heart disease has a cause, rather than simply being part of getting older, then I am of the view that we understand very little.

The approach to identifying causation has been to study people with coronary heart disease and then compare them with similar people without coronary heart disease with respect to clearly defined characteristics. In this way risk indicators can be identified, without jumping to premature conclusions that risk indicators are causative. It has been noted, for example, that men are more at risk than women and that risk increases with age.

As well as comparing individuals there have been comparisons of populations, and, as we shall see, there is a striking geographical variation between the south-east of England and the north and west of England, where there is a much higher risk. The risk seems to be even greater in Scotland and Northern Ireland, and we will be considering geographical variations in more detail later.

The identification of risk indicators has been a major industry and, even by 1981, 246 risk indicators had been identified [1]. These might provide clues regarding causation but they cannot be assumed to be directly causative. It has been noted that the risk of women developing coronary heart disease increases after the menopause, but hormone replacement therapy has been disappointing in preventing this [2]. It has also been noted that men who are bald are at a greater risk of coronary heart disease than those with a good head of hair [3], but providing wigs for bald men has never been the subject of a clinical trial. Although baldness might provide a clue to causation it is not regarded as causative in itself.

This leads us to the important observation that we have risk indicators that are simply indicators; modification of them cannot be expected to confer any benefit. There are also risk indicators that can be modified with benefit to the individual, but separating the two types is difficult. Ideally each becomes a hypothesis of the causation of coronary heart disease and therefore each requires an intervention study in the form of controlled clinical trial. It is not always possible to achieve this and so we must form a judgement regarding whether a risk indicator is likely to a cause of the disease or merely indicative of something else. The word judgement implies a process of making a decision without the necessary information to form a robust conclusion. The term risk factor can be misleading and lead people to form a premature conclusion that it is causative. I prefer the term risk indicator, which I believe is more appropriate in epidemiological understanding.

As well as geographical and biological indicators of coronary heart disease there are also social indicators. It has been noted in many studies that those who go to church regularly enjoy better health in general and a lower risk of coronary heart disease in particular [4]. No particular denomination of Christian church appears to be unique in this respect, and only Christian church-going seems to indicate good health outcome. It has been noted in Johannesburg, South Africa, that Jewish people appear to have an increased risk of coronary heart disease, and we shall see shortly that this is also true of South Asians living in the UK [5], although this is not obviously linked to the frequency of religious attendance. Church-going is likely to only be a risk indictor, or could compulsory church attendance improve the outcome of current non-church-goers with coronary heart disease? Common sense (i.e. judgement) would suggest that the former is true, but the latter option has not been subjected to a clinical trial: imagine the obstacles!

An even more powerful indicator of good health than church attendance is eating a meal sitting around a table with the family when a child. Once again there is the feeling that this is just an indicator of a variety of other lifestyle factors. Undertaking a clinical trial would be a daunting task.

There are also ethnic issues. We have already seen that South Asian ethnicity is associated with an increased risk of rickets/osteomalacia and tuberculosis when living in the UK and the USA; we will see that there is also an increased risk of coronary heart disease and diabetes. The details of ethnicity need to be identified and we will revisit this subject later.

It is important to realise two things regarding the identification of more than 240 risk indicators of coronary heart disease. The first is that somehow they are all pieces of a puzzle that must be assembled in a way to produce a coherent picture. Secondly, we must ask ourselves why medical science has gone to so much trouble to assemble so many risk indicators for coronary heart disease. This is unprecedented in medical investigation and really points to the fact that the cause of the disease is simply unknown. If it were known, investigation of this magnitude would not be necessary.

Causal thinking throughout the latter half of the 20th century concerning coronary heart disease has been dominated by two major contenders: diet and psychological factors, in particular stress. Like other risk indicators, they need to be explored in detail to understand them. Those responsible for public and individual health wish to intervene for the benefit of health but we sometimes see titles or headlines such as *Dietary Selenium: Time to Act* when a research intervention study would be more appropriate [6]. Evidence is often elusive; it might take many years to undertake appropriate clinical trials, and so judgement will be necessary regarding how and when to intervene. As in the case of John Snow, who removed the handle from the Broad Street pump in London in 1837, intervention might be effective but he had a good understanding of the cause of the cholera epidemic. The problem with coronary heart disease is that we do not have good understanding of it, but this is not generally acknowledged.

There are many dissenters from the accepted wisdom of coronary heart disease, one in particular being the Swedish researcher Uffe Ravnskov [7]. Within the conventional model there too many paradoxes, and we will be investigating these because paradoxes are an important opportunity to find the truth: as Thomas Kuhn comments, 'Discovery commences with awareness of anomaly' [8]. If interventions based on incomplete understanding are not shown to be effective then they should be withdrawn, but there is rarely the enthusiasm to do so: professionals are very ready to apply their dogma to the population, even for the best of motives, but are very reluctant to reverse it. This has been described well as 'the tyranny of health' [9].

# 21

# PSYCHOLOGICAL FACTORS AND CORONARY HEART DISEASE

With the apparent decline in importance of the obvious microbial diseases by the middle of the 20th century, it was the middle classes who enjoyed the most benefit. This was probably a reason why coronary heart disease appeared to emerge first in this group, aided by the fact that they had better access to health care and specialist services. We must not forget that before the inception of the National Health Service (NHS) in 1948, specialist services were only found in the teaching hospitals of the major cities; the infirmaries of smaller towns were run mainly by general practitioner (GP) specialists. It was the new funding system of the NHS that allowed salaried specialist services to be available everywhere and to everyone. The specialists around the time of 1950 were therefore centred in the cities of the land, mainly in London, and they had a large private clientele from whom they obtained a clinical experience that was not based upon the full social spectrum.

Coronary heart disease became recognised as an illness of the businessman, of the executive, in exactly the same way that duodenal ulcer was recognised earlier in the century. Coronary heart disease was thus seen to be the result of working too hard and the stress associated with this. The response was sympathy, a recognition that the individual was devoting more of his or her time to work than he or she should have been, and a reduction of work was the reward for developing the disease. It became almost a mark of respect, a sign of professional success. Life was full of comments regarding people working so hard that they were 'bound to become ill', 'heading for a coronary' and 'a typical heart attack-type of person'. The recent history of 'disease as a reflection of the psyche' was particularly well reviewed in 1985 by the American physician and author Marcia Angell, writing in an editorial in *The New England Journal of Medicine*, of which she was the first woman to be Editor-in-Chief [1].

The psychological model of coronary heart disease was refined into two personality types, type A and type B. Type A was seen as the go-getter, the enthusiast, the leader of society, the person who would drive himself with hard work. Women were effectively excluded from discussion at this time, with coronary heart disease appearing to be a male-dominated disease and women being barely represented in professional and executive life. Some might argue, however, that virtually all women are by nature type A. The type B personalities were seen to be rather more work-shy, the followers rather than the leaders and people who did not appear to be working under what might be called stress.

Personality type A and the external factor of stress were seen to be the culprits of coronary heart disease, and this fitted in well with the reward system of illness enjoyed by executives. As with duodenal ulcer, work-blaming was a useful professional concept.

We have already touched upon social issues and the social stratification of society: a very important health issue. I should point out at this stage that in the UK there has been for many years a social definition used by the civil service and based on the occupation of the population. Although it can be criticised, it is surprisingly robust in identifying those in society who are at particular risk. The categories are as follows: (1) professional and executive workers; (2) managerial workers; (3) office workers and skilled manual workers; (4) semi-skilled manual workers; (5) unskilled labourers and unemployed people.

The process of social investigation culminated in the studies of the late Sir Douglas Black, former Professor of Medicine at the University of Manchester, Chief Scientist to the Department of Health and President of the Royal College of Physicians of London, and Peter Townsend, Professor of International Social Policy at the London School of Economics. Their work was published as the influential book *Inequalities in Health* [2], originally a government report [3] that was somewhat embarrassing to the conservative government as it identified a major problem to which politicians had no answer. Black and Townsend showed that the best health profile within the UK was orientated towards the professional and executive groups and the worst health was clearly with the manual working classes and the unemployed. This made particularly uncomfortable reading for the government, which was responsible for the maintenance of public health, but it also upset the idea that professional people and business executives (including politicians) were working themselves into early graves.

Research has been particularly valuable in respect of personality type and coronary heart disease, as both are quite easily defined. British cardiologists were generally more sceptical of the personality type as a cause of coronary heart disease than their counterparts in the USA. An early assault upon what was accepted wisdom came from the departments of psychological medicine and cardiology at King's College Hospital, London, UK [4]. This paper was published in 1982 in *The Lancet* under the topic 'Dogma Disputed'. The authors studied 99 patients with coronary heart disease who had the extent of their disease defined by coronary angiography. Their personality types were assessed blind, that is with no observer knowledge of the angiography findings, using a psychological measurement technique called the Bortner score [5]. The results were surprising: the 26 men with normal and minimally diseased arteries had significantly higher type A scores than the 41 men with important coronary artery occlusions. The results were thus just the opposite of conventional wisdom; the authors 'question the value of the use of type A and coronary-prone behaviour as interchangeable terms'.

The study also looked at the social profile of their subjects, divided simply into manual and non-manual workers. There was a strong tendency for male non-manual workers to have personality scores closer to the type A end of the spectrum but this was not apparent in women. Psychiatric illness was considered to be present in 61% of those with normal or minimally diseased arteries and in only 23% of those with important coronary occlusions. This was also in conflict with the idea that coronary heart disease might be in some way psychosomatic.

In 1985, the USA Multicenter Post-Infarction Research Group published the results of a study on the influence of personality factors on the course of coronary heart disease [6]. The study of 516 patients found that there was no relation between personality factors and total mortality, coronary mortality or long-term outcome following acute myocardial infarction.

A further study, from St George's and the Royal Free Hospital Medical schools, London, UK, investigated, prospectively over a period of more than 6 years, 5936 men aged 40–59 years, recruited from general practice in 19 British towns [7]. Once again the Bortner scoring system was used and once again the non-manual workers were predominantly towards the type A end of the personality spectrum. And type A behaviour did not predict the incidence of the clinical events of coronary heart disease.

The School of Public Health at the University of California, Berkeley,

USA, provided another well-researched study [8]. This was a retrospective study of 257 men who had been studied over a period of 8.5 years as part of the Western Collaborative Group Study. There was a lower mortality among those with type A behaviour, in both older and younger groups.

These studies should have put an end to the concept of a type A coronary-prone individual but, although this has probably been the case amongst most medical professionals, the idea appears to linger on in lay circles. This leads to the subject of stress and the heart, reviewed in a *British Medical Journal* editorial with characteristic thought and clarity by the late Tony Mitchell, who died very shortly after retiring from his position as Professor of Medicine at the University of Nottingham, UK [9]. He felt that the traditional terminology of physics indicated that stress was something applied from outside, whereas strain was an internal response. The problem with stress is that, within health thinking, it lacks a clear definition. It is usually meant to indicate something external, 'a person is working under great stress'. This leads to the erroneous view that health is more fragile in the executive but, as suggested in 1954 by Sir Melville Arnott, at the time Professor of Medicine at the University of Birmingham, UK [10]:

> The life of a physician in Birmingham is surely less stressful than that of a peasant in the Yangtse valley with the ever present menace of flood, famine, pestilence, and war or of the tribesman in equatorial Africa tortured by the taboo and sanction of primitive belief.

A study of 270 000 men working for the USA Bell Telephone Company indicated quite clearly that it is not the 'stress' of the business executive that predicts coronary heart disease, but poor education of other members of the workforce [11]. This study was published in 1968 and its lack of impact indicates that such an objective study was no match for misdirected conventional wisdom. Stress had to be redefined to accommodate the facts.

Mitchell pointed out that a number of social factors indicate a high risk of coronary heart disease, if only in men. They include social isolation, lack of membership of a club or religious group, lack of contact with family and friends, lack of educational achievement, lack of employment, low status of employment, job dissatisfaction, family difficulties and financial difficulties [9]. With these factors we could state that the least educated have the highest levels of stress and the best educated have the lowest levels, contrary to the traditional view. It has become clear in recent years that lack of education is a major factor in health and something that can possibly be influenced by government action.

Several studies have indicated that low levels of education are associated with a range of poor health measures, more than just a high risk of coronary heart disease, but the reasons for this are not known. It is probable that there is a biological link but, if so, an intermediary mechanism has not been identified or even proposed. The alternative view is that it is behavioural, that education helps the individual who is ill to penetrate health services, or that perhaps health professionals take more notice of and provide better care to the educated.

To try to separate these factors, a study was undertaken in four metropolitan areas in the USA to investigate the health impact of education in young adults aged 33–45 years. The study aimed to look at subclinical coronary heart disease, that is disease in a 'latent' form present within the body that has not created any symptoms or other features of illness. This would remove the impact of behavioural factors [12]. We have seen the pathology of coronary heart disease, with atheroma in the arteries. Like so many tissues with chronic inflammation, over time atherosclerotic coronary arteries become calcified, thus becoming visible on X-ray films. This feature was used in the study, which involved the radiological measure of coronary artery calcification in asymptomatic individuals. In men and women, in white and black racial groups, there was a particularly high incidence of disease in those whose education did not take them to high school, with a 25% prevalence of coronary artery calcification. In contrast, those whose education took them beyond college had an overall prevalence of about 5%.

This five-fold higher risk in those with only minimum educational is clearly an alarming issue for those with responsibility for public health. Public investment in education is likely to deliver greater health benefits than investment in the 'illness service', and this fits in well with UK initiatives to expand higher education at university level. The study shows that the phenomenon itself is clearly biological: the measurement was only of asymptomatic disease. But behind the increased susceptibility of those with only minimal education there are likely to be behavioural factors. We still need to understand what they might be; the need for intervention will need to be something other than education for those for whom higher education is simply not appropriate.

The list of social issues that correlate with coronary heart disease includes many that are indicative rather than causative. The link between these and the disease is not clear, nor is it necessarily useful to link them all together under the term stress. Using the term stress implies that psychological factors are active in the production of the disease, but this may not be the case. There are certain anecdotes whereby an acute stressful event might precipitate myocardial infarction and perhaps sudden death, as in the example of the World Cup football match broadcast on the television that we saw earlier [13]. However, it must be remembered that although this might be a critical or even terminal event, it is a specific rather than a general feature. It is not the same as the development of the disease over a period of 20 years or more.

We must review the model presented earlier, that illness is a combination of disease and behavioural factors. Acute psychological trauma can be regarded as a behavioural factor. If this is added to a disease that has reached a critical level, with, for example, a 90% occlusion of a coronary artery, then an acute life event, even watching a football match, could result in clinical illness or sudden death. The mediation of this might be a spasm of the coronary arteries, a contraction of the muscle of the artery wall leading to narrowing of the lumen. It is instantaneous and usually reversible, but perhaps fatal if coronary artery circulation is already severely compromised by atherosclerotic disease.

There are associations between depressive illness and the outcome of a variety of diseases. The link between them is far from understood but must be something of fundamental biological importance for a range of illnesses to be associated, not only coronary and other atherosclerotic diseases but also cancers [14]. Evidence is generally conflicting but mind–body interactions must not be disregarded. They might be important in the management of individual patients but, if we are looking for the cause of coronary heart disease, then I believe we must look somewhere other than the minds of the population.

On the day of the transit of Venus, 8 June 2004, three extremely interesting health reports appeared in the UK national press. The first was a report of a new book by Michael Holick, Professor of Medicine in Boston, Massachusetts, USA, who proposed that sunshine is helpful to health and that many people are relatively deficient of vitamin D [15]. We have already come across some of the work of Holick and we shall be meeting more of his work later.

The second report was that statin drugs used for reducing blood cholesterol level seemed to result in a lower risk of cancer [16], and we shall be revisiting this work in more detail later. The final report concerned the publication of a book by Sir Michael Marmot, Professor of Epidemiology at Imperial College, University of London, UK [17].

Marmot had spent his working life investigating the epidemiology of heart disease, particularly regarding social groups. We will be reviewing much of his work later, but the main finding of his work over many years is that the poor and under-educated have the highest risk of heart disease.

He expressed the view that an improvement in health is helped by an improvement in the socio-economic status of individuals, emphasising the process of improvement rather than the absolute wealth of the individual as being of critical importance. His further conclusion was that the process is mediated by psychological factors, specifically being in control of life events.

So here we see once again the idea that psychological factors might have an influence on disease, but Marmot left it at that. He did not attempt to identify the final stage of plausibility and he did not suggest a mechanism. We are therefore left with his assertion that:

$$\text{psychological factors} \longrightarrow \text{disease}$$

However, I would certainly challenge this view and, based on a knowledge of pathology, my reasoning would indicate that there must be an intermediary mechanism along the following lines:

$$\text{psychological factors} \longrightarrow \text{behavioural and biological processes} \longrightarrow \text{disease}$$

But the model is probably not quite as simple as this. Professor Ami Schattner, of the University-Hadassah Medical School, Jerusalem, recently reviewed the interesting and real association of psychological and psychiatric factors with a variety of diseases, not just coronary heart disease [14]. Marmot also indicated that increased mortality as a result of 'not being in control' went beyond coronary heart disease and appeared to be associated with a variety of diseases.

We must remember the work of Paracelsus (see Chapter 1) [18], who defined the basis of disease recognition in western society, suggesting that each disease has a specific pathology. It is therefore difficult to envisage a psychological factor that would result directly in a variety of different pathologies, by which we mean diseases. My interpretation of the reviews by Schattner [14] and Marmot [17] is that the psychological factors do not give rise to disease itself but may give rise to an increased susceptibility to disease, a very different thing. I would therefore suggest the following model:

$$\text{psychological factors} \longrightarrow \text{behavioural and biological processes} \longrightarrow \text{susceptibility to disease}$$

At this point we leave objective evidence and it is appropriate to think about the possibilities that present themselves. How might depression or a major lack of self-esteem and social isolation result in an increased susceptibility to disease? I suggest that it could be through a mainly indoor existence with lack of sunshine and vitamin D production, leading to immunodeficiency. We will be exploring this in more detail later, but so far we have noted the historic association of social deprivation with vitamin D deficiency. The suggestion that students revising for exams in the spring and early summer have a high susceptibility to infections could be based on relative vitamin D deficiency because of their excessive indoor lifestyle at that time during their lives, rather than the stress of the exams.

In the spring of 2005 an interesting article appeared in the *New Scientist*, written by Kevin Tracey from New York, USA, who has spent 20 years trying to understand the nature of the inflammatory process [19]. We will be looking at details of this subject later, but one aspect of Tracey's work must be mentioned at this point. Chemicals released from inflammatory and immune cells control the inflammatory process, and the modulation of this is of critical importance. Tracey indicates that this is in part controlled by the vagus nerve. This, the 10th cranial nerve, originates in the brain stem and has a long course (vagus = wanderer), travelling through the chest and the abdomen. Its branches have contact with immune cells within the abdomen, and thus it provides the link between the brain and immune competence. This is a mechanism whereby psychological factors might have an influence on disease. I will be stressing the importance of control of immunity and the inflammatory process in subsequent chapters.

There may be people who still consider that the major atherosclerotic component of coronary heart disease is psychological in origin, but such thought defies the experience of more than a century of pathology. It would be necessary for such proponents to explain a plausible mechanism whereby psychological factors result in coronary artery disease. Taking into consideration all that we know about the biology of the atherosclerotic process within the coronary and other arteries, we need to ask the question: does it make sense? Plausibility increases if we separate psychological factors from the cause of coronary artery and other diseases but accept that they could increase susceptibility by acting through behavioural factors, as described. The importance of inflammation must not be forgotten.

# 22
# DIET AND CORONARY HEART DISEASE

The discovery of vitamins in general gave impetus to the view that unexplained diseases might be the result of the deficiency of an essential component of our food. In addition to this, there were two particular strands of thought that led people to consider that coronary heart disease might be dietary in origin.

The first was the observation by early pathologists that cholesterol is present within the atheromatous tissue of diseased coronary arteries. In the 1950s and 1960s, it was noticed that autopsies performed on young men who had died as the result of trauma revealed what were called fatty streaks in the aorta [1]. It was thus concluded that the disease starts in early life with deposition of fat, ultimately leading to narrowing of arteries. This was effectively a physical process, similar to the way in which domestic pipes might become furred-up by rust. Indeed the concept of 'furring-up by fat' was the message being delivered by the British Heart Foundation to the population of the UK through an advertising campaign as recently as the beginning of 2004.

It had been determined that cholesterol was a component of blood plasma and it was also discovered that cholesterol was present in food, in particular in animal fat and dairy products. A simple model was therefore presented that the more dietary fat eaten, the greater the blood level of cholesterol, and the inevitable development would be atheroma with the ultimate clinical expression of coronary heart disease. The scene was thus set for the 'diet–cholesterol–heart' hypothesis that has dominated thinking during the past half century.

The effects of this have been profound. In the 1950s, children were encouraged to eat dairy products and eggs, a continuation of the public health considerations of the 1930s and concern about under-nutrition, particularly vitamin D deficiency. Things changed in the 1970s, when full-fat milk was discouraged, so that the market is now dominated by skimmed and semi-skimmed milk. Butter has been replaced by margarine, which is allegedly better for our health and is advertised as such, but the evidence to support this statement is lacking. It has become part of conventional wisdom and politico-industrial propaganda that foods containing cholesterol are dangerous. Margarines, low-fat butter substitutes, are said to be good for us because they contain unsaturated hydrocarbons that are alleged to have protective properties.

The diet–cholesterol–heart hypothesis has been based to a major extent on simple comparisons that appeal to popular imagination, but with a powerful underlying propaganda campaign. For example, comparisons have been made between nations such as the UK, with a high prevalence of coronary artery disease, and mainly developing countries, in which the disease is effectively unknown. The dietary excesses of Europe and north America are obvious and, therefore, under the principle of 'we are what we eat', it is concluded that we who enjoy plenty of meat and dairy products are responsible for our illnesses and that we are eating our way towards an early grave. But the number of variable factors that differ between such locations is immense and it is not appropriate to draw conclusions from such uncontrolled comparisons. This is really the problem with the dietary hypotheses: scientific method means controlling all factors other than the one to be tested, but to do this with human populations is difficult or impossible.

Later chapters will look at the geography of coronary heart disease in more detail, but we need to recognise certain variations at this stage. One of the earliest studies to investigate geographical variations in the incidence of coronary heart disease was undertaken by Ancel Keys (1904–2004), a professor a the University of Minnesota, USA, mainly within Europe and published in 1980 as the Seven Countries Study [2]. This was a long-term study that started in 1958 and we will review it later. It demonstrated an association between national levels of animal fat intake and coronary heart disease and it thus provided a considerable impetus for the diet–cholesterol–heart hypothesis. But this study could not exclude a number of factors that differed between the countries under investigation.

Dietary stereotypes have usually not been subjected to proper evaluation. For example, there is a higher incidence of death from coronary heart disease in the north of England than in the south. It is automatically assumed in the south of England that people living in the north of the country eat the wrong foods, especially fish and chips. But is this popular view valid? Is not fish supposed to be good for us?

A research project performed in 1988 looked at the populations of Ipswich in the south-east of England, Stoke-on-Trent in the midlands, and Wakefield in the north: the Three English Towns study [3]. The study demonstrated that, during the years 1968–78, the lowest mortality rate from coronary heart disease was in Ipswich, with a standardised mortality ratio (SMR) of 86. The population of Stoke-on-Trent had a higher rate, at 119, and the highest was 123 in Wakefield. The pattern of overall mortality was similar when deaths from all causes were investigated.

The main purpose of the study was to look at food consumption to try to find a dietary explanation for these differences, and this is an excellent example of a very detailed dietary study of a modest number of people. Looking at the average intakes of fat, carbohydrates and protein, we can see that there were no significant differences between the diets of the population samples in the towns, as shown in Table 22.1.

**Table 22.1 Diet and coronary heart disease in three English towns [3].**
Mean daily intakes of nutrients are expressed as grams per day; death is expressed as SMR; the age range was 35–74 years; CHD = coronary heart disease

|  | Number | Energy (MJ) | Fat (g) | Carbohydrate (g) | Sugar (g) | Protein (g) | Fibre (g) | CHD deaths |
|---|---|---|---|---|---|---|---|---|
| *Men* | | | | | | | | |
| Ipswich | 119 | 10.8 | 107.9 | 308.7 | 120.3 | 85.4 | 20.7 | 89 |
| Stoke | 128 | 11.6 | 107.9 | 315.1 | 117.0 | 94.5 | 20.2 | 115 |
| Wakefield | 110 | 10.1 | 96.5 | 271.2 | 106.0 | 84.1 | 17.9 | 117 |
| *Women* | | | | | | | | |
| Ipswich | 129 | 7.1 | 73.0 | 192.2 | 76.5 | 64.3 | 15.1 | 79 |
| Stoke | 150 | 7.3 | 72.4 | 205.0 | 78.2 | 66.2 | 15.8 | 128 |
| Wakefield | 120 | 7.0 | 71.9 | 189.4 | 73.0 | 63.1 | 14.0 | 137 |

*Adapted with permission from the British Medical Journal Publishing Group.*

There was clearly no dietary explanation for the very significant mortality differences. The authors' comment was that, in relation to the relatively high level of fat consumption in Ipswich, the relatively low mortality rate from coronary heart disease was 'paradoxical'. Please note that this term will keep appearing as further studies are reviewed. A paradox or anomaly is very important in assessing how robust or otherwise a theory might be.

The conclusion of the authors of the study was [3]:

*Our findings suggest that the geographical inequalities in mortality in Britain, in particular mortality from ischaemic [coronary] heart disease, cannot be attributed to differences in consumption of energy or fat during middle life.*

The northern dietary stereotype was not upheld by this study, what we might call the 'three English towns paradox'. Present-day attitudes make it obvious that this well-researched and important study, from the Medical Research Council Environmental Epidemiology Unit at the University of Southampton, UK, had no influence whatsoever on public and professional attitudes towards the diet–cholesterol–heart hypothesis and the stereotype of northerners. The paradox was completely ignored by the medical–nutritional–scientific community because it did not fit in with existing dogma.

Another approach to the problem was to identify a group of people, record their dietary habits, blood cholesterol concentration and a variety of other factors, and then observe their subsequent health. This was undertaken by Professor Jerry Morris, from the Department of Community Health, London School of Hygiene and Tropical Medicine, UK. Morris and colleagues undertook dietary studies of 337 healthy men working for banks and London transport during 1956–66 [4]. During the following 10 years the incidence of coronary heart disease was assessed in relationship to a baseline diet, and the conclusions were as follows:

*The coronary attack rate among the men was related to their energy intake but not in the way expected: high intake was associated with a low risk of coronary heart disease ... The analysis of dietary cholesterol against coronary events showed no association at all ... Evidently in these data the association between energy intake or cereal-fibre intake or the ratio of P:S (polyunsatuarated:saturated fatty acids) in the diet and CHD is not mediated or explained in any simple way through plasma cholesterol concentrations.*

Here we have what is a very important observation, what we might call the 'London banking and transport paradox'. Like many other paradoxes, it casts serious doubt on the prevailing conventional wisdom. A high intake of energy in the diet was associated with a lower risk of death from coronary heart disease and cholesterol appeared to be unimportant. Once again this study had no effect on existing dogma and it was ignored.

There was an indication in this study that the fibre content of the diet was higher in those with a low incidence of coronary heart disease. The group was distributed into tertiles, the lowest third, middle third and highest third, regarding fibre intake. The incidence of coronary heart disease was 22, 16 and 7 in the respective groups, and this was related only to fibre from cereals. There was no apparent effect of fibre from fruit, vegetables, pulses and nuts, for which the incidence of coronary heart disease was 14, 18 and 13 (Figure 22.1). There was no relationship between consumption of sugar and subsequent coronary heart disease.

**Figure 22.1 Relationship between diet fibre intake and deaths from coronary heart disease [4].**

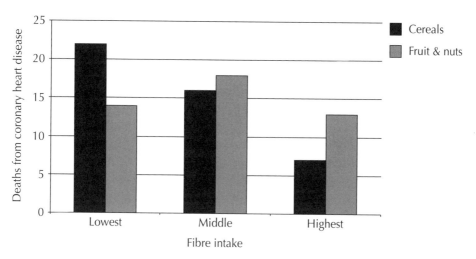

*Adapted with permission from the* British Medical Journal Publishing Group.

There was another interesting observation from this study. The men were grouped into the shortest third, middle third and tallest third; the incidence of coronary heart disease was, respectively, 22, 14 and 8. The observation that short stature was related to an increased risk of coronary heart disease led to the suspicion that under-nutrition gives an increased risk, against the conventional wisdom that over-nutrition causes heart disease.

A more recent study from the Harvard School of Public Health, USA, reported a 14-year follow-up of 43 732 men aged 40–75 years [5]. Diet was assessed in detail, and in particular the content of total fat, saturated fat, mono-unsaturated fat, polyunsaturated fat, *trans*-unsaturated fat, cholesterol, red meat, dairy products, nuts and eggs. There was no association between dietary factors and the subsequent development of stroke, the other main clinical manifestation of atherosclerotic disease.

It is important to appreciate that the work of Keys in the Seven Countries Study looked at death rates from coronary heart disease and dietary characteristics of the various countries. His work provided major support for the developing diet–cholesterol–heart hypothesis, as his findings were that the countries with a high incidence of age-adjusted deaths from coronary heart disease, mainly in northern Europe, tended to have a diet relatively high in animal fats. However, diet is only one of a large number of factors that can vary between countries. The national diet variations that showed an association with coronary heart disease have been extrapolated to variations of the diets of individuals, which is not quite the same thing. We have already seen a number of studies in which the expected associations based on the findings of Keys are not found when individuals are studied, and the association between saturated fat/cholesterol intake and coronary heart disease is thus inconsistent.

Another study from the Harvard School of Public Health, USA, appeared in 1996, reporting a 10-year follow-up study of 43 757 health professionals who were free from diagnosed cardiovascular disease at the onset [6]. There appeared, on first analysis, to be a positive association between a high saturated fat intake and subsequent coronary heart disease. However, this association disappeared when the fibre content of diet was taken into consideration; the conclusion was that there was no association between saturated fat intake and coronary heart disease. But, as with the London banking and transport study, there was a strong suggestion that the fibre content of diet might in some way be protective.

The diet–cholesterol–heart story has been based on observations of coronary heart and other atherosclerotic diseases, but other investigators concerned with determining the causation of the disease and possible links with nutrition have looked at the bigger picture. It is not only coronary heart disease that varies in incidence between different countries, localities and social groups, but also a number of other diseases and overall survival. There was therefore an attempt to look at diet in a more comprehensive way; although the diet–cholesterol–heart hypothesis has a certain simple attraction and superficial plausibility, it is very specific and it is not an appropriate model regarding susceptibility to a range of diseases. The big picture that will become clear as the book progresses, shows disease patterns of western countries to have a high prevalence of coronary heart and other diseases that are unknown or rare in underdeveloped countries. The diet–disease hypothesis has therefore looked at the relationship between what have been called the diseases of civilisation and the industrialisation of food production.

Refined sugar was thought by John Yudkin, Professor of Nutrition at Queen Elizabeth College, University of London, UK, to have a potential for disease production [7,8]. Sugar is clearly related to diabetes, which is itself closely related to coronary heart disease. Yudkin noted that sugar is converted by an industrialised process from a raw vegetable form into a highly refined soluble form. It therefore has the property of being absorbed by the gastrointestinal tract very rapidly, potentially causing metabolic disruption inside the body. Refined sugar provides a high calorie intake but, because of its highly soluble nature, they are calories that do not satisfy the appetite, and Yudkin felt it obvious that this would lead to over-consumption. This was an interesting theory, difficult to test, but it probably influenced the decline in sugar consumption per capita during the latter part of the 20th century. Yudkin reported in 1964 what he described as 'the first published evidence that people with atherosclerotic disease differ in diet from other people' [9]. He and his dietician colleague noted a higher intake of sugar by men with peripheral arterial disease and first myocardial infarction compared with controls (Table 22.2). Although the association between sucrose (table sugar) consumption and coronary heart disease has been confirmed, sugar is also associated with cigarette smoking and socio-economic deprivation [10]. A causal link between sugar and coronary heart disease cannot therefore be assumed.

**Table 22.2 Sugar intake and occlusive atherosclerotic disease [9]**

|  | Number | Age, years (mean) | Sugar intake, g/day (mean) |
| --- | --- | --- | --- |
| Myocardial infarction | 20 | 56.4 | 132 |
| Peripheral arterial disease | 25 | 56.5 | 141 |
| Controls | 25 | 56.0 | 77 |

© 1964, adapted from The Lancet with permission from Elsevier.

However, Yudkin was a scientist and cautious. He did not wish to jump to conclusions concerning the association between an external factor such as sugar consumption and disease on an international scale. He drew attention to the fact that, as far as he could determine, the strongest association between the emergence of coronary heart disease in the UK and an environmental factor was with ownership of a radio or television set, emphasising that associations could only generate hypotheses and not conclusions.

The other aspect of the industrialisation of food production was the milling of wheat, from a coarse wholemeal product to a highly refined white product with a virtual absence of fibre. We have just seen two important studies, the London banking and transport [4] and the USA professional men [6], in which it emerged that the fibre content of the diet might be protective against coronary heart disease. The fibre depletion hypothesis was promulgated by several people in the 1970s, mainly Surgeon Commander T. L. Cleave, a Royal Navy surgeon, Dr Hugh Trowell, who worked in Uganda, and Professor Denis Burkitt, who also worked in Africa. They arrived at their conclusions semi-independently [11].

Perhaps the first suggestion that disease might be caused by the refinement of carbohydrate with a reduction of its fibre content was made by Arthur Rendle Short, Professor of Surgery in Bristol, UK, in the early years of the 20th century [12]. He described the emergence of appendicitis and summarised the various theories that had been proposed for its causation. He noted that it tended to run in families, some families having a 'special liability'. He also noted that it was more common in privileged persons of higher socio-economic status and he concluded that a diet depleted of fibre was the most likely cause. The fibre story that developed later in the 20th century had a major influence on dietary patterns that continues at the present time. However, critical evaluation has not occurred and studies have been based on association without intervention.

A study from Zutphen in the Netherlands investigated a 10-year follow-up of 871 middle-aged men with a baseline assessment of diet [13]. For the purpose of the analysis, the subjects were divided into five groups (quintiles) based on their fibre intake. Mortality from coronary heart disease was four times higher in those with the lowest intake of fibre compared with those with the highest (Figure 22.2). Deaths from cancer were similarly three times higher in the lowest dietary fibre group. This is an example of looking at the big picture but, as mentioned earlier, the problem is the number of confounding variables, as the authors indicate. They comment: 'A diet containing at least 37g dietary fibre per day may be protective against chronic disease in Western societies'.

**Figure 22.2 Dietary fibre and mortality [13].**

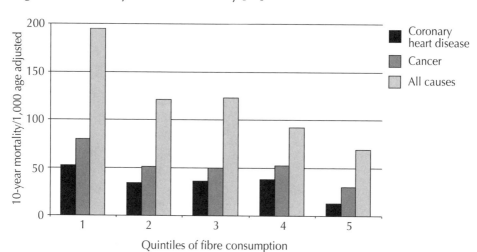

A problem with the dietary fibre hypothesis has been the lack of a robust and plausible intermediary mechanism. One attempt was made by Kenneth Heaton, working in the Department of Medicine at Bristol University, UK. His major research was concerned with the cause of gall-stones, a condition that remains unexplained. Gall-stones are formed mainly from cholesterol, which is secreted by the liver into bile. Bile also contains bile salts or acids that are synthesised in the liver from cholesterol and have a detergent function, keeping cholesterol in solution in bile. Heaton suggested that a high fibre content in a diet would bind bile salts within the intestine, thus preventing their re-absorption by the terminal ileum. As a consequence the liver would need to synthesise more bile salts, thus consuming more of the substrate cholesterol, leading to a reduction of the blood level of cholesterol. He demonstrated that wheat bran as a dietary fibre supplement did indeed lead to a reduction in the serum triglyceride and cholesterol concentrations [14]. The weakness of this as a mechanism is that it depends upon the diet–cholesterol–heart hypothesis, and this is far from robust.

A more recent attempt to provide plausibility to the fibre hypothesis has been along the following lines. Enterolactone is a fibre product, a lignan, that is produced from fibre in the diet by the action of bacteria in the large intestine, and it is absorbed into the blood. It is thought to be protective against cancer, but the active research group from the Finnish Institute of Public Health wondered if it might be the factor by which dietary fibre protects against coronary heart disease. The research group undertook a 7.7 year follow-up study of 167 men who had survived an acute coronary event and a similar number of matched controls [15]. The blood enterolactone level was lower in those with coronary heart disease than in controls. During follow-up, those men with the highest levels of enterolactone in the blood had the lowest risk of heart events. Enterolactone has a number of metabolic effects and, although much research is yet to be undertaken, it is possible that it has a protective role against the development of coronary heart disease.

The association between dietary fat and coronary heart disease is very weak and lacks consistency [16]. Dietary sugar shows a slightly stronger association, but also with other factors that have not been eliminated in subsequent studies. Dietary fibre shows a stronger association but there is no plausible intermediary mechanism. There is a fourth dietary factor that has been linked to coronary heart disease, and that is the apparent protective action of fish oils.

We have already seen that the health of Scottish people deteriorated during the processes of urbanisation and industrialisation of the 18th and 19th centuries. This has been ascribed to lack of sunlight but also the cessation of the traditional diet of fish. Similarly, the Inuit people of Greenland have had a low incidence of coronary heart disease and this is thought to be because of the traditional high fish diet [17]. The recent emergence of coronary heart disease among the Inuits might be to the result of a decline in fish consumption rather than exposure to what is usually called a western diet.

To investigate the relationship further between fish consumption and coronary heart disease, the very active researcher Daan Kromhout and his colleagues from the Netherlands, working in the University of Leiden, who had been responsible for the fibre study, undertook another dietary study in Zutphen [18]. A baseline study was made in 1960, recording the diet of 852 well middle-aged men. After 20 years of follow-up, the mortality from coronary heart disease was more than 50% lower among those who consumed at least 30 g of fish per day than among those who did not eat fish. This shows a more powerful association than any of the other dietary surveys. A similar result emerged from further research from the Harvard School of Public Health, USA, a 16-year follow-up study of 84 688 nurses [19].

Each of the dietary hypotheses of causation of coronary heart disease has a certain amount of plausibility and is supported by a certain level of observational evidence. However, there are obvious individual exceptions in that people consuming a high-cholesterol, high-sugar, low-fibre or low-fish diet might survive to an old age with no evidence of heart disease. On the other hand, people who are completely virtuous in their dietary patterns can develop coronary heart disease. This is the striking weakness of each hypothesis: none is rigorously consistent and none can be considered to provide the answer to the riddle of coronary heart disease. There seems to be no other explanation on offer and, despite their weaknesses, the dietary theories have become popular and filled the intellectual vacuum. People are being persuaded to eat a diet low in fat, low in sugar and high in fibre, with fish rather than meat. The healthy eating campaign is part of our lives.

It must be emphasised that the dietary theories are only theories: there are suspicions but there is no proof, the meaning of which we will leave until later in this book. Dietary experiments should be undertaken, but there are major difficulties in mounting controlled trials of dietary change in human populations. In clinical trials of tablets, those in the control group are given a placebo or dummy tablet, and tablets are easily taken. Tablet counting is part of the management of a trial and the opportunities for cheating by the participants are very much reduced. But with diet, things are different: can people be persuaded to avoid fat and sugar and to take a high-fibre diet? Can the control population be persuaded not to do so when the advertising in the media suggests that the active diet is generally considered to be safer? How can cheating be identified?

Therefore natural experiments are necessary, observing the fate of people who by choice undertake a diet change. The strength of this as a scientific process is extremely limited, as such people are self-selected, being either extremely virtuous or extremely careful in respect of health. Either way, they are likely to change several lifestyle factors simultaneously in order to achieve good health and a long life. Thus many confounding variables are introduced and it is difficult to separate one factor from another.

One natural experiment that has been described was the imposition of dietary change in the UK during the Second World War. It has been observed that death rates from coronary heart disease appeared to decline during this time and it has been suggested that it was because of a change in the national diet, in particular with less sugar as a result of import restrictions and at the same time flour was refined to a lesser degree. The weakness of this approach is that the epidemiology of coronary heart disease was poorly developed, and the causes of illness and death of the population were not of the greatest interest to a government that was concerned with national survival. Furthermore, it can be argued that one way to reduce mortality from one cause, such as coronary heart disease, is to introduce a high mortality rate from another cause, on the basis that humans are mortal and must die of something. During wartime, death rates from various types of injury rise dramatically, mainly in the younger members of the population, and so death rates from disease later in life will decline. This, once again, shows the limited value of natural experiments but, on the other hand, natural experiments do provide a good opportunity for observation, if not actual proof.

Despite all the difficulties, there must be clinical experiments, clinical trials, to attempt to determine whether dietary manipulation is helpful. Intervention and alteration of the national diet should not take place without some objective evidence of benefit. Many trials have been undertaken, but the results are generally inconsistent and inconclusive; despite this, healthy-eating initiatives have continued. A review of 27 studies in which dietary fat or cholesterol consumption was modified was undertaken by a group in the UK [16]. The conclusion was that a modification of fat intake results in a small reduction of cardiovascular events but has little effect on mortality.

It has been suggested that, if there is to be an approach to a national diet, step one would be as follows: total fat less than 30% of total calories; ratio of polyunsaturated fat to saturated fat 1:1; cholesterol less than 300 mg daily; calories reduced to achieve a desirable weight. The authors then reviewed five trials of this diet at a level of intervention of individual people [20]. There was a reduction in serum cholesterol of between 0% and 4%; population education reduced serum cholesterol by between 0.6% and 2%. When the population approach and individual dietary advice were combined, then the change in serum cholesterol varied from a fall of 2.1% to a rise of 1.0%. It was concluded that this was of no value and the change in serum cholesterol was inadequate to produce any significant benefit in those at risk [20]. This must be taken into context with the observations that the fall in coronary heart disease deaths in the UK and USA during the past 30 years has not been associated with a reduction of dietary fat intake.

The only trial that has shown a significant advantage in the diet treatment group is the Diet And Re-infarction Trial (DART) undertaken by the Medical Research Council Epidemiological Unit in Cardiff, UK [21]. This was a secondary prevention study in that it recruited men who had survived a myocardial infarction, with the purpose of preventing a second attack and early deaths. Because those recruited already had coronary heart disease, more end-points of death or myocardial infarction could be expected over a short follow-up of 2 years than if healthy people had been recruited. The study advised subjects to increase consumption of fat, fish or fibre intake, each with a control group. The results can be seen in Table 22.3.

**Table 22.3 Effects of changes in fat, fish and fibre intake on death and myocardial re-infarction [21].**
Deaths expressed as percentage deaths at 2 years; CHD = coronary heart disease; MI, myocardial infarction

| Diet group | All deaths | CHD deaths | Non-fatal MI | CHD events |
|---|---|---|---|---|
| Fat advice | 10.9 | 9.5 | 3.4 | 13.0 |
| No fat advice | 11.1 | 9.6 | 4.6 | 14.2 |
| Fish advice | 9.3 | 7.7 | 4.8 | 12.5 |
| No fish advice | 12.8 | 11.4 | 3.2 | 14.6 |
| Fibre advice | 12.1 | 10.7 | 4.0 | 14.7 |
| No fibre advice | 9.9 | 8.4 | 4.0 | 12.4 |

© 1989, adapted from The Lancet with permission from Elsevier.

Fat advice appeared to be ineffective regarding cardiovascular and death outcome. Fish advice was beneficial, but fibre advice appeared to be detrimental. Those receiving fish advice had a total mortality of 9.3% at 2 years compared with the controls with no fish advice whose mortality was 12.8%. The corresponding figures for deaths from coronary heart disease were 7.7% and 11.4%, a clear benefit.

The health advantage of consumption of oily fish is generally accepted. It is usually felt that the fatty acids in fish, especially the omega-3 fatty acids, are in some way protective. The parallel with tuberculosis is generally forgotten and there is no general view that it might be the high vitamin D content of oily fish that is protective, and which might have helped the Inuit people until the recent adoption of a western diet.

It seems to be impossible for medical science to stop and rethink the conventional wisdom that animal fats cause heart disease. Uffe Ravnskov is the independent Swedish researcher whose work we have already met in Chapter 20, and we will meet it again. He commented (thinking in the way of the scientific philosopher Karl Popper) [22]: 'The diet/heart disease hypothesis is unfalsifiable and should therefore be classified as non-science'.

The point is that the diet–cholesterol–heart hypothesis is so ingrained in western, and indeed in international, society that evidence to the contrary is systematically ignored. Any pretence at science was lost long ago. Apart from the addition of oily fish, and possibly cereal fibre, diet is of no relevance to the development of coronary heart disease but, in all reviews, that option is never expressed.

Overall, 21 studies, including more than 150 000 participants with and without coronary heart disease, have failed to find an eating pattern that would support the diet–cholesterol–heart hypothesis [23]. Many intervention studies have failed to demonstrate a consistent benefit from reducing dietary fat, and only fish supplements seem to be helpful.

But new life was breathed into the diet hypothesis by Professor Ram B. Singh, based in Moradabad, India. He and colleagues produced a number of impressive papers, the first of the series being published in the *British Medical Journal* in 1992 [24]. His 2002 paper in *The Lancet* describes a study in which he and colleagues undertook 'a randomised controlled trial in 1000 patients with angina pectoris, myocardial infarction, or surrogate risk factors for CAD [coronary artery disease]. 499 patients were allocated to a diet rich in whole grains, fruits, walnuts, and almonds. 501 controls consumed a local diet similar to the step 1 National Educational Program (NCEP) prudent diet' [25]. The results showed a considerable advantage to those receiving dietary treatments compared with controls, as is shown in Figure 22.3.

**Figure 22.3  Effect of Indo-Mediterranean diet [25].**
MI = myocardial infarction.

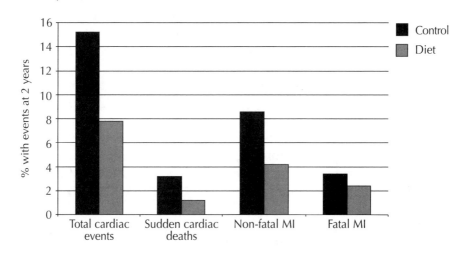

© *2002, adapted from* The Lancet *with permission from Elsevier.*

The benefit of Singh's Indo-Mediterranean diet is clearly extremely impressive, with a 50% reduction of cardiac event rates after only 2 years and an almost two-thirds reduction of sudden cardiac deaths, from 3.2% in the control group to 1.2% in the diet group. The results have been widely quoted, for example in an influential editorial in the *New England Journal of Medicine* [26].

In reality the results are too good to be true; no diet trial has achieved anything like such an impressive result. Scepticism was expressed in private to the editor of the *British Medical Journal* following the 1992 paper and further private correspondence following the 2002 paper in *The Lancet*. A public statement was made in both these journals in July 2005 [27,28], with the intimation that the results are suspect and almost certainly fraudulent. *The Lancet* also carried a letter from Dr C. R. Soman, Health Action by People, India, providing a critical analysis of the 2002 paper [29]. Singh was requested to provide the original data for re-examination but he informed the investigators that the documents had been eaten by termites.

All work by Singh and colleagues should be disregarded but its effects are not easily undone. The diet–cholesterol–heart hypothesis has been fraudulently strengthened and the great majority of those who have been impressed by Singh's results are unlikely to read the subsequent detailed accounts in the *British Medical Journal* and *The Lancet*. We can thus appreciate why it is so important to read and analyse original papers, a process that I hope to achieve in this book.

The important conclusion of this chapter is that the diet–cholesterol–heart hypothesis appears to be unsustainable. If we are looking for the cause of coronary heart disease, then diet, and in particular a high-fat diet, does not provide the answer.

# 23
# THE LENINGRAD PARADOX

In the previous chapter we have seen that no single dietary component appears to be the cause of coronary heart disease. Fish consumption is probably protective, but protective against what? We still cannot identify the cause, the factor that initiates the pathological process that ultimately leads to the clinical manifestations of the disease.

But the feeling that diet is in some way the cause of coronary heart disease remains the basis of public health initiatives. The diet–cholesterol–heart hypothesis lives on, and conventional wisdom now tells us that the important dietary factor is gluttony, that is over-nutrition. We are being warned against the over-feeding of children leading to obesity, and in the summer of 2004 the UK national press warned us of dire consequences. We are told that we are a sitting on a time bomb of an epidemic of coronary heart disease resulting from childhood obesity. We are warned of the dangers of eating 'fast food', the translation of *Schnell Imbiss*, which has been popular and perfectly respectable in Germany for many years.

There is nothing intrinsically harmful about prepared food for which the customer need only wait a few minutes in a take-away rather than half an hour or so in a restaurant. I think there must be general feeling that food prepared in our own kitchen from natural ingredients is somehow better for us, or at least more virtuous, than food which has been prepared in a restaurant or fast service in a takeaway shop. There is probably the poorly expressed view that toiling in the kitchen slows down and therefore minimises food production whereas our affluence leads to the purchase of far more food than we could be bothered to prepare for ourselves. The truth of this assertion is most doubtful.

The time taken for food to be served is of no relevance to the development of coronary heart or perhaps any disease. It would, however, be appropriate to look at the quantity of food, and its energy density in particular, for ideas regarding how disease might result.

Calorie consumption per person increased during the first half of the 20th century and levelled off during the second half. So during the first half of the 20th century, calorie intake increased in parallel with deaths from coronary heart disease but during the second half there was no dietary change that might be responsible for the decline of the epidemic. Over-nutrition did not appear to be the cause of the 20th century epidemic of coronary heart disease, and so why should it be expected to cause a 21st century epidemic?

The concern about fast food is that its energy density is higher than home-made food, but people will queue up for a 'fast salad' that is thought to be nutritious. There is no doubt that supermarkets and lunch-time fast-food outlets sell large amounts of prepared imaginative salads that are very low in energy content. It is the take-away shops selling beefburgers that are regarded with disdain and distaste by middle-class and middle-aged commentators. The average beefburger contains rather less fat than the average Greek meal but, to fit in with conventional wisdom, it must somehow be different because Greeks are healthy, even if they have a tendency to become overweight.

We are told that over-nutrition will lead to early death. There is no question that morbid obesity is to be avoided; body weight in excess of 20 stones will lead to serious impairment of mobility and respiratory difficulties. Obesity is sometimes associated with diabetes and can lead to serious metabolic problems, but it is the milder form of obesity that is much more common and much more benign. We are told that our children are becoming more obese, but perhaps this is because of the restricted ability to exercise and the domination of their lives by the television and computer. The freedom of children to play outside is prohibited by a combination of real and perceived social and traffic dangers.

There are, however, serious questions that might lead us to doubt the diet–heart hypothesis, a simple relationship between over-nutrition and the subsequent development of heart disease. Let us not forget that present concerns are that children who are over-fed and obese today will develop life-threatening heart disease tomorrow. The comparisons with Greece lead us to question the wisdom of this simple assertion and there are further doubts that must be taken seriously.

St Petersburg in Russia was called Leningrad at the time of the siege by Nazi troops in 1941–44. As a result of this siege, the population suffered from severe food shortage, leading to the death of approximately 630 000 citizens from hunger-related causes.

Study of the survivors has been undertaken, in particular a study that was carried out in 1975–77 of 3905 men who lived in St Petersburg and of whom one-third had experienced the siege. It was therefore possible to assess the health outcome of those who experienced the severe famine of the siege compared with other Russian citizens who did not [1]. Conventional wisdom that over-nutrition in childhood and early adult life leads to heart disease and a shorter life would lead us to expect that the survivors of the famine would have subsequently enjoyed long and healthy lives. This has not been the case.

During the follow-up period of study, 2048 of the 3905 men died, 662 from coronary heart disease and 333 from strokes. Those who had experienced the siege had a death rate from coronary heart disease 28% in excess of what would be expected for an age-matched Russian population. Adjustments for occupation, education and smoking had no impact on the risk estimate, although they did have an effect on absolute risk of dying during the follow-up period. Those who were exposed to famine at the time of puberty seemed to have the greatest risk of subsequent death from coronary heart disease. The authors, from St Petersburg and Stockholm, concluded: 'Starvation, or accompanying chronic stress, particularly at the onset of or during puberty, may increase vulnerability to later cardiovascular disease' [1].

The explanation of this conclusion is not immediately obvious but clearly the assertion that over-nutrition in adolescents will lead to coronary heart disease in later life must be seriously questioned. The well-documented experience of the siege of Leningrad must present a serious paradox to the diet–heart hypothesis and must lead us to look afresh at the cause of coronary heart disease.

The Leningrad paradox is in direct contrast to what we are told. We must add this to the Barcelona paradox, three English towns paradox and London bank and transport paradox, which we have examined in previous chapters. The diet component of the diet–cholesterol–heart hypothesis is looking far from robust but it will be necessary for us to look at the cholesterol–heart link in more detail.

There is another aspect to the siege of Leningrad. The citizens were under almost constant bombardment and had to seek shelter. This demanded an indoor existence, usually in cellars, with minimal exposure to the sun. For the same reason the opportunities for fishing must similarly have been negligible. The survivors must have been deficient in vitamin D and this might be the explanation for their poor health outcome in later life.

Before we leave this chapter, it is important to note the lesson we can learn from the siege of Leningrad. Starvation, through mechanisms that are not clear, leads to significant impairment of immunity and predisposition to infection. Perhaps this might have something to do with the subsequent development of coronary heart disease.

# PART 5

# CHOLESTEROL

# 24
# CHOLESTEROL AND CORONARY HEART DISEASE

One of the most important health-care developments during the mid-20th century was clinical chemistry, the ability to measure the chemical constituents of blood in the hospital laboratory. The rather complicated Van Slyke process enabled the measurement of chloride, which was important in the determination of the acid–base balance, but was ultimately superseded in the mid-1960s by the Astrup method, which allowed estimation of the blood pH, partial pressure of carbon dioxide in the blood and bicarbonate concentration simultaneously. Flame photometry was developed in the 1950s, enabling the measurement of sodium and potassium in the blood.

Measurement of the cholesterol concentration of the serum component of blood became routinely available in hospital laboratories in the 1950s, although its measurement had been possible in specialised scientific laboratories since early in the century. The measurement of serum cholesterol was initially expressed in milligrams per 100 millilitres (mg/100 mL) of serum. This expression of concentration is still in use in the USA, something that causes international confusion because European laboratories have converted to standard international (SI) units, expressed as millimols per litre (mmol/L). The conversion factor is 38.4, meaning that a serum cholesterol level of 5.2 mmol/L is approximately 200 and exactly 199.68 mg/100 mL (or 199.68 mg/dL; dL being decilitre and 1 dL = 100 mL). It is this conversion that determines the widespread use of 5.2 mmol/L in epidemiological and clinical practice.

The ability to measure serum cholesterol provided the opportunity for exploring further the hypothesis that had been presented, namely that a high dietary intake of cholesterol would lead to a high blood level of cholesterol and then to cholesterol deposition in the arteries. The diet–cholesterol–heart hypothesis is basically that cholesterol is toxic, but this is never stated clearly. A toxic substance is one in which damage is done in direct relationship to the amount consumed and in direct relationship to the concentration that it achieves in the blood. It will affect all people exposed in a similar way, and this is the alleged mechanism in respect of cholesterol.

The alternative reaction to an external substance is an idiosyncrasy or allergy, which cannot be foreseen, affects only a few people exposed, its effect is not related to the blood concentration and it is not dose related (a small amount can cause the same damage as a large amount). It is important to remember that a toxic effect is the result of a direct link between the toxic substance and the individual or population damaged, whereas an idiosyncrasy is indirect, often through an allergic process.

It was necessary to explore the proposed relationship between blood (serum) cholesterol and coronary heart disease in the general population by looking at the illness outcome as predicted by the serum cholesterol level. There have been two particularly well-publicised studies that looked into this, one from the UK and one from the USA.

The Multiple Risk Factor Intervention Trial (MRFIT) was conducted in the USA and published in 1986 [1]. It analysed the mortality of 361 662 men aged between 35 and 57 years after 6 years of follow-up. The serum cholesterol concentrations can be seen in Figure 24.1 to be 'normally' distributed, which means that the average is in the middle and the distribution curve is symmetrical. The average (mean) level of cholesterol was about 5.8 mmol/L or 223 mg/dL. The majority of those studied had a cholesterol level greater than 5.2 mmol/L (200 mg/dL), at present the level above which it is said that intervention should take place. This will be discussed in more detail below.

**Figure 24.1  Distribution of serum cholesterol in 361 662 USA men aged 35–57 years [1].**

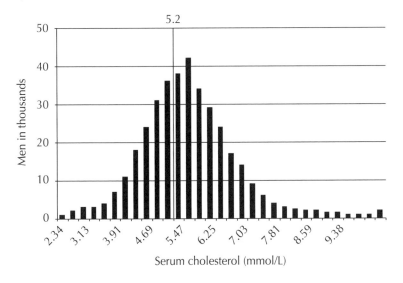

Figure 24.2 indicates that in the study group the death rate increased with serum cholesterol. Mortality from coronary heart disease and also from 'all causes' was highest in the top 15% of the serum cholesterol range but there was little difference within the great majority of subjects.

**Figure 24.2  Six-year death rate per 1000 men according to serum cholesterol [1]. CHD, coronary heart disease.**

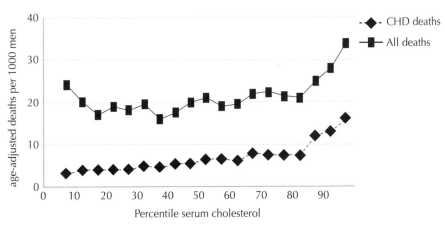

To simplify the display of data, the subjects were divided into quintiles based on the serum cholesterol level, from the lowest to the highest groups, each being 20% of the study group. The relative risk of death from coronary heart disease was expressed for each quintile compared with the lowest quintile, as shown in Figure 24.3.

We can see that the risk of death from coronary heart disease appears to increase progressively with the serum cholesterol concentration, in keeping with a pattern of toxicity. The study also quotes the National Institutes of Health (Bethesda, USA) consensus development conference on lowering cholesterol to prevent heart disease, which called for 'aggressive treatment of patients with cholesterol concentrations within the 90th percentile' (that is the top 10%), a modest aim compared with present-day policies that include all those with a serum cholesterol level above 5.2 mmol/L, which is most people [2].

**Figure 24.3  Relative risk of death at 6 years [1].**

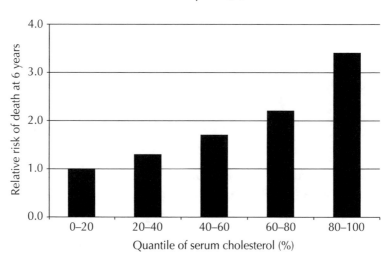

© 1986, adapted from The Lancet with permission from Elsevier.

The Whitehall study, undertaken in the UK, investigated the relationship between serum cholesterol and subsequent death from coronary heart disease [3]. The study was undertaken by Professor Geoffrey Rose and Dr Martin Shipley from the Department of Epidemiology at the London School of Hygiene and Tropical Medicine, London, UK. They studied 17 718 male civil servants aged between 40 and 64 years and, for the purpose of the analysis, also grouped the participants into quintiles in relationship to the serum cholesterol concentration. The results can be seen in Figure 24.4.

**Figure 24.4 Morality at 10 years based on quintile of serum cholesterol [3].**

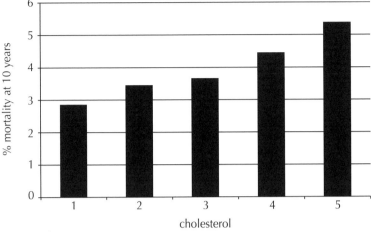

*Adapted with permission from the British Medical Journal Publishing Group.*

There is a clear gradient of risk, with the lowest quintile having the lowest risk of death from coronary heart disease at 10 years, namely 2.72% of those initially recruited. The highest cholesterol quintile had the highest death rate, with 5.98% at 10 years. The serum cholesterol concentration thus predicted the likelihood of death from coronary heart disease. The authors went on to make the assumption that by reducing the serum cholesterol level of the population, the death rate from coronary heart disease would be reduced and that this was 'a public health imperative'. They were acting on the basis of accepted wisdom and not scientific objectivity, but the scene was being set for population intervention and dietary manipulation: the tyranny of health professionals acting on the basis of flimsy evidence.

At this point it is worth hesitating to think about what a normal serum cholesterol level actually means. Most biological variables, such as height and weight, form a normal distribution from which an average can be determined. Measurements are arranged symmetrically around the mean but there can be outliers who are clearly in a disease state. With height, conditions that interfere with natural growth, for example pituitary underactivity or chronic disease, can cause people to be abnormally small or, for example because of over-activity of pituitary growth hormone secretion during the growing phase, abnormally tall. We can generally identify these extremes, which turn out to be very rare.

Figure 24.5 shows the distribution of serum cholesterol level in the UK population, specifically of men aged between 40 and 59 years, published in 1998 by the NHS Centre for Reviews and Dissemination (London, UK) [4]. It demonstrates quite clearly a 'normal' distribution of serum cholesterol but also something else of great importance. It compares the serum cholesterol distribution of men with and without coronary heart disease and the difference is surprisingly little, about 0.6 mmol/L.

**Figure 24.5  Distribution of serum cholesterol levels among British men aged 40–59 years [4].**

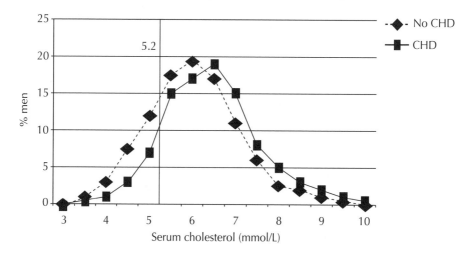

*CHD, coronary heart disease. Crown © 1998, adapted with permission.*

An important point is the number of men, with or without coronary heart disease, who have a serum cholesterol above 5.2 mmol/L, which is today regarded as the maximum permissible. The size of the perceived public health problem is immense, and massive action will be necessary to meet the challenge of reducing the serum cholesterol levels of about 70% of middle-aged men. I will also point out that more men in the UK have a serum cholesterol level above the 5.2 threshold than the men in the USA MRFIT study. We will revisit the geography of cholesterol in a later chapter.

Another way of looking at these data is that the difference in serum cholesterol between those with and those without coronary heart disease appears to be modest. It does not deliver the message that serum cholesterol is the major 'cause' of cardiovascular death in the way that we have been led to expect by the MRFIT and Whitehall studies [1,2]. But the question remains whether serum cholesterol is toxic or damaging in itself or merely an indicator of some other biological or disease process.

With most biological data, we take a normal range (statistically two standard deviations each side of the average) and identify the people within it as being normal, but we must appreciate that normal is not the same as perfect, which is rarely attainable. Rose and Shipley [2] noted that perfection and normal are different things, and they were instrumental in developing the idea that serum cholesterol should not be regarded as having a normal range but that simply 'the lower the better': perfection is as low as possible. This idea has been emphasised in more recent years, and it basically means that the majority of people are ill, whether we know it or not. We know that we might be summoned to see our family doctor for a 'routine check'. We can go in under the impression that we are well, but come out with a diagnosis, an illness, often of a high serum cholesterol.

For many years, the early features of aortic atherosclerosis have been observed at autopsies of healthy individuals who had died as the result of violence. As early as 1936, Lande and Sperry had observed that such changes bore no relationship to the serum cholesterol level recorded immediately after death [5]. This did not conform to the diet–cholesterol–heart hypothesis that had already developed but, as usual, there was a vaguely plausible explanation for this paradox, that cholesterol might disappear from the blood stream immediately after death. This objection was easily discounted by subsequent experiments. However, somehow these observations were conveniently ignored and the flawed hypothesis continued to become widely accepted. A more detailed review of this subject has been undertaken by Uffe Ravnskov, an independent researcher from Sweden [6].

There is a clear family pattern to coronary heart disease, and the reason for it has not been clear. The family incidence of tuberculosis was similarly not clear but considered to be constitutional (that is inherited), until the microbial and thus transmissible nature of the condition was realised. The question surrounding family risk of coronary heart disease is whether it is mediated by environmental factors or by a metabolic abnormality determined by genetic mutation, although the two are not mutually exclusive. Family members initially have the same social class and thus lifestyle, but this might not last long with access to higher education and career development.

It has been considered generally that the family risk of coronary heart disease is somehow constitutional, and this is obvious in practical clinical medicine today: a person suspected of having coronary heart disease is asked about family history as a risk factor, regardless of variables such as social class. It has been recognised that a component of family risk, but by no means all of it, can be explained on the basis of serum cholesterol levels, and this is given credence by the recognition of families with a particularly high serum cholesterol level, familial hypercholesterolaemia (FH). This condition has supported the hypothesis that a high level of cholesterol in the blood leads to coronary heart disease. However, the vast majority of people with a family clustering of coronary heart disease do not have familial hypercholesterolaemia, and so the nature of inheritance is not clear.

The development of atherosclerotic disease in people with familial hypercholesterolaemia does not always occur, and the simple genetic model does not appear to be as straightforward as was initially thought. There are other factors at play that cast doubt on the model that a high serum cholesterol per se is toxic or damaging.

It is important to note that families with hypercholesterolaemia have usually been investigated because one family member, the index case, presented with cardiovascular disease at a young age. The other family members would then be identified through community tracing. In this circumstance it is impossible to separate the genetic from the environmental factors, known and unknown, that might be present in a family and that might lead to the development of coronary heart disease.

From the point of view of research, familial hypercholesterolaemia can be regarded as a natural experiment. It is genetically determined and 700 different mutations have been identified. We rely on observations of people with particularly high serum cholesterol to help test the hypothesis that high cholesterol in the blood causes cholesterol deposition in the tissues and particularly the arteries, leading to coronary heart disease.

An important study took place in the Netherlands, recording details of a large family with hypercholesterolaemia, identified not through the end points of coronary heart disease but through population screening for serum cholesterol [7]. In other words the family did not appear to have a particular susceptibility to coronary heart disease for whatever reason, and therefore the influence of environmental factors within the family was minimised. Screening had identified two members of the family with serum cholesterol levels of 9.20 and 10.24 mmol/L. A further family member came to light following myocardial infarction at the age of 51 and he was found to have a serum cholesterol of 12.78 mmol/L.

The complete family tree was constructed over seven generations, with causes of death identified from records, and a total of 412 ancestors and descendents was traced. It was noted that during the 19th and early 20th centuries mortality was not increased in carriers of the mutation, in keeping with the fact that coronary heart disease had not emerged to a significant level at that time and of course estimation of serum cholesterol levels were then unknown.

It can be seen in Figure 24.6 that before the epidemic of coronary heart disease the family had a mortality rate significantly lower than the national average, in other words they had a biological advantage. There are more recent examples of health advantages of a high serum cholesterol that we will meet later. The mortality rate in the family increased after 1914, reaching its peak between 1935 and 1964, and it fell thereafter. There were two major branches of the family carrying the abnormal gene, the relative risk in one branch being 3.26 and in the other branch 1.78, a significant difference in itself.

**Figure 24.6  All causes of mortality of 250 members of a family with familial hypercholesterolaemia [7].**

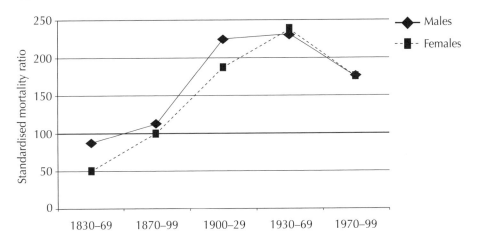

*Adapted with permission from the British Medical Journal Publishing Group.*

If genetically determined familial hypercholesterolaemia was the cause of coronary heart disease, then clearly deaths and other expressions of the disease would have been constant during history, unless members of the family died prematurely from other more prevalent conditions. This was not the case in this family, and in the 19th century family members were recorded as having lived to remarkable old age. We would also expect family members to have exhibited a fairly uniform pattern of disease, but it turned out that the risk of death varied very significantly among family members. The development of the disease matched perfectly the epidemic of coronary heart disease that emerged throughout the 20th century, as we saw Chapter 18. In the 20th century there was an excess mortality among the family members compared with the background population and so it would appear that there was an increased susceptibility to coronary heart disease or early death from it, but nevertheless most of the family members did not die from this condition.

The conclusion of this important and unique study is that the major cause of coronary heart disease in people with familial hypercholesterolaemia is an environmental factor and not a genetic factor, and it is obviously important that this environmental factor should be recognised. There is nothing in this study or any other study of familial hypercholesterolaemia to suggest a damaging effect of cholesterol in the diet.

The experience of familial hypercholesterolaemia initially suggested that an elevated level of cholesterol in the blood might be important in the development of coronary heart disease. The fact that it was only in the 20th century that coronary heart disease became a cause of death in people with familial hypercholesterolaemia indicates that cholesterol cannot be the prime moving factor but only a possible co-factor. Similarly, different families with familial hypercholesterolaemia have a very variable incidence of coronary heart disease, once again indicating that cholesterol is not the prime mover. This, of course, is very much against the overall diet–cholesterol–heart hypothesis, which is based on the premise that cholesterol is the prime mover.

It is also important to recognise that the members of the family from the Netherlands survived to comparatively old age, especially in earlier generations, indicating that hypercholesterolaemia may have provided a survival advantage at a time when deaths from infectious diseases were more common. We will investigate this possibility again in further chapters that will be looking at the elderly paradox and the relationship between cholesterol and inflammation.

Doubt about the direct relationship between cholesterol and coronary heart disease also emerges from observations of another group of people who are known to have a very high serum cholesterol level. These are people with primary biliary cirrhosis (PBC), a chronic liver disease of unknown cause. It is rare and affects mainly middle-aged women. Whereas at one time it caused a great deal of illness and was often fatal, it can now be treated by liver transplantation. It is characterised by jaundice and associated itching but also by xanthelasma, cholesterol deposits in the skin, particularly in the creases of the palms of the hands and around the eyes. The deposition of cholesterol in the tissues can be very dramatic in primary biliary cirrhosis and it is the result of a very high level of cholesterol in the blood. However, despite marked hypercholesterolaemia and against all expectations based on the cholesterol–heart hypothesis, there is no excess cardiovascular mortality in patients with primary biliary cirrhosis [8].

This observation undermines the proposal that coronary heart disease is the result of cholesterol being deposited into the arterial tissues in relationship to its concentration in the blood. Primary biliary cirrhosis provides one of those natural experiments of immense importance, namely a group of people in whom the serum cholesterol level is raised to a very high level with tissue deposition. In this case there is no effect on the heart and, as a result, a direct damaging effect of a high serum cholesterol level causing coronary heart disease must be seriously questioned. Similarly, this study suggests that the excess coronary heart disease deaths among those with familial hypercholesterolaemia might be mediated by a mechanism other than the elevated cholesterol level in the blood. We also need to ask ourselves about the role of cholesterol in atheroma. Is it just an accident of evolution?

A problem with the prediction of coronary heart disease is that it appears to have a very long development time, perhaps several decades, before it is finally expressed as a clinical illness. Therefore when an individual is examined or assessed, if there is no history of a previous coronary event then there is no way of determining with relative ease whether the individual does or does not have coronary artery disease. The only way of determining this would be to undertake a radiological imaging process, a coronary angiogram, which is at present almost always an invasive procedure, not without risk and certainly not to be performed for the sake of curiosity. The two studies mentioned, MRFIT and Whitehall, looked at individuals within the study population without knowing at the point of entry whether those individuals had coronary heart disease or not.

Another important population survey took place in Framingham, Massachusetts, USA, and we have already looked at aspects of this. The distribution of serum cholesterol levels among men aged 35–49 years, displayed in Figure 24.7, showed higher cholesterol levels in those with coronary heart disease [9].

**Figure 24.7 Distribution of serum cholesterol in men aged 30–49 years [9].**

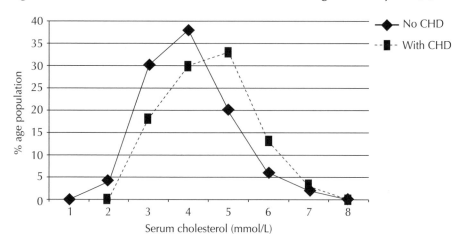

*CHD, coronary heart disease. Adapted from the Annals of Internal Medicine with permission from the American College of Physicians.*

But there are further data of great importance. Whereas men below the age of 50 with coronary heart disease had on average a higher serum cholesterol, this was not the case for men aged 50 years and older. Figure 24.8 shows the corresponding data for the 50–62 year age group.

**Figure 24.8 Distribution of serum cholesterol in men aged 50–62 years [9].**

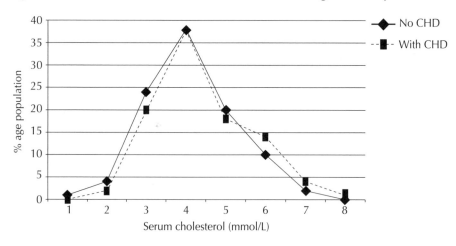

*CHD, coronary heart disease. Adapted from the Annals of Internal Medicine with permission from the American College of Physicians.*

There was no significant difference between those with and those without coronary heart disease, clearly indicating the unimportance of serum cholesterol as a predictor of disease above the age of 50 years. We are not usually told this. Most episodes of and deaths from coronary heart disease occur at an age greater than 70 years and it is uncommon below the age of 50. These data from Framingham are not widely quoted because they do not fit in with the diet–cholesterol–heart hypothesis.

We have already looked at the Whitehall and MRFIT studies, which showed a relationship with serum cholesterol level in men below the age of 60 years, indicating that the higher the serum cholesterol, the greater the risk of death from coronary heart disease. A refinement of this was a re-analysis of data collected initially by the Lipid Research Clinic's follow-up study in the USA [10]. This very important study was published in 1990 and has been undertaken by three highly respected cholesterol workers, Jacques Rossouw, Barry Lewis and Basil Rifkind [11]. They started by analysing the data relating to all the men in the original study, showing an increasing risk of death from coronary heart disease with increasing serum cholesterol. They then took the critical step of subdividing the men into those known to have coronary heart disease and those who were not known to have it. The difference was quite dramatic, as can be seen in Figure 24.9. The increased risk of death with an increase in serum cholesterol in those with coronary heart disease was very significant. However, the important observation was in those without coronary heart disease: the increasing death rate with increasing cholesterol was very small.

**Figure 24.9  Mortality from coronary heart disease (CHD) based on groups of serum cholesterol [11].**

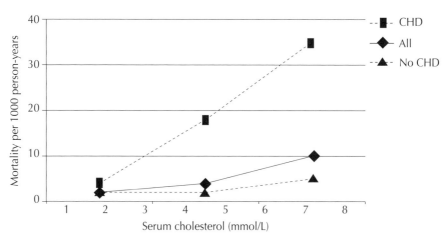

There are three possible conclusions to be drawn from this study that escaped the attention of the authors. First, if cholesterol has a causative role, it can only have a secondary accelerating effect on people with established heart disease and cannot be a prime mover. Secondly, if cholesterol is not the prime mover of coronary heart disease, could the elevated level be the result of the disease process rather than its cause? We will look into this possibility in a later chapter. Finally, we must remember that people who are considered to be normal and who have no evidence of disease might have coronary heart disease but in a latent form that cannot be identified at the time. The main message from this study is that serum cholesterol concentration appears to be of little importance in people who are well and do not have coronary heart disease.

It is important to point out that the authors of this paper made the curious comment in their conclusion that 'the causal role of cholesterol in re-infarction has been demonstrated'. This is a conclusion that does not appear to be related to the findings. They seem to have missed the point that the main conclusion of their study is, if anything, that cholesterol has a secondary rather than primary role in the development of coronary heart disease.

If we are looking for the cause of coronary heart disease we must look beyond cholesterol, but it would be premature to leave the cholesterol story at this point. There is clearly a relationship between cholesterol and coronary heart disease that must be understood, because there is likely to be a hidden truth. The relationship could be causal but, on the other hand, the relationship could be like so many other risk indicators, simply an indication of people who are at risk without the cholesterol being the cause in itself.

The diet–cholesterol–heart hypothesis is well established but some words of warning have been issued. For example Edward H. Ahrens stated in 1976 [12]:

*The lipid hypothesis is the postulate that reduction of the level of plasma cholesterol in an individual or in a population group would lead to a reduction in the risk of suffering a new event of coronary heart disease. It is a premise based on the undisputed fact that people with higher plasma cholesterol levels have more and early coronary heart disease than do others with lower cholesterol levels; but the premise has not yet been proved true to the satisfaction of epidemiologists and biostatisticians or of the medical community at large. Though the hypothesis has been put to the test repeatedly in the past two decades, completely satisfactory evidence has not yet been advanced, either pro or con.*

This was written more than 30 years ago and many more studies have been published during this time; we will be looking at several of them. We must not lose sight of the fact that the relationship with cholesterol is not specific for coronary heart disease; for example, the MRFIT study showed a relationship between serum cholesterol and mortality from all causes. This points to a fundamental truth about cholesterol of which we are at present unaware but must try to understand.

In this chapter we have looked at the associations between serum cholesterol and coronary heart disease. The next step is to look at the effect of reducing the cholesterol content of the blood by medical interventions. Does reducing serum cholesterol concentration reduce the risk of subsequent coronary events and is it of benefit to those treated? Before we move to this subject, it would be as well to take a look at the metabolism of cholesterol within the body.

# 25

# THE METABOLISM OF CHOLESTEROL

The synthesis of cholesterol is very similar to that of vitamin D, in that the immediate precursor of both is 7-dehydrocholesterol, which itself is synthesised from squalene, the long-chain fatty acid that is also known as shark oil (see Chapter 16). The synthesis of squalene and its derivatives 7-dehydrocholesterol and cholesterol takes place mainly in the liver but it can also occur in other tissues, including the skin. The structure of cholesterol is shown in Figure 25.1, and its similarity to the various vitamin D molecules is clear.

Cholesterol that is produced inside the body is endogenous and cholesterol derived from food is, of course, exogenous. Fatty substances taken in the diet are digested in the small intestine under the influence of enzymes called lipases. These are secreted by the pancreas and are also found in the surface membrane of the cells lining the small intestine.

Fats are usually in the form of long-chain fatty acids. These can be saturated, which means that no other atoms can be added to them, or unsaturated, which means they have the potential for the addition of other atoms, most simply hydrogen. Unsaturated fatty acids are generally liquid, for example vegetable oils. When they are saturated, they are more solid. Margarines are produced from oils by adding hydrogen atoms in the industrial process of hydrogenation, resulting in a more solid end product.

**Figure 25.1 The structure of fatty acids and cholesterol.**

Squalene

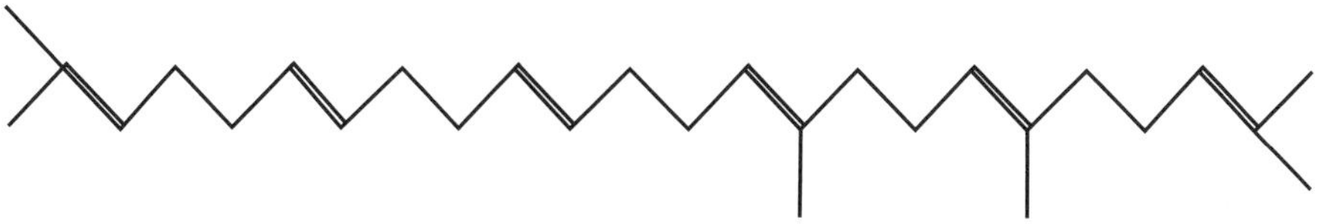

Cholesterol

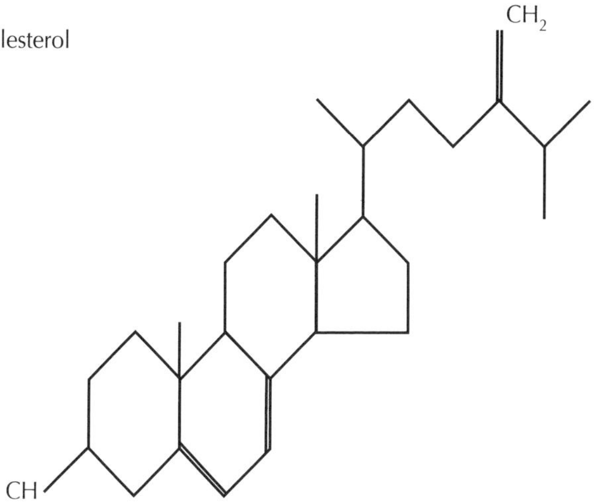

Unsaturated fatty acids can be mono- or polyunsaturated, depending on the number of additional hydrogen atoms that can be added to the molecule. We have also seen the term *trans*-unsaturated fatty acids, which effectively is concerned with the symmetry or isomerism of the molecule (*trans*- means across or on the other side of, in this case, the molecule, but it could be the Atlantic Ocean, as opposed to *cis*-, which means on the same side of; but these details are not of importance at present). We have encountered an unsaturated fatty acid called omega-3, which is found in fish oils. It is also called linoleic acid and is shown in Figure 25.2. The double bond indicates that the molecule is unsaturated, with two double bonds in this case. Squalene is also unsaturated (Figure 25.2).

**Figure 25.2 The structure of fatty acids.**

Squalene (shark oil)
*This is poly-unsaturated and the unsaturated double bonds are trans*

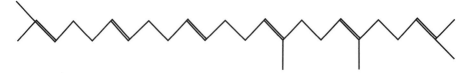

Linoeic acid (omega-3)
*This is poly-unsaturated and the two unsaturated double bonds are cis*

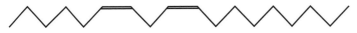

Palmitic acid
*This is a saturated fatty acid*

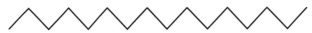

During the process of digestion, long-chain fatty acids, either saturated or unsaturated, are broken down by lipases into shorter chains that can be absorbed by the intestine. Cholesterol and related sterol compounds such as vitamin D are not digested but are absorbed as such by active transport systems across the small intestinal membranes. They enter lymphatic channels in the small intestine or, alternatively, the portal venous blood stream to the liver. The lymphatic channels, in which fatty substances are transported as chylomicrons, by-pass the liver and enter the systemic circulation by the major lymphatic channel, the thoracic duct.

Cholesterol is a fatty substance and therefore will dissolve in organic hydrocarbon solvents but will not dissolve in water. This is a feature of most biologically active compounds within the body, the vast majority of which are only lipid soluble, a property that enables them to enter cells through the lipid-based membrane. Most medications are similarly lipid soluble. A major function of the liver is to convert lipid-soluble substances into water-soluble substances by conjugating them with glucuronic acid, a process that makes them biologically inactive and enables water-based excretion through the kidneys. Lipid-soluble substances will not dissolve in blood and are transported within the blood attached to albumin, the major blood protein. Cholesterol is similarly attached to protein and is transported through the blood in the form of lipoproteins.

Studies of lipoproteins indicate that there are basically three types: high-density (HDL), low-density (LDL) and very low-density (VLDL) lipoproteins. Since the late 1970s it has been possible to identify these and an interesting observation has been made; whereas the largest component, LDL, is like total cholesterol in that it appears to have a direct association with coronary heart disease, HDL is different and appears to have an inverse relationship with coronary heart disease [1]. The higher the HDL concentration in the blood, the lower the risk of myocardial infarction. Using lay terms, some documents refer to 'good cholesterol' (HDL) and 'bad cholesterol' (LDL). The interactions producing lipoproteins are shown in Figure 25.3.

The MRFIT and Whitehall studies [2,3], and also most of the cholesterol-lowering therapies that we will visit in the next chapter, are based on total serum cholesterol and not its LDL fraction. Recent studies have looked at lipoprotein groups as well as total cholesterol and, although these add to the understanding of cholesterol metabolism, they do not seem to add a great deal to clinical practice or even to the development of the diet–cholesterol–heart hypothesis.

We have already encountered familial hypercholesterolaemia. As with all genetic disorders, the vast majority of people with familial hypercholesterolaemia are heterozygous; it has been reported that this applies to 1 in 500 of the populations of Europe and the USA [4]. The homozygous state, when both of the pair of genes are abnormal, has an incidence of about 1 in 1 000 000 live births, surprisingly lower than expected given the incidence of the heterozygous state. Homozygous familial hypercholesterolaemia is associated with a serum cholesterol above 15 mmol/L. It was discovered in 1974 that the genetic defect is the tissue receptor for LDL, which means that the LDL component of cholesterol spends more time in the circulation and as a result blood concentrations of LDL and total cholesterol increase.

Although it is generally felt that HDL cholesterol is beneficial to health and in some way protective against coronary heart disease, it appears that things are not quite so straightforward. It has been reported from Finland that, in a population with a heavy alcohol intake and when there is liver damage, a high level of HDL cholesterol is not associated with reduced coronary disease or total mortality [5].

**Figure 25.3 Lipoprotein metabolism.**

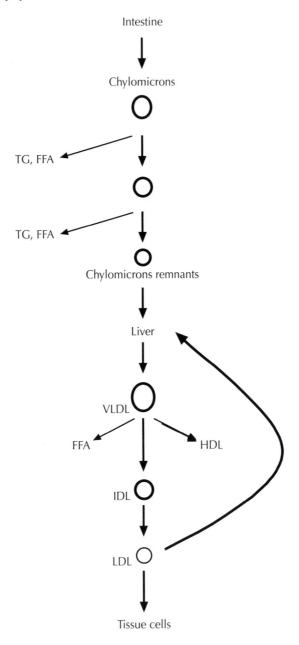

*TG, triglyceride; FFA = free fatty acid; VLDL = very low-density lipoprotein; HDL = high-density lipoprotein; IDL = intermediate density lipoprotein; LDL = low-density lipoprotein.*

There is another lipid compound called triglyceride. Its structure, shown in Figure 25.4, is three fatty acid chains linked by a glycerol base, and it is the main form in which fatty acids circulate in the blood stream. It is usually short term (just a few hours) following a meal, delivering fatty acids around the body for storage or metabolic purposes. The presence of triglyceride in large amounts in the blood when fasting is generally associated with dietary excesses and diabetes. It has a relationship with coronary heart disease, particularly when combined with a high cholesterol level, but it has not been the subject of any major clinical trials regarding the treatment or understanding of the disease process.

**Figure 25.4 The structure of a triglyceride.**

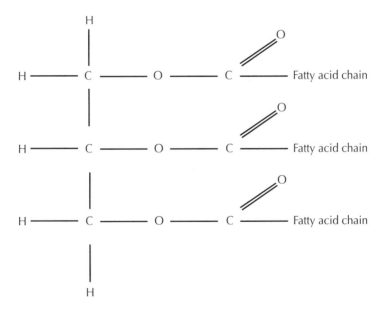

An enormous amount of research work has been concentrated on understanding the metabolism of cholesterol within the body. However, it remains enigmatic regarding how these complex processes might result in the disease that we recognise as atherosclerosis and coronary heart disease. We must not lose sight of the fact that more than 50% of people with coronary heart disease have a normal serum cholesterol concentration and no evidence of disordered cholesterol metabolism.

# 26
# SEASONAL VARIATION OF VITAMIN D AND CHOLESTEROL

We have already noted the seasonality of disease, in that several conditions, including the clinical manifestations of coronary heart disease, appear to be more common in the winter months. I have suggested that the burden of illness in the winter might be the result of inadequate sunlight exposure and thereby vitamin D insufficiency.

The observation that rickets occurs mainly in the winter and spring led to the idea that there was a seasonal variation in vitamin D synthesis by the body. It was not possible to verify this until vitamin D in the blood could be measured. This became possible with the development of the process of photo-stereo-assay, which demonstrated quite clearly that there is a reduced synthesis of vitamin D in the winter, with blood levels being about half of those during the summer [1].

Traditionally the vitamin D content of diet has been based on international units of activity of vitamin D, standardised to promote healing of rickets in rats whose diets had been depleted of vitamin D and with no sun exposure. Ten micrograms of vitamin D (measured) is equivalent to 400 international units (assayed) and is about half the minimum daily requirement. The measurement of vitamin D itself is very different from measuring its biological activity, which is now possible. Calcidiol is measured in tiny quantities of nanograms per litre of blood; calcitriol is present in the blood in only picograms per litre.

At certain temperate latitudes, vitamin D synthesis will only take place during the months of April–September. The reason for this is that during the winter the days are short and the sun is low in the sky; the intensity of the sun, the ultraviolet wavelength reaching sea level, is reduced because the sunlight must pass through more atmosphere before reaching ground level. In north-western parts of the UK, cloud cover is greater in the winter months than the summer months, adding to the insufficiency of sunlight. Figures 26.1 and 26.2 demonstrate the sunshine recorded daily at Myerscough in central Lancashire, UK, during the months of December and June; the differences are very considerable.

**Figure 26.1 Hours of sunshine per day, June 2002, Myerscough, Lancashire, UK.**

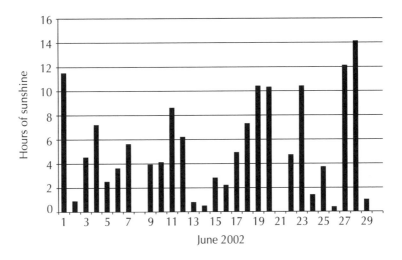

*Data supplied by the UK Meteorological Office. Crown © 2005.*

**Figure 26.2  Hours of sunshine per day, December 2002, Myerscough, Lancashire, UK.**

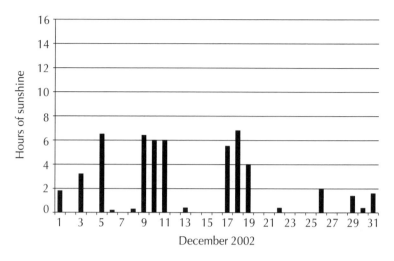

*Data supplied by the UK Meteorological Office. Crown © 2005.*

It must be remembered that the latitude of Myerscough is 53°45' north, which results in very significant seasonality and variation of day length between December and June. For example, in June the day length is about 16 hours and therefore there are potentially 500 hours of sunshine during that month. The reality of a 10-year mean of 185 hours, and 145.6 in 2002, is the result of cloud cover being present most of the time. In December the day length is less than 8 hours and so there are potentially only about 250 hours of sunshine, albeit at low intensity. The reality of a 10-year mean of 44.8 hours, and 52.9 in 2002, once again indicates a great deal of cloud cover in this location in the north-west of England. Scotland and Ireland have a similar climate and it must be remembered that the Romans called Ireland 'Hibernia', which is translated as 'winter', indicating the Roman view of what they considered to be winter weather all of the year. Could it be that the climate and low level of sun exposure of the populations of Ireland, Scotland and north-western England is responsible for their poor health?

Research investigating in more detail the influence of latitude on vitamin D synthesis was undertaken in Boston (Massachusetts, USA) and Edmonton (Alberta, Canada) [2]. Boston is located 42°36' north of the equator and Edmonton 55°34' but at an altitude of 668 metres, or 2192 feet, above sea level, which gives a rather more intense sunlight (ultraviolet energy) at ground level. Central Lancashire, UK, is located at latitude 53°45′ north, Belfast, UK, at 54°36′ and Glasgow, UK, at 55°52′. All are at a similar latitude to Edmonton but all are effectively at sea level and therefore receive sunlight at lower intensities. Boston is on a latitude between Rome (41°54′) and Florence (43°46′) in Italy.

In order to undertake this study the researchers required specimens of skin, and for this purpose they used foreskins obtained from the circumcision of newly born boys. The nature of the resident population meant that only white skin was used; it would have been interesting to see the results in pigmented skin. The advantage of studying a skin specimen detached from the body is that all the vitamin D synthesised can be measured, because it does not disappear into the blood circulation.

The skin specimens studied were kept moist in a dish and exposed to sunlight on a cloudless day. After exposure for 1 hour, the amount of 7-dehydrocholesterol was measured and also its photo-products, including pre-vitamin D and vitamin D. The results of the study are shown in Figure 26.3.

**Figure 26.3 Photo-synthesis of vitamin D after 1 hour exposure to sunlight by month of year [2].**

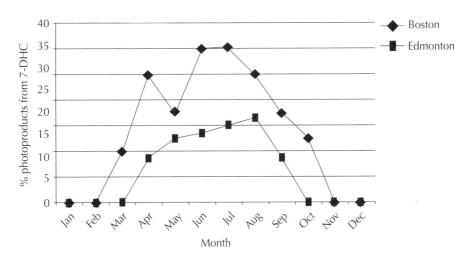

*Adapted with permission from the Journal of Clinical Endocrinology Metabolism.*

We can see that in January, February, November and December in Boston and Edmonton, no photo-synthesis occurred. In Edmonton, at a higher latitude, there was also no photo-conversion in March and October. The study demonstrates an increasing amount of photo-synthesis of vitamin D during the summer months and that the amount is greater in Boston than in Edmonton, the peak levels being about twice as great.

In Figure 26.4, we can see the annual sunshine in Myerscough, Lancashire, UK. The pattern is virtually the same as that in Edmonton but the intensity of ultraviolet energy will be less in Myerscough because of the lower altitude, close to sea level.

**Figure 26.4 Hours of sunshine per month 1991–93, Myerscough, Lancashire, UK.**

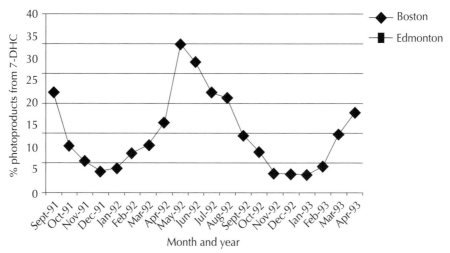

*Data supplied by the UK Meteorological Office. Crown © 2005, adapted with permission.*

I have undertaken studies in Blackburn, Lancashire, that have shown that, during the winter months, vitamin D levels in the blood (measured as calcidiol) are lower than in the summer months [3,4]. The studies also showed that people with gardens had a higher vitamin D level in the blood during the summer and winter, suggesting that incidental outdoor leisure, as opposed to sunbathing, is effective in the synthesis of vitamin D. The results are shown in Table 26.1.

**Table 26.1 Vitamin D levels (as calcidiol nmol/L) in people from Blackburn [3,4]**

|        | Garden | No garden |
|--------|--------|-----------|
| Summer | 27.08  | 24.19     |
| Winter | 24.25  | 18.62     |

We have already seen that tuberculosis is linked to insufficiency of vitamin D. It therefore seems plausible that the seasonality of other diseases, in particular respiratory disease and coronary heart disease, might also be the result of a reduced exposure to sunlight, and thereby immunosuppression resulting from reduced vitamin D synthesis.

Robert Scragg is a community health researcher who has been working mainly in Australia and New Zealand. When he was working in Adelaide, Australia, in 1981 he proposed that the seasonal variation of deaths from coronary heart disease might be the result of variations of sunlight exposure and protection by vitamin D [5]. Further research conducted in Auckland, New Zealand, tested this hypothesis further by looking at 179 patients who had survived myocardial infarction, comparing them with a control group of people of the same age and sex who were apparently well [6]. Those with myocardial infarction had lower blood vitamin D levels than controls, and this was more pronounced in the winter months, as shown in Figure 26.5.

**Figure 26.5 Mean vitamin D levels in patients with myocardial infarction (MI) and controls [6].**

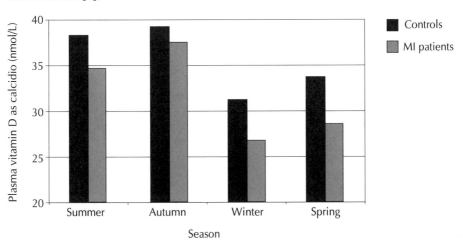

*Adapted from the* International Journal of Epidemiology *with permission from the Endocrine Society.*

It was at this stage in my personal research into the geographical variation of disease in general and coronary heart disease in particular that I became aware of the similarity of structure of vitamin D and cholesterol, and furthermore that they both have the same precursor, 7-dehydrocholesterol. This was a clear metabolic link between the two, as well as both being associated with coronary heart disease, vitamin D being protective and cholesterol apparently harmful. It is clear that the metabolic production of vitamin D from 7-dehydrocholesterol is suppressed during the winter because of low levels of sunlight. Therefore I wondered whether during this time the metabolic pathway in the skin might be directed towards cholesterol production. This model would predict a higher serum cholesterol level in the winter months, and I set out to explore this possibility.

Table 26.1 shows that the blood level of vitamin D is higher in the summer than in the winter and higher in people with gardens than those without. As part of the same study, my colleagues and I measured the serum cholesterol levels of the same subjects (Table 26.2). In August 1992, a group of 37 people who had gardens had a mean serum cholesterol of 5.84 mmol/L, compared with a similar group without gardens who had a mean cholesterol of 6.34. This supported the hypothesis being tested, that incidental exposure to the sun would lead to a reduction of serum cholesterol level.

**Table 26.2  Blood cholesterol levels (mean serum cholesterol as mmol/L) in people from Blackburn [3,4]**

|        | Garden | No garden |
|--------|--------|-----------|
| Summer | 5.84   | 6.34      |
| Winter | 6.68   | 6.59      |

I had also predicted that cholesterol levels would be higher in the winter and that the difference as a result of garden ownership would then be lost. This proved to be the case; the cholesterol levels were 6.68 and 6.59, not a significant difference but higher than in the summer. This supported the model that, in the absence of sunlight, sterol synthesis in the skin is directed to cholesterol, as shown in Figure 26.6. Whereas the synthesis of pre-vitamin D and vitamin D as cholecalciferol requires energy input from ultraviolet light to open the molecular ring structure, the synthesis of cholesterol does not require this external source of energy.

**Figure 26.6 Sunlight and sterol synthesis in the skin.**

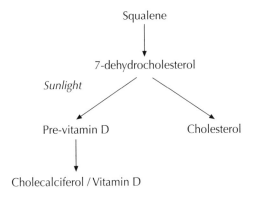

My research would not have been possible without my colleagues Eric Hindle and Terry Dyer, senior biochemists in the Royal Blackburn Hospital, Blackburn, UK. We tested the seasonality of cholesterol further by grouping the serum cholesterol measurements undertaken in our laboratory and displaying the average month by month. We were analysing about 1500 specimens per day, not from a random population base but from blood samples sent into the laboratory for a variety of reasons. We did not anticipate any seasonal change in the nature of the patients investigated. The results are shown in Figure 26.7. There was a very significant variation throughout the year, with higher levels in the winter and lower levels in the summer. These mirrored the results of the vitamin D studies from Edmonton, which is at about the same latitude as Blackburn (shown in Figure 26.3).

It was only after we had undertaken this work that I realised that the seasonality of cholesterol had been identified in a number of earlier studies; it was first recognised as long ago as 1924. As there is no conventional explanation for this phenomenon it has not been given much airing; few people seem to know of it or regard it as of great significance. In 1973, it was stated in a letter to *The Lancet*: 'We now know that there is a pronounced seasonal variation in cholesterol – low in the summer and high in the winter' [7].

**Figure 26.7 Mean serum cholesterol (mmol/L/month) in 1992–93 in Blackburn.**

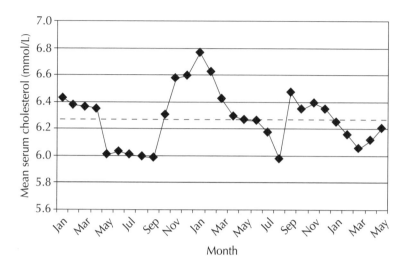

*Mean = 6.28 [3,4].*

The author was referring in particular to earlier work that was not readily accepted and evidence became conflicting [8]. In a review of 19 studies, Robert Ripley, working for the American Heart Foundation in New York, USA, felt that the variations were probably 'mathematical artefacts' [9], an example of how to dismiss data that do not fit in with the hypothesis.

Further studies were undertaken at the University of Helsinki, Finland, and these included investigation of the diurnal variation of cholesterol, the variation throughout the course of the day rather than the year. The blood level of cholesterol was found to be highest during the night, reaching a peak soon after midnight, and at its lowest during the morning and mid-afternoon [10]. This has been confirmed in a further study that stated [11]:

*In summary, although regulatory mechanisms responsible remain to be characterized, daily periodicity in rates of free and total cholesterol formation is indicated in humans. In particular, a pronounced depression of synthesis is observed during the daytime period.*

It is difficult to explain the daytime variation on the basis of diet, and I have seen no attempt to explain it on the basis of sunlight exposure. However, the above observation is compatible with a reduction of the synthesis of cholesterol when vitamin D is being synthesised, that is, during the hours of daylight. It might be predicted that this diurnal variation would diminish during the winter, but I have not yet seen this investigated.

More recent studies of the seasonal variation of serum cholesterol have been carefully controlled with much larger sample sizes, and they have confirmed the pattern. The Lipid Research Clinic's coronary primary prevention trial placebo group comprised 1446 men aged 35–59 years with hypercholesterolaemia. Over a 7-year study period the winter peaks of cholesterol were obvious, as shown in Figure 26.8 [12].

**Figure 26.8 Mean plasma cholesterol levels, 2-month groups [12].**

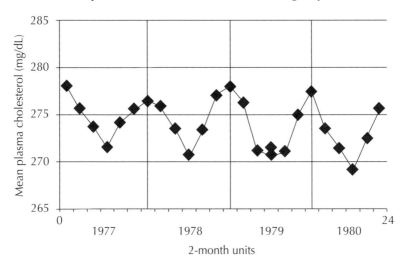

*Adapted from Circulation with permission from Lippincott, Williams and Watkins.*

This study also looked at the amplitude of variation in relation to the town of residence in the USA. The conclusion was that: 'latitude rather than climate (i.e. temperature) appeared paramount' [12].

A health screening programme of 140 000 men and 32 000 women in the UK, and 30 000 men and 12 000 women in Japan, also showed serum concentrations of cholesterol to be higher in the winter than in the summer [13]. The authors related this to temperature but there is no known effect of temperature on cholesterol synthesis in the human and it would be most unlikely in an isothermic (warm-blooded) species. There was no consideration given to sunlight, which is by far the major controlling factor of air temperature at a given latitude, but the authors came very close to realising that the key factor is sunlight:

*A genuine correlation could be due either to a direct effect of temperature on cholesterol levels or the effect on cholesterol of some other seasonal parameter which itself is strongly correlated with temperature.*

Could this be anything other than sunlight?

It might be argued that the seasonality of cholesterol is related to diet but this is not supported by the facts. There is a change of diet in the summer but serum cholesterol levels diminish in April, which happens to be the time at which vitamin D levels rise at the same latitude in Edmonton. Diet does not change in April, according to evidence from the UK general household survey (Table 26.3) [14].

**Table 26.3  Household consumption of various foods, ounces per person per week [14]**

|  | January/ March | April/ June | July/ September | October/ December |
|---|---|---|---|---|
| Milk and cream | 3.87 | 3.73 | 3.61 | 3.76 |
| Cheese | 3.93 | 4.28 | 4.19 | 4.05 |
| Meat and meat products | 32.97 | 35.06 | 33.76 | 33.87 |
| Fish | 4.64 | 4.96 | 5.23 | 4.76 |
| Fats | 8.95 | 8.95 | 7.92 | 9.20 |
| Sugar and preserves | 7.28 | 7.95 | 7.50 | 7.96 |
| Vegetables | 82.13 | 76.77 | 74.36 | 80.48 |
| Fresh fruit | 19.97 | 21.86 | 24.39 | 19.90 |

*Crown © 1991, adapted with permission.*

It can be seen that at the present time there is not a great deal of seasonality to dietary patterns; we are now in an era of air transport, with world-wide food production available all the time. Fifty years ago it would have been unimaginable for most northern European households to eat strawberries at Christmas, but this is perfectly possible in the UK today. However, if we examine Table 26.3, we can see that, although there is an increase of consumption of fresh fruit in July, this could not explain the reduction of serum cholesterol in April. The Lipid Research Clinic's coronary primary prevention trial also failed to find a dietary explanation for the winter peak of serum cholesterol; the study recorded the paradox (another one) of a slightly higher dietary cholesterol intake during the summer months [15].

The phenomenon of a seasonal variation of serum cholesterol might be regarded as a curiosity but it is something that requires explanation and it might contain an important truth. It suggests that there is an environmental factor that has an influence on serum cholesterol level. The question is whether climate might have a direct effect on cholesterol metabolism or whether the mediation is through seasonal effects on agriculture, despite the lack of evidence from the UK general household survey [14] and the failure of Gordon and colleagues [15] to find such an explanation.

If people insist that diet is the explanation of the seasonal variation of serum cholesterol, they do so in the absence of evidence. Seasonal changes of cholesterol levels have been demonstrated in studies that have controlled diet, in both humans and other animals, and we must look for explanations other than diet. Seasonal variation in cholesterol has been observed in the rat, monkey, baboon, woodchuck and badger. An environmental factor is obvious, and I would propose that it is sunlight and not air temperature.

Something that seems to have escaped other investigators is the fact that cholesterol and vitamin D are both derived from 7-dehydrocholesterol, which forms the basis of the metabolic solution to the seasonal variation of serum cholesterol, as shown in Figure 26.6. Although I have indicated that the winter peak of serum cholesterol cannot be because of dietary change, and although I have suggested that it might be because of a metabolic diversion in the absence of sunlight, there is another possible explanation. The intermediary between winter and serum cholesterol could be the occurrence of winter diseases, such as respiratory infections and coronary heart disease. Could an elevated serum cholesterol be the result of coronary heart disease rather than a cause or epiphenomenon? We will consider this later when we look at the relationship between cholesterol and inflammation.

# 27
# CHOLESTEROL-LOWERING THERAPIES

S o far the diet–cholesterol–heart hypothesis has appeared to be far from robust. There is no consistent association between diet and serum cholesterol level. The association between serum cholesterol and risk of coronary heart disease is not as convincing as the initial Whitehall and MRFIT studies first suggested [1,2]. Reduction of the cholesterol and saturated fat content of food shows no consistent benefit and some paradoxes. The diurnal and seasonal variations of serum cholesterol cannot be explained on the basis of diet. All these uncomfortable observations must lead us to question the diet–cholesterol–heart hypothesis, and one crucial experiment appears obvious: does reduction of the serum cholesterol level through diet or pharmacological means benefit the subjects concerned, and does the incidence of coronary heart disease thereby diminish?

In Chapter 22 we saw that dietary fat intake cannot be regarded as causative of coronary heart disease, although fish oils might be protective. In 2001, the conclusion of Hooper and colleagues, from the universities of Manchester, Teesside, Bristol and Edinburgh, Southampton General Hospital, Princess Royal Hospital, Telford, and the Institute of Child Health, London, UK, was that a modification of fat intake results in a small reduction of cardiovascular events but there is little effect on mortality [3]. The paper suggests that:

*Despite decades of effort and many thousands of people randomised, there is still only limited and inconclusive evidence of the effects of modification of total, saturated, mono-unsaturated, or polyunsaturated fats on cardiovascular morbidity and mortality.*

We can take this no further: dietary restriction does not appear to help people with or without coronary heart disease. We are uncertain how these dietary trials influenced serum cholesterol levels but this is not of great importance in itself. Serum cholesterol is only a proposed intermediary mechanism linking diet and coronary heart disease: it is the influence on the disease and its mortality that is fundamental. There is no conclusive evidence that reducing cholesterol by dietary means has any beneficial effect, and it has been demonstrated that the effect of diet on serum cholesterol levels is very modest. Most cholesterol is synthesised within the body, mainly in the liver.

Although studies aimed at reducing dietary fat and cholesterol have not shown consistent benefit, this has not stopped low cholesterol diets from being actively promulgated throughout society and in particular upon people who are known to have coronary heart disease. The reason for this is that the application of so-called science is generally based on paradigms rather than proof, but more of this later. The whole process has been driven by evangelism, which is more powerful than truth or reason. It has been observed consistently that there is no benefit to be gained from treating women with cholesterol-reducing diets, and so there has been a certain, but only transient hesitation, when it comes to population intervention, individual intervention being a more modest approach [4]. When it comes to identifying the cause of coronary heart disease, it can hardly be realistic to suggest that it is diet cholesterol in men and something different in women. There are very definite male–female differences in incidence and we will look at possible explanations for these later.

I have already mentioned that the only dietary manipulation that has been shown to have benefit has been fish oil supplementation (the DART study) [5] but this is not a test of the diet–cholesterol–heart hypothesis. It is information that does not fit in with our understanding of the causation of coronary heart disease, but there is general encouragement to eat fish rather than meat. If fish oils protect against coronary heart disease, what sort of disease is it?

The first medication used to reduce the cholesterol concentration of blood was clofibrate, which ICI marketed as Atromid-S. I remember it being used widely and rather indiscriminately when I was working as a very junior doctor in the late 1960s. It was given to people who had suffered from myocardial infarction or angina based on the idea that cholesterol was the cause of the disease. This was before the publication of controlled trials to assess its effectiveness and safety. In fact in the late 1960s clinical trials were still in their infancy and treatment was given, as indeed is still often the case, on the basis of what seemed to be sensible, that is it was paradigm-based.

There is no question that clofibrate reduces serum cholesterol levels but our knowledge of cholesterol metabolism had not developed very far and nobody really knew the mechanism whereby cholesterol levels were reduced. It was not known whether it was an inhibition of synthesis or an enhancement of excretion; it had to be one or the other and it turned out to be the latter. In the early 1970s it was noted that more people with gallstones seemed to be taking clofibrate than would be expected in the general population. This was later clearly demonstrated to be the case and it appeared that clofibrate was increasing the excretion of cholesterol by the liver, leading to a supersaturated state of bile with precipitation of cholesterol as gallstones [6]. This side-effect of clofibrate had to be balanced against the benefits in respect of cardiovascular mortality, but these benefits remained unknown.

A clinical trial of clofibrate therapy was instigated by WHO in the mid-1960s and the initial results were published in 1978 [7]. It was a primary prevention trial, which meant that at the time of recruitment into the trial the subjects had no clinical manifestations of coronary heart disease, the purpose of the treatment being to prevent it. The results indicated that if healthy middle-aged men with moderately elevated serum cholesterol were treated with clofibrate, there was a lower incidence of non-fatal myocardial infarction than in comparable controls. There was, however, no reduction in mortality from coronary heart disease, clearly the most important outcome when we consider that it is a major cause of death. The results also indicated that in the treated group there was a higher mortality from non-cardiovascular disease than in the control group. These observations cast doubt not only on the diet–cholesterol–heart hypothesis but also on the safety of cholesterol-lowering clofibrate.

A second, more comprehensive, report followed in 1980 [8]. This study was of more than 15 000 men followed up for a maximum of 11 years, a total of 150 000 person-years of observation. This included time spent in the trial itself and 4 or more years of follow-up after the trial was completed. If the subjects had high serum cholesterol, they were allocated to one of two groups, treatment with clofibrate or placebo control. Those with low serum cholesterol were untreated and also served as controls. The results can be seen in Table 27.1.

**Table 27.1 Primary prevention using clofibrate [8].**
CHD = coronary heart disease

| | Group 1<br>High cholesterol<br>Clofibrate | Group 2<br>High cholesterol<br>Control | Group 3<br>Low cholesterol<br>Control |
|---|---|---|---|
| Number | 5331 | 5228 | 5117 |
| Deaths | | | |
| All causes | 396 | 317 | 198 |
| CHD | 157 | 138 | 46 |
| Non-CHD | 239 | 179 | 152 |
| Cancers | 125 | 99 | 82 |

© 1980, adapted from The Lancet with permission from Elsevier.

We can see that the coronary heart disease mortality was similar in the two high cholesterol groups, slightly higher at 157 in those treated with clofibrate, and 138 in the controls. In other words, the treatment was not preventing cardiac death. However, the all-causes death rate was highest in the clofibrate-treated group and this group also had the highest death rate from cancers.

Clofibrate immediately went out of use as a treatment of coronary heart disease because it was regarded as a pointless and perhaps dangerous treatment. From a scientific rather than a clinical viewpoint, the trial did not support the hypothesis that lowering cholesterol levels in the blood reduces deaths from coronary heart disease.

There followed an interlude of several years during which pharmacological reduction of serum cholesterol lapsed. John Yudkin, Professor of Medicine at University College London Medical School, UK, stated in 1993 [9]:

*Studies to date have shown little impact of drugs that lower cholesterol concentration and blood pressure on either coronary heart disease or total mortality. Although new treatments for hypercholesterolaemia or hypertension might help prevent coronary heart disease, other approaches to reduce the burden of premature death are required.*

This was a time when the surgical treatment of coronary heart disease was developing but not dealing with causative factors, whatever they might be. Surgery could only provide secondary prevention, treatment for people who had already experienced and survived a clinical episode of coronary heart disease.

Things changed 3 years later; 1994 saw the publication of the results of the first clinical trial of simvastatin, the first of a new class of medications generally called statins. Statins inhibit the synthesis of cholesterol and an outline of the mechanism is shown in Figure 27.1.

**Figure 27.1 The mechanism of action of statin drugs.**

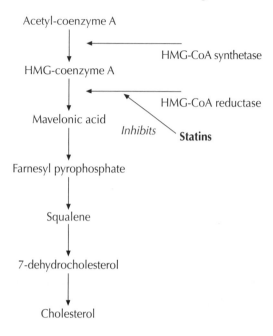

The first trial was called 4S: the Scandinavian Simvastatin Survival Study [10]. It was a secondary prevention trial; the 4444 recruits were men and women aged between 35 and 70 years who at the time of recruitment were known to have coronary heart disease, either angina or a previous myocardial infarction. Treatment was with a so-called lipid-lowering diet and either simvastatin or placebo, with follow-up for a median of 5.4 years.

The results are shown in Table 27.2 and it can be seen that 256 deaths (12%) occurred in the placebo group and 182 (8%) in the simvastatin-treated group. In other words, if 100 people known to have coronary heart disease are treated with simvastatin for about 5 years, 4 (i.e. 12 minus 8) who would otherwise have died within this time will not do so. The number needed to treat (NNT) to prevent one death is thus 25 (i.e. 100/4).

The cardiac deaths were similarly reduced. There were major reductions in the serum total cholesterol and LDL cholesterol levels, with an increase in the HDL cholesterol level, the good cholesterol.

This trial clearly indicated that simvastatin reduces serum cholesterol and also reduces deaths from coronary heart disease. I choose these words carefully for reasons that I will explain in more detail shortly. However, others have not chosen their words so carefully to describe these results, and the evangelistic fervour suggested that the diet–cholesterol–heart hypothesis had been proved.

**Table 27.2 Result of the 4S study of simvastatin [10].**
CHD, coronary heard disease

|  | Placebo | Simvastatin treatment |
|---|---|---|
| Number | 2223 | 2221 |
| Total cholesterol (%) | +1 | −25 |
| LDL (%) | +1 | −35 |
| HDL (%) | +1 | +8 |
| Triglycerides (%) | +7 | −10 |
| All deaths, *n* (%) | 256 (12) | 182 (8) |
| CHD deaths, *n* (%) | 189 (8.5) | 111 (5) |
| CHD events, *n* (%) | 622 (28) | 431 (19) |
| Cancer deaths, *n* | 35 (1.6) | 33 (1.5) |

© *1994, adapted from The Lancet with permission from Elsevier.*

4S was followed by the publication in 1995 of a primary prevention trial undertaken in the west of Scotland using the statin drug pravastatin [11]. This study has become known as WOSCOPS (West Of Scotland COronary Prevention Study). The subjects were 6595 men aged 45–64 years with no history of coronary heart disease and the follow-up period was an average of 4.9 years. The serum cholesterol level had to be at least 6.5 mmol/L to qualify for entry, so the risk of death was expected to be higher than for the total male population of that age. A serum cholesterol level above 5.2 mmol/L is currently regarded as undesirable and to be treated; strictly speaking the results of WOSCOPS should not be extrapolated to include people with a serum cholesterol below 6.5 (the minimum level to qualify for entry into the trial) or people outside the age range studied or even women, but in practice extrapolation is inevitable.

The detailed results are shown in Table 27.3. It is clear that pravastatin reduced serum cholesterol levels by 20% and also reduced deaths from coronary heart disease without increasing deaths from other causes. Pravastatin, like simvastatin, is a successful treatment. It follows from this study that out of 100 men with a serum cholesterol of 6.5 mmol/L or above but no known coronary heart disease treated with pravastatin 40 mg daily for almost 5 years, one death will be prevented (i.e. 4.1% – 3.2%). The NNT is therefore 100. Additional gains are two fewer non-fatal coronary events (6.5% – 4.6%) and about one fewer surgical intervention (2.5% – 1.7%), either percutaneous transluminal coronary angioplasty (PTCA) or coronary artery bypass grafting (CABG). At the end of 2006, the price of pravastatin 40 mg, produced by Squibb Pharmaceuticals was approximately £1. The cost of treating 100 people for 5 years at that unit cost was thus close to £200,000. However, when generic pravastatin became available in 2003, the price reduced to 16 pence and the cost of treating 100 people for 5 years fell to £29,000. The health gain for this cost is one fewer fatality, two fewer non-fatal coronary events and one fewer coronary artery revascularisation procedure; whether this is good value for money is a matter of judgement but it is obviously better value for money at the cheaper price.

**Table 27.3 Prevention of coronary heart disease (CHD) events with pravastatin (WOSCOPS) [11]**

|  | Placebo | Pravastatin |
| --- | --- | --- |
| Number | 3293 | 3302 |
| Serum cholesterol change (%) | 0 | −20 |
| LDL cholesterol change (%) | 0 | −26 |
| HDL cholesterol change (%) | 0 | +5 |
| Triglyceride change (%) | 0 | −12 |
| All deaths, n (%) | 135 (4.1) | 106 (3.2) |
| CHD deaths, n (%) | 52 (1.7) | 38 (1.2) |
| CHD events (not fatal), n (%) | 204 (6.5) | 143 (4.6) |
| Cancer deaths, n (%) | 49 (1.5) | 44 (1.3) |
| Surgical intervention (PTCA or CABG), n (%) | 80 (2.5) | 51 (1.7) |

The gain from treatment in this study was less than in 4S. Whereas in 4S the participants were known to have coronary heart disease, which is the most important risk indicator for a subsequent cardiac event, WOSCPS recruited lower risk people without evidence of disease. As in any treatment, targeting those with disease is going to produce a greater return than a less discriminatory approach.

A further study of pravastatin showed a similar benefit, this time a secondary prevention trial of people known to have coronary heart disease, the Cholesterol And Recurrent Events (CARE) study from the USA [12]. The treatment resulted in a reduction of serum cholesterol, LDL cholesterol and triglyceride and an increase in HDL cholesterol, with a reduction of total deaths and deaths from coronary heart disease. Whereas WOSCOPS directed treatment at men with a high serum cholesterol level of more than 6.5 mmol/L, the CARE study selected recruits on the basis of a serum cholesterol less than 6.25 mmol/L (240 mg/dL).

A further trial indicated that 'aggressive lipid-lowering therapy', this time using atorvastatin, was at least as effect as coronary angioplasty in low-risk patients with stable angina [13]. Another study using atorvastatin looked into the effect on the pathology of atherosclerotic disease rather than clinical outcome [14]. The carotid arteries in the neck were used for the assessment because of their ease of access using ultrasound techniques. It is interesting to note that the thickening of the wall of the carotid arteries decreased by an average of 0.031 mm in patients taking atorvastatin 80 mg daily taken for 2 years, whereas it increased by an average of 0.036 mm in a similar group taking simvastatin 40 mg daily. This is paradoxical in respect of the diet–cholesterol–heart theory and suggests that perhaps all statins are not equal. It suggests that although they all inhibit the enzyme HMG-CoA reductase (see Figure 27.1) and they all reduce serum cholesterol concentration, the effect on the carotid artery is because of a different action of certain statins, perhaps a direct action rather than via cholesterol lowering.

Simvastatin therapy was also given to assess a possible effect on the secondary prevention of stroke, in a randomised controlled trial of 20 536 people known to have cerebrovascular disease or be otherwise at high risk of stroke [15]. Although there is no consistent association between serum cholesterol and stroke, the study claimed to investigate 'cholesterol-lowering with simvastatin'. What the group was really investigating was the effect of simvastatin on stroke incidence; not quite the same thing. There was a benefit in the treated group, with a stroke rate of 4.3% compared with 5.7% in the placebo group. As expected, the average serum cholesterol concentration fell in those treated with simvastatin.

It is interesting to note that this is reported as a 25% reduction in the stroke event rate, but to understand this we must know about the stroke event rate itself. The only number that is usually mentioned in the national press is 25%, but this is meaningless regarding translating the results from a clinical experiment into clinical practice. The vital information is the reduction of 25% of the event rate (5.7%) of the placebo group. The NNT provides a much more realistic appraisal of clinical usefulness; in this case it is 1.5 (5.7 – 4.3), meaning that three events would be prevented by treating 200 people with simvastatin 40 mg daily for 5 years (a total cost of £349,727 at the 2006 price of proprietary simvastatin at £1 per tablet at the dose used, or £58,400 if generic simvastatin at 16 pence per tablet was used at the same dose; this represents about £120,000, or about £19,000, to prevent one cerebrovascular event, depending on the cost of the simvastatin used.

Michael Oliver, formerly Professor of Cardiology at Edinburgh University, UK, and more recently at the National Heart and Lung Institute, London, UK, was one of the major organisers and authors of the clofibrate trial. He maintained for many years almost a lone voice of caution regarding the relationship between cholesterol and coronary heart disease, and he was particularly concerned that the therapeutic evangelism might do more harm than good [16]. However, after publication of 4S and WOSCOPS, his words of scientific caution were lost to the vast majority accepting the cholesterol–heart hypothesis, when he declared that '[these trials] show benefit from reducing hypercholesterolaemia' [17]. His conclusion was flawed by assuming equivalence between statin therapy and cholesterol lowering. An editorial in the *British Medical Journal* suggested in its headline that lipid lowering is now indicated for patients with normal cholesterol concentrations [18].

A leading lipid researcher in the UK is Paul Durrington, Professor of Medicine at the University of Manchester. In a recent excellent review of disorders of cholesterol and lipid metabolism, he fell into the same trap of equating statin therapy with cholesterol lowering [19]. He stated:

*The past eight years have brought about a transformation in clinical trial evidence for the effects of lowering serum cholesterol. Earlier scepticism was so great that proof was demanded that lipid lowering decreases not only mortality but also morbidity from coronary heart disease and all cause mortality … Statin treatment now presents the greatest likelihood that a physician engaged in general medical practice can routinely prolong life.*

The latter two sentences of Professor Durrington are entirely different as he moves from the expression 'lipid lowering' to 'statin treatment' without differentiating between the two. Statin therapy introduces a number of variable factors, some known and some unknown, into a treatment group compared with a control group. A reduction of serum cholesterol is only one of the actions, and the beneficial outcome from statin therapy cannot be concluded to be the result of that action. His final statement is correct, that statin treatment gives the opportunity to prolong life, but, as always, at a cost; and the better the therapy is targeted, the lower that cost will be. The beneficial effects of statin therapy are real but they must not be equated with cholesterol lowering.

The trials described have all been flawed regarding scientific discipline and the conclusions reached. They have all been designed to test the three respective statin preparations, with the subjects being carefully randomised to either treatment or placebo. Tables were published to provide evidence that randomisation had been successful and that the treatment and placebo groups were identical in all respects except the treatment itself. The conclusion to be drawn was that treatment with the statin drugs is effective. The observation that there was a reduction in average serum cholesterol in the treated groups was, of course, expected.

Figure 27.1 displays what is generally regarded as the action of statins, HMG-CoA reductase inhibitors to use the correct scientific name. If statin therapy had only this one metabolic action, then there would be scientific justification for assuming that statins were acting through serum cholesterol reduction. However, the trials themselves show quite clearly that there are other metabolic consequences of statin therapy. A reduction of LDL cholesterol might be expected to equate to total cholesterol reduction, but there was also a reduction of serum triglyceride concentration, an unforeseen event, and an increase in HDL. Neither of these obviously result from HMG-CoA reductase inhibition and indicate that that there are more metabolic actions of statins than are known. In other words, the cholesterol-lowering effect was not controlled in the studies and cannot be equated with statin therapy.

The result of the statin intervention studies can be represented as in the first model in Figure 27.2. This is factual and indicates two of the outcomes of the trials. To move to the second model in Figure 27.2 is not automatic and is most certainly not proven by the clinical studies described above. In these studies there were three variable factors active simultaneously: statin therapy, cholesterol lowering and clinical outcome. Only the statin therapy was under experimental control. Cholesterol lowering itself was not under experimental control and therefore no conclusions can be drawn from it. I am afraid that equating cholesterol lowering with statin therapy shows a medical disregard for scientific thinking that has been present for half a century.

**Figure 27.2 Possible relationships between statin therapy, cholesterol lowering and clinical outcome.**
CHD = coronary heart disease.

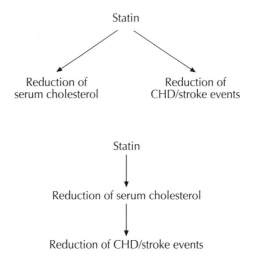

It is pertinent to go back to the late 19th century and consider the treatment of epilepsy. Medical thought follows fashions, and the fashion in the 1890s, continuing into the early part of the 20th century, was that masturbation, the solitary vice, was a cause of all sorts of ailments, one of which was epilepsy. The logic therefore was that the treatment of epilepsy should be based upon suppression of sexual desire, and treatment with bromide was instituted. It turned out to be effective and remained in use until barbiturates were introduced in the 1920s. In Figure 27.2, think of bromide in place of statin therapy, masturbation in place of cholesterol lowering and epilepsy in place of coronary heart disease/stroke. The model and the thinking are identical.

The example of bromide treatment for epilepsy illustrates how a medication can be effective through a mechanism that had not been anticipated. Did bromide suppress epilepsy because of a direct effect of bromide on brain function, or rather malfunction, or was bromide effective because of the anticipated and planned effect of suppressing sexual desire? With hindsight we know that bromide is effective because it is a cerebral depressant, thus suppressing epileptic discharges by the brain. We realise now that 'excessive' sexual desire and masturbation are not the cause of epilepsy, and masturbation as the cause of the condition has fallen from fashion. Let us not forget the strength of fashion in determining medical therapy, and the clothing devices introduced at the end of the 19th century to prevent the solitary vice. Cholesterol lowering is the fashion at present and is promulgated by evangelists similar in their mission to those who attempted to suppress masturbation a century ago.

Do statins reduce the clinical events of coronary heart disease and cerebrovascular disease because they lower serum cholesterol levels, or is it through an entirely different and unforeseen mechanism? We now know that statins do much more than lower serum cholesterol, and the many unforeseen actions might help us uncover the truth. We need to look more closely at the relationship between statins, serum cholesterol level and coronary heart disease. Additional information is available from the WOSCOPS publications, as shall be discussed in the next chapter.

# 28

# THE SCOTTISH PARADOX AND THE ACTIONS OF STATINS

In the previous chapter, we looked at WOSCOPS, the pravastatin trial conducted in the west of Scotland, a region with perhaps the highest death rate from coronary heart disease in the world. The result was a significant benefit from pravastatin 40 mg daily given to men with serum cholesterol of at least 6.5 mmol/L. There was a reduction in the 5-year mortality rate from 4.1% to 3.2% [1]. Both mortality and serum cholesterol were reduced, but not correspondingly.

We have already looked at Framingham, the town in Massachusetts, USA, in which a great deal of information has been generated concerning the development of coronary heart disease. From the data published, it could be expected that the serum cholesterol reduction achieved in WOSCOPS (25%) would have achieved a reduction in the rate of coronary events of 24%. In practice the reduction of coronary events was 35% (from 6.5% to 4.6%) [2]. It is interesting to reflect on the opening paragraph of the WOSCOPS paper [2]:

*Clinical trials testing the 'lipid hypothesis', that lowering plasma cholesterol leads to decreased risk of CHD, were first conducted in the 1970s and 1980s. Results were generally positive and led with increasing conviction to the conclusion that MI could be prevented by lipid-lowering therapy. However, definite proof that such treatment could reduce cardiovascular mortality and improve overall survival was not forthcoming until the recent publication of landmark studies in primary and secondary prevention [the authors refer here to 4S and WOSCOPS].*

I emphasise again that the clinical trials were testing the specific medication and not the lipid hypothesis. The authors failed to appreciate the empiricism of the scientific method and they made the same mistake as those who successfully treated epilepsy with bromide a century earlier.

In WOSCOPS, the effect of pravastatin was much greater than anticipated: how could this be explained? It is, of course, in keeping with Figure 27.2a, that pravastatin has two independent actions. The first is to reduce serum cholesterol and the second is to reduce coronary heart disease events; the two effects need not be equal. It would not be in keeping with Figure 27.2b, that cholesterol reduction is the necessary intermediary of the effect of statins on coronary heart disease. Furthermore, the effectiveness of pravastatin was not related to the serum cholesterol levels of the subjects at the start of the trial.

To explore these effects further, the researchers took the results of the reduction of serum cholesterol of the subjects taking pravastatin and divided them into five groups, quintiles, in a way that we have encountered previously [2]. The results are shown in Figure 28.1. Those in whom the serum cholesterol (LDL cholesterol in the paper) did not change [1] were considered not to have taken the tablets prescribed, and this is an inevitable part of normal human experience. The total coronary heart disease event rate in this group was 11%, similar to those taking placebo.

**Figure 28.1 Cholesterol lowering and coronary heart disease event rate [2].**

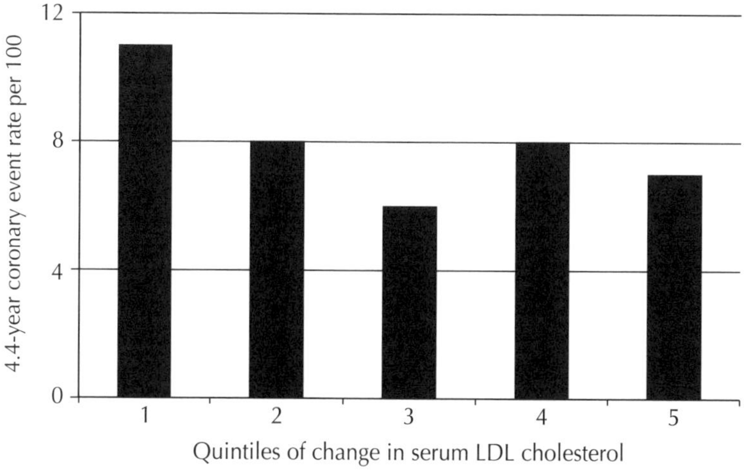

Quintiles of change in serum LDL cholesterol

*Adapted from Circulation with permission from Lippincott, Williams and Watkins.*

The subjects in quintiles 2–5 were assumed to have taken the tablets as directed, and reductions of serum LDL cholesterol were 12%, 24%, 31% and 39%. However, they all had a similar reduction of coronary event rate at between 6% and 8%. This was clear evidence that the effect of pravastatin on coronary heart disease was independent of its cholesterol-lowering property, what we might call the West of Scotland paradox. Figure 28.2 shows an absence of an association between cholesterol lowering and clinical effect, with an $R^2$ of only 0.052 (this will be explained in more detail shortly; for now note that a result of close to 1 indicates a significant effect and close to 0 no significance). This result obviously does not fit in with the diet–cholesterol–heart hypothesis and casts serious doubt on it. The paradox does not, of course, detract from the therapeutic benefit of pravastatin, which is the result of the WOSCOPS clinical experiment.

**Figure 28.2 Effects of pravastatin on cholesterol and coronary events [2].**

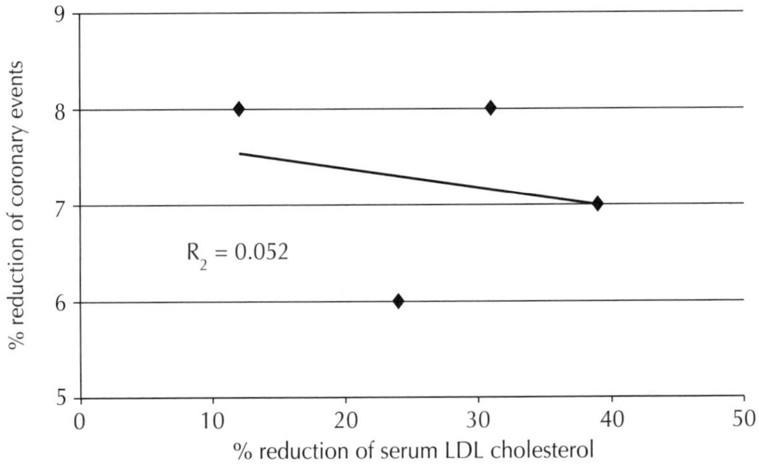

*Adapted from Circulation with permission from Lippincott, Williams and Watkins.*

It would appear that there is more to statin therapy than was initially thought. The authors considered this, suggesting that 'pravastatin may, through pathways not involving lipid lowering, beneficially affect atherosclerosis' [2]. They noted a few effects of pravastatin other than lipid lowering, which immediately invalidates WOSCOPS as a scientific experiment of lipid lowering: it was simply a clinical experiment to test the effectiveness of pravastatin.

WOSCOPS produced a wealth of data and subsequent analysis revealed other surprises. The development of new diabetes during the course of the trial was investigated; unexpectedly a predictor of diabetes was not taking pravastatin. Diabetes developed in 3.5% of those taking placebo but in only 2.8% of those taking pravastatin [3]. This indicates an additional effect, reducing risk of diabetes, through an unknown mechanism.

The diet–cholesterol–heart hypothesis has always proposed that deposition of cholesterol within the walls of the coronary and other arteries would take place over several decades, starting in childhood. Ultimately, because of the deposition of cholesterol together with added surface blood clots, a critical narrowing of a coronary artery would occur and the result would be a clinical expression of coronary artery disease. As the disease takes so long to develop, it would be expected that regression of the changes would also take a long time. It was therefore anticipated that statin therapy, undoubtedly reducing the serum cholesterol level, would arrest the process and hopefully reverse it over a long period of time, allowing cholesterol to re-enter the blood stream once the serum cholesterol level became lower. A reduction in arterial wall thickness in people taking atorvastatin has been demonstrated, as described in the previous chapter with the example of people with familial hypercholesterolaemia [4]. Such processes would have long time horizons, and a benefit within just 2 years was quite surprising.

The general pattern of care given to patients with myocardial infarction in hospital has been to provide emergency care to stabilise heart function and resuscitation measures as necessary. Later care has been secondary prevention: advice on lifestyle and diet, possibly referral for surgical intervention and finally cholesterol-lowering therapies. It had been conventional wisdom that the serum cholesterol estimation during an acute attack is not be a true indicator of the patient's natural serum cholesterol and that blood for this purpose should be taken during the convalescence phase, usually following discharge from hospital. In this way those patients with high serum cholesterol could be identified and dietary treatment started. Only if this failed to lower serum cholesterol significantly, as was usually the case, would statin treatment be prescribed. There was no urgency for statin therapy to be started because the time for it to have an effect would be very long.

Evidence that statin therapy is effective irrespective of serum cholesterol level led to it being used earlier in the course of acute myocardial infarction. One unexpected result of WOPSCOPS was that there appeared to be an early beneficial effect of pravastatin, earlier than was expected from the diet–cholesterol–heart hypothesis.

The first week in April 2001 saw the publication of two studies looking at the short-term effects of statin therapy. An international group, from the USA, UK, Canada, Hungary and France, re-examined data from previous clinical trials of thrombolytic therapy given to treat myocardial infarction [5]. The trials left other treatments, including statins, to the discretion of the treating physician. The study divided the patients into those who were prescribed statin therapy early and who were thus taking it at the time of discharge from hospital, and those who were prescribed statin therapy at a later date. The mortality rate at 30 days was 1.7% in those prescribed statin therapy early and taking it at 30 days, and 3.5% in those not doing so. There was clearly a very early benefit from statin therapy.

The Myocardial Ischaemia Reduction with Aggressive Cholesterol Lowering (MIRACL) study was a prospective randomised controlled trial of the treatment of patients with an acute coronary event [6]. It was a multi-centre study undertaken in 122 centres in Europe, North America, South Africa and Australasia; 3086 patients were allocated to receive either placebo or atorvastatin 80 mg daily, starting 24–96 hours after the acute coronary event. Assessment was at 16 weeks. Table 28.1 shows that there were no significant differences in deaths (4.2% and 4.4%) but there were fewer non-fatal coronary events in the atorvastatin group, 6.2% as opposed to the 8.4% in the control group. There were also fewer strokes in the atorvastatin group.

**Table 28.1  Effects of atorvastatin on early recurrent ischaemic events after acute coronary events [6]**

|  | Placebo | Atorvastatin |
| --- | --- | --- |
| Number | 1548 | 1538 |
| Deaths, n (%) | 68 (4.4) | 64 (4.2) |
| Coronary events, n (%) | 130 (8.4) | 95 (6.2) |
| Strokes, n (%) | 24 (1.6) | 12 (0.8) |

Such an early benefit is beyond the predictions of the diet–cholesterol–heart hypothesis. It suggests that statins have a very early effect, within a matter of hours, because of a mechanism that is independent of the well-established cholesterol lowering. This point was brought out by Carl Vaughan and his colleagues from the Department of Pharmacology and Therapeutics at University College, Cork, Ireland, commenting on the 4S study and WOSCOPS [7]. They observed that:

*The clinical benefit of the drugs used in these studies is manifest early in the course of lipid lowering therapy before plaque regression could occur.*

The more numerous the clinical effects of statin therapy, the less reliable the intervention trials are in supporting the diet–cholesterol–heart hypothesis.

Not only is there a rapid onset beneficial effect but there is also a rapid rebound effect when statins are stopped. In a study from Germany, it was noted that of 1616 patients who were admitted to hospital because of acute coronary syndromes, those taking statins at the time of admission had only half the risk of death of those not taking stains [8]. The most surprising and unexpected finding was that if statins were stopped on admission to hospital, the risk of cardiac death and non-fatal event during a period of just 30 days rose three-fold, as shown in Figure 28.3. These effects indicate a direct effect of statins on the heart, not a cholesterol-lowering effect.

**Figure 28.3 Coronary event rates and statin therapy [8].**

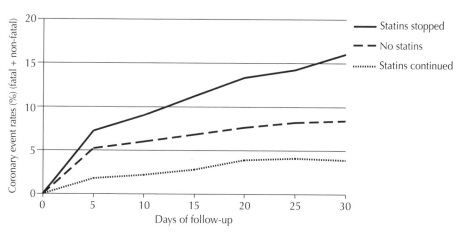

*Adapted from Circulation with permission from Lippincott, Williams and Watkins.*

Experimental evidence from the laboratory has shown that statins given to rodents might increase bone formation [9]. A study to assess this in the human was undertaken by reviewing women in Chingford, UK, who were part of a long-term study of post-menopausal osteoporosis; 31 of the 1003 women under review were taking statins and they had greater bone density than comparable women not taking statins [10]. This points to another unexpected but beneficial effect of statins.

One of the main problems after heart transplantation is the development of rapidly progressive coronary artery disease, reducing the length of survival. In an attempt to prevent this, 47 recipients of heart transplantation were given pravastatin and the outcome was compared with 50 controls. There was a significant and immediate benefit from pravastatin; the development of cardiovascular disease was less in the treated group, three compared with 10. However, and completely unexpectedly, those patients receiving pravastatin had only three transplant rejections, compared with 14 in the control group. The survival rate was 94% for those receiving pravastatin and 78% for the controls [11]. Pravastatin was thus acting in an anti-rejection fashion, again indicating that pravastatin has properties other than cholesterol lowering. A subsequent paper indicated a variety of anti-inflammatory actions of pravastatin and effects on immunity [12]. A further study from the same group in Sacramento, California, USA, indicated that pravastatin has a similar anti-rejection effect following kidney transplantation [13].

It has been noted by many researchers that statins have an anti-inflammatory action entirely different from the cholesterol-lowering action. An attempt to assess this led to a study published recently that was a trial of atorvastatin in the treatment of 116 patients with rheumatoid arthritis [14]. Rheumatoid arthritis is a chronic disabling condition, the major pathological process of which is inflammatory but the cause of which is unknown. Treatment of 58 patients with atorvastatin 80 mg daily produced a clinical improvement compared with the 58 controls who received placebo.

There are also suggestions that statins might be helpful in multiple sclerosis and trials are apparently in progress. A preliminary study has looked at the effect of simvastatin treatment on the characteristic (gadolinium-enhancing) lesions seen with magnetic resonance (MR) scanning. Thirty patients were treated and the outcome was a 44% reduction in the number of lesions, with a 41% reduction in their volume [15].

However, the several unforeseen benefits of statins as a result of a range of cellular effects suggest caution because there could be unanticipated disadvantages. If blocking an enzyme such as HMG-CoA reductase always has an advantage, it might have happened as an evolutionary development. Statins appear to be remarkably safe but side-effects do occur. Muscle damage (rhabdomyolysis) can be a side-effect of statin therapy, and one statin (cerivastatin, Bayer Pharmaceuticals Division) was removed from use in August 2001 because the occurrence of this has been more frequent than is acceptable [16]. There is also a suspicion that statins have a detrimental effect on memory [17,18]. On the other hand, there is a suggestion of a reduced incidence of Alzheimer's disease in people taking statins [19].

A more fundamental effect of statins was reported to the American Heart Association in Dallas, Texas, in November 2005 [20]. John Canty and his colleagues from the University of Buffalo had given statins for 1 month to pigs with damaged hearts. Subsequent examination showed 10 times as many stem cells in the damaged areas in those given statin compared with controls, and this helped the process of repair. They also observed more stem cells in healthy pigs given statins, indicating a very important and generalised beneficial effect of statins [20].

The Scottish paradox is that the beneficial effect of statin therapy is unrelated to the cholesterol-lowering property of this class of drugs. Statins were introduced to reduce serum cholesterol, following the diet–cholesterol–heart hypothesis. It is clearly the case that statins have many more actions, and therefore their clinical benefit cannot be used to verify the diet–cholesterol–heart hypothesis, which therefore remains weak and untested.

It has been demonstrated that statin drugs (originally derived from a fungus) are clearly of benefit in a number of clinical situations, and their introduction appears to be an example of serendipity, a chance development that has taken clinical science in an unexpected direction. We must look beyond cholesterol to understand the causation of coronary heart disease, but before doing so I would like to examine another paradox.

# 29
# THE ELDERLY PARADOX

Many people who consider themselves to be in normal good health are no longer left alone. 'The last well person' in the USA was a fictional professor of algebra; despite extensive medical investigation the doctors had been unable to find anything wrong with him [1]. We are in an era of preventative medicine, something that is often confused with early detection of subclinical illness. The theme of the day is HPDP ('Hippie-Dippie'), Health Promotion Disease Prevention, which in practice means very intrusive medicine and the medicalisation of society. It seems to be readily accepted in what W. H. Auden called 'the age of anxiety'.

Immunisation is an acceptable aspect of preventative action, as long as there is a balance between the safety of the process and avoidance of a serious illness. Occasionally the balance is confused by the possible but rare risk of immunisation being borne by an individual with the benefit being to the community as a whole. There is, for example, some concern about possible damage to a few children from measle immunisation, but immunisation undoubtedly prevents potentially serious illness in large numbers of children. Breast cancer screening is based on making the diagnosis earlier than if symptoms (usually a lump) were allowed to develop. The success depends on the outcome of the cancer being determined more by the treatment process than the biology of the cancer, and this remains controversial.

With coronary heart disease, there is no suitable method of detection of the disease before its clinical manifestations develop: angina, myocardial infarction or sudden death. Because it is common and because conventional wisdom tells us that it is the result of diet and other lifestyle characteristics, prevention means in practice attention to the national diet and exhortations for us all to eat less fat. This population approach has been said to be like tackling alcoholism by persuading all the population to drink slightly less alcohol: it will do nothing to help those with alcoholism and it will be a minor irritant to those without [2].

Clearly a more targeted approach is necessary, and therefore, if subclinical coronary heart disease cannot be detected, those at high risk must be identified. This must not appear to be discriminatory, particularly to the high-risk groups of the socially underprivileged and South Asian immigrants, who we shall consider in detail in later chapters. This is particularly relevant because conventional wisdom, which is very influential but almost entirely wrong, tells us that coronary heart disease is effectively self-induced, in particular by eating the wrong foods. The diet–cholesterol–heart hypothesis is unchallenged and therefore the key to identifying individuals at particularly high risk is cholesterol screening.

This works on the basis that a high serum cholesterol level is an indicator of cardiovascular death, and we have seen some evidence that this is true. However, an individual does not necessarily want to know that his or her life will be short unless something can be done to prolong it. Like all population screening exercises, the identification of high serum cholesterol will always produce considerable anxiety in some individuals; it will always give someone something else to worry about. Before creating national anxiety (although it is probably already too late), it is as well to make certain how useful the serum cholesterol level of an individual is for predicting the future: we need to look critically at its predictive value.

The early work of relating serum cholesterol to future risk was undertaken using working men as the subjects. In Chapter 24 we considered the MRFIT study, which looked at men aged between 35 and 57 years [3], and the Whitehall study, whose subjects were men aged between 40 and 64 years [4]. However, only about 30% of men suffering from a heart attack fall into this age group; the majority are older than 70 years. Is it reasonable to assume that what is found in middle-aged men is equally applicable to older people?

Doubt concerning this has been present for some time. We have seen data emerging from the long-term study of coronary heart disease in the town of Framingham, Massachusetts, USA, organised by the National Heart, Lung and Blood Institute of the USA. A publication recording 30 years of follow-up was entitled 'Cholesterol and mortality' [5]. Its conclusion was quite remarkable and has been followed by what might be called a stunned silence: 'After age 50 years there is no increased overall mortality with either high or low serum cholesterol levels'.

I use the term 'stunned silence' because this finding has received no publicity and has had no practical impact whatsoever. Remember that more than 90% of coronary heart disease presents after the age of 50 years. Think how many people older than 50 years have had their serum cholesterol level tested to try to predict coronary risk when it does not. Of course this finding does not fit in with the diet–cholesterol–heart hypothesis, and therefore cholesterol screening continues without critical assessment.

The data to support the statement from the Framingham study are shown in Figures 29.1 and 29.2, indicating the relationship between serum cholesterol and overall survival in men aged 31–39 and 56–65 years. It is clear that, in the younger men, high serum cholesterol is related to poor survival not just from coronary heart disease but from all causes.

**Figure 29.1 Thirty-year mortality by serum cholesterol in men aged 31–39 years [5].**

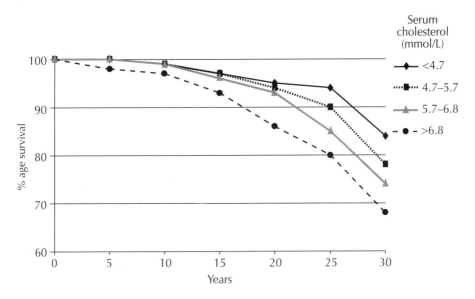

**Figure 29.2 Thirty-year mortality by serum cholesterol in men aged 56–65 years [5].**

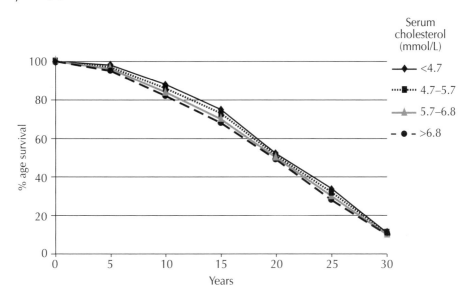

Please note that in these two figures the scales are different, but the purpose is to demonstrate survival related to serum cholesterol. Figure 29.1 indicates that, after 30 years, 70% of 35-year-old men with a serum cholesterol of greater than 6.8 mmol/L will still be alive, as will 85% of men with a serum cholesterol of less than 5.7. The follow-up for 30 years of men who were aged 60 at the beginning of the study cannot expect the same survival. The point is that 10% are alive after 30 years, they will reach their 90th birthday, irrespective of the serum cholesterol at the start of the study.

So in young men in whom the risk of death is relatively low, high serum cholesterol is a predictor of what is, on average, a relatively poor survival. In older men, in whom the risk of death is much higher, serum cholesterol is of no predictive value. Measuring the serum cholesterol of middle-aged men cannot be expected to provide any useful information.

We also see from this important study from Framingham that serum cholesterol is of very little predictive value in young women, as shown in Figure 29.3. Compare this with Figure 29.1, which illustrates men of the same age, 31–39 years; in men of this age the average 5-year survival was about 78% and in women about 88%.

In Figure 29.3 the lines run much closer together, indicating a much less predictive value of serum cholesterol regarding women. Furthermore, it can be seen that the life expectancy of women of this age is better than that of men. In older age groups of women, as with men, the survival curves are close together, as in Figure 29.2. This indicates that serum cholesterol has no predictive value in these age groups. But think again of how many women have their serum cholesterol measured!

**Figure 29.3 Thirty-year mortality by serum cholesterol in women aged 31–39 years [5].**

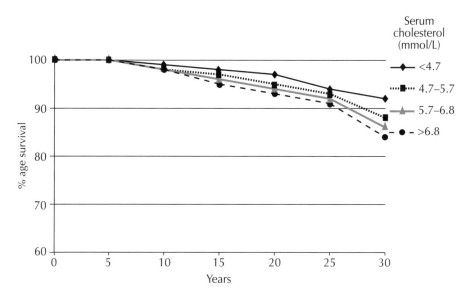

The other point to note again is that the survival rate is based on death from any cause and these data do not refer just to death from coronary heart disease. The predictive value of serum cholesterol and death in young men remains an enigma and we will return to it later.

The relationship between serum cholesterol and survival was investigated further in a group of 92 women aged 60 years and older who were living in a nursing home in Paris [6]. The women were selected as being free of cancer because it had been recognised previously that serum cholesterol is generally low in people with cancer (or that cancer is more common in people with low cholesterol) [7]. The subjects were followed up for 5

228

years and it was quite clear that those with the lowest serum cholesterol had the worst survival. The death rate in those with a serum cholesterol of 4 mmol/L was 5.2 times the death rate in those with a serum cholesterol of 7 mmol/L.

The relationship between death rate and serum cholesterol is what is called U-shaped, or J-shaped if asymmetrical, as in Figure 29.4. Although the optimum serum cholesterol in this group of women was 7 mmol/L, those with serum cholesterol greater than 8 mmol/L had a slightly higher death rate. Those with the lowest serum cholesterol had the highest death rate of all.

**Figure 29.4 The relative death rate and serum cholesterol of women aged 60+ years [6].**

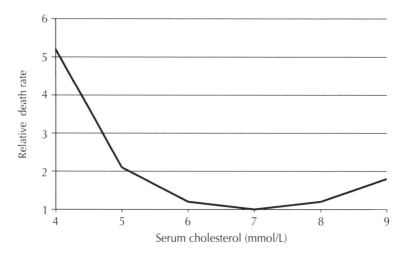

© 1989, adapted from The Lancet with permission from Elsevier.

There are two ways of looking at death rates: one is to look at the number or percentage surviving, as in the Framingham data described above, and the other is to look at the number or percentage dying, and that was the method chosen in the study from Paris. Figure 29.5 shows the death rates for 5 years based on serum cholesterol. The death rate, that is the risk of dying, increased with increasing age, as would be expected. The important and unexpected fact emerging from the figure is that the highest death rate was in those with the lowest serum cholesterol; this is the elderly paradox.

**Figure 29.5 Five-year mortality by serum cholesterol in women aged 60+ [6].**

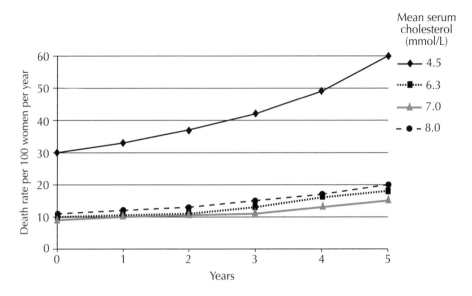

The evangelists of the diet–cholesterol–heart hypothesis might argue that the reason for the high death rate in those women with low serum cholesterol was that they were already, but unknowingly, dying of cancer, but this possibility had been eliminated as far as possible at the start of the study. The authors commented that cancer mortality declined after the age of 70 years, and during the 5-year follow-up, during which 53 of the 92 women died, autopsy revealed cancer to be the cause of death in only one.

Another interesting result, and again paradoxical, is that at the onset of the study the mean serum cholesterol of women known to have coronary heart disease was 5.9 mmol/L; it was higher, at 6.3 mmol/L, in those who were not known to have coronary heart disease.

A further study of elderly subjects was undertaken in New Haven, Connecticut, USA, in a community-based study of 997 people aged more than 70 years with a follow-up of 4 years [8]. The coronary heart disease mortality was once again paradoxical in that a higher level of serum cholesterol was associated with a lower death rate from coronary heart disease. This is shown in Figure 29.6.

**Figure 29.6 Four-year coronary heart disease (CHD) mortality based on serum cholesterol (age > 70 years) [8].**

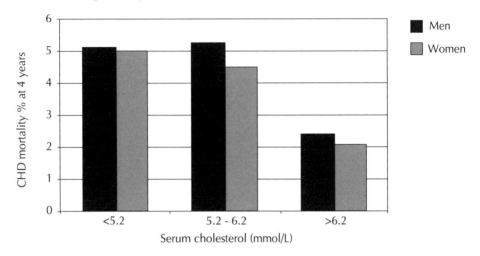

A similar result came from the Honolulu Heart Program, a study of 3572 men aged 71–93 years [9]. This study looked at survival, as did the Framingham study, and two ways of looking at the same data are shown in Figures 29.7 and 29.8. The figure shows survival over a period of 6 years in four groups based on serum cholesterol. Those with the lowest serum cholesterol level had the worst survival, that is the highest mortality; another example of the elderly paradox. The results were unchanged when first-year deaths were discounted, the purpose of this being to avoid the possible effect of low serum cholesterol and death being to the result of present but undiagnosed cancer.

**Figure 29.7 Six-year survival by serum cholesterol in men aged 71–93 years [9].**

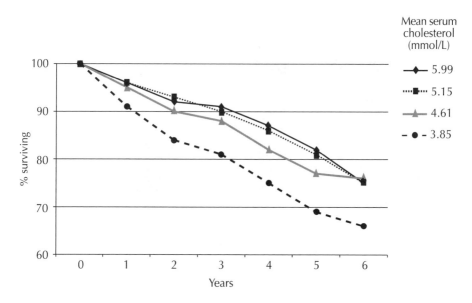

© 2001, adapted from The Lancet with permission from Elsevier.

**Figure 29.8 Death rate based on serum cholesterol in men aged 71–93 years [9].**

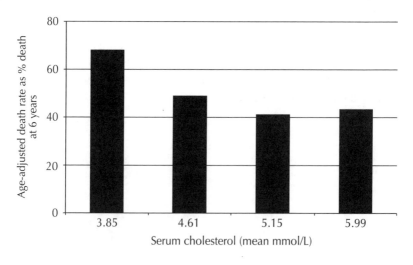

© 2001, adapted from The Lancet with permission from Elsevier.

Another interesting observation came out of this study. For the purpose of analysis, the subjects were divided into two groups, those with risk indicators of coronary heart disease (smoking, hypertension, diabetes or pre-existing coronary heart disease) and those without. In both of these groups the mortality rate was lowest in those with the highest serum cholesterol.

In those with risk factors, the risk of death for those in the highest cholesterol quartile (mean 5.99) was only 75% of those in the lowest quartile (mean 3.85). If we look at those without risk factors, those in the highest cholesterol quartile had only a 56% risk of death compared with those in the lowest quartile. Clearly, in this age group above 70 years, low serum cholesterol cannot be regarded as a good thing. It is worth noting some of the statements and conclusions of the authors [9]:

*A generally held belief is that cholesterol concentrations should be kept low to lessen the risk of cardiovascular disease. However, studies of the relation between serum cholesterol and all-cause mortality in elderly people have shown contrasting results … Only the group with a low cholesterol concentration had a significant association with mortality … We have been unable explain our results. These data cast doubt on the scientific justification for lowering the cholesterol to very low concentrations in elderly people.*

It is difficult for medical professionals and society to absorb the observation that low serum cholesterol is associated with a worse health outcome, but the evidence is strong. Although high serum cholesterol in younger men appears to be associated with an increased risk of coronary heart disease, it does not appear to be associated with an increased risk of stroke. This has been noted in several studies over the years but it has been difficult to understand as, in the majority of cases, both are manifestations of underlying atherosclerotic disease. Why is there no link between serum cholesterol and stroke?

An investigation into this was undertaken in Glasgow, UK, studying 977 patients admitted to the Acute Stroke Unit in the Western Infirmary [10]. The objective was to investigate the relationship between serum cholesterol and the type of stroke, 3-month outcome and long-term mortality. The result was a surprise: 'After adjustment for known prognostic factors, higher serum cholesterol concentrations were associated with reduced long term mortality after stroke.'

In other words, the higher the cholesterol, the lower the risk of death after stroke; another paradox. The survival curves based on three of the quintiles of serum cholesterol are shown in Figure 29.9. Only about 54%

of those with a serum cholesterol of less than 4.8 mmol/L survived for 500 days, compared with about 74% of those with a serum cholesterol of greater than 7.

**Figure 29.9 Survival after stroke by serum cholesterol [10].**

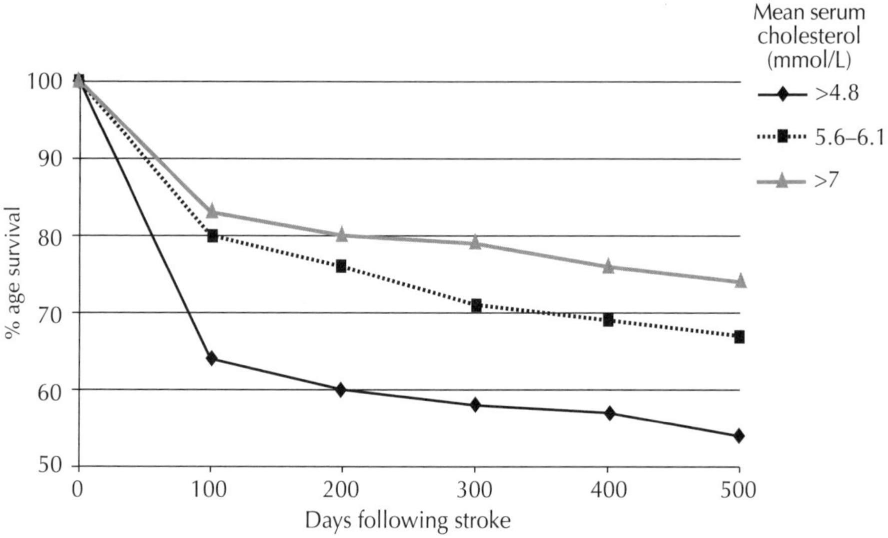

*Adapted with permission from the British Medical Journal Publishing Group.*

Although this can be seen to be an extension of the elderly paradox, the observation was in all age groups. The term stroke implies something sudden, and that something is brain damage because of a disruption of its blood supply, cerebral infarction. Within the brain, the process can be a haemorrhage as a result of a spontaneous rupture of an artery, or alternatively, and more frequently, the occlusion of an artery. The part of the brain damaged by infarction can vary, and damage to the frontal lobes because of occlusion of the anterior cerebral artery carries a higher mortality than occlusion of the middle cerebral artery. This would give rise to what is termed a lacunar infarction with a characteristic left- or right-sided paralysis (hemiplegia).

The data presented in Table 29.1 show the outcome for these two types of stroke, and for both types and both age groups outcome was better for those with the higher serum cholesterol.

**Table 29.1 Survival after stroke (%) [10]**

|  | Age 50 years | Age 75 years |
|---|---|---|
| Anterior circulation infarction |  |  |
| Cholesterol 5.2 mmol/L | 54 | 31 |
| Cholesterol 7.5 mmol/L | 62 | 40 |
| Lacunar infarction |  |  |
| Cholesterol 5.2 mmol/L | 88 | 61 |
| Cholesterol 7.5 mmol/L | 91 | 69 |

*Adapted with permission from the British Medical Journal Publishing Group.*

The authors describe the unexpected finding as a 'counter-intuitive effect of cholesterol', another term for paradox. They comment that it must challenge attempts to lower serum cholesterol, and so it would appear. But here we encounter yet another paradox.

The UK Medical Research Council (MRC) and the British Heart Foundation (BHF) together sponsored a placebo-controlled trial of simvastatin 40 mg daily involving 20 536 adults aged between 40 and 80 years [11], which we reviewed in detail in Chapter 27. It was a secondary prevention study as all patients had known expressions of coronary heart disease or other occlusive arterial disease. The death rate from coronary heart disease during the 5 years of follow-up was 5.7% in the treated group compared with 6.9% in the placebo group, in keeping with other statin trials. The occurrence rate of stroke (fatal or non-fatal) was 4.3% in the treated group compared with 5.7% in the placebo group. Simvastatin therapy therefore reduced the incidence of stroke.

If a high serum cholesterol is a good thing in respect of a stroke, as is shown in the Glasgow study [10], and if statin therapy is helpful, then clearly we can see once again that the clinical benefit from statins is nothing to do with the cholesterol-lowering properties. The title of the MRC/British Heart Foundation paper was: 'MRC/BHF heart protection study of cholesterol lowering with simvastatin in 20 536 individuals' [11]. Scientific bodies such as these ought to have been more careful with the use of language; by 2002 it was clear that cholesterol lowering and statin therapy cannot and must not be equated. The title should not have mentioned cholesterol lowering as that was not what was being investigated; it was a clinical trial of simvastatin therapy.

Other studies have shown a benefit from statin therapy regarding stroke prevention. The conclusion of these trials, the elderly paradox and the Glasgow study on the favourable effect of a high serum cholesterol on outcome from stroke once again casts serious doubt on the diet–

cholesterol–heart hypothesis, which is continuing to look unsustainable. The studies also indicate that there is much more to statin therapy than lowering serum cholesterol, and we shall be revisiting this later.

# 30

# THE GEOGRAPHY OF CHOLESTEROL

S o far we have looked at the significance of serum cholesterol level for individuals, but for a public health perspective it is necessary to look at the significance of cholesterol in respect of populations. This is very similar to the research undertaken by John Snow in identifying the source of cholera in London, recognising the location at which cholera had the greatest incidence and relating that to an environmental factor, namely the water pump in Broad Street. It is necessary in respect of coronary heart disease and cholesterol to use the same approach to identify the populations who are most at risk.

I have already indicated a close link between cholesterol and vitamin D. I have proposed that 7-dehydrocholesterol in the skin is converted into cholesterol in the absence of sunlight and into vitamin D in the presence of sunlight. I would therefore predict that the average cholesterol level of a population in the northern hemisphere would be higher in more northern latitudes, where ultraviolet light at ground level is less, and that, correspondingly, serum cholesterol levels would be lower in locations closer to the equator, where there is more exposure to sunlight.

We noted in Chapter 22 that the first major investigation into the incidence of coronary heart disease in different populations was undertaken by Professor Ancel Keys of the University of Minnesota, USA [1]. He started the study with a baseline examination of 17 763 apparently healthy men aged 40–59 years and the follow-up was for a maximum of 25 years. During this time of observation about 6000 men died, 1500 from coronary heart disease. The importance of the work of Keys cannot be underestimated. He motivated a large number of people in several countries to take a major interest in the collection of data concerning various aspects of health and coronary heart disease. The impetus and motivation had to be sustained for 25 years.

The data are available for us to examine, perhaps leading to conclusions that Keys and his colleagues would not appreciate. The data are spread throughout the book but I have collated much of it in tabular form and an extract can be seen in Table 30.1. The cholesterol data were originally presented as mg/dL, as is the USA tradition, but I have transposed them into the equivalent mmol/L. Keys also studied USA railway workers but I have omitted these data as they lack the geographical precision of the European and Japanese data.

**Table 30.1 The Seven Countries Study [1].**
CHD = coronary heart disease

| Country | Region | Annual death rates per 10 000 men All causes | CHD | Mean cholesterol mmol/L | Mean % calories from fat |
|---------|--------|------------|-----|-----------|----------|
| Finland | East Finland | 186 | 99 | 6.82 | 23 |
| Slovenia | Slovenia | 165 | 21 | 5.16 | 14 |
| Finland | West Finland | 148 | 35 | 6.54 | 17 |
| Italy | Crevalcore | 138 | 25 | 5.00 | 10 |
| Japan | Ushibuka | 136 | 7 | 5.96 | 3 |
| Yugoslavia | Zrenjanin | 122 | 15 | 5.44 | 10 |
| Netherlands | Zutphen | 122 | 42 | 5.21 | 18 |
| Yugoslavia | Velika Krsna | 119 | 8 | 4.19 | 9 |
| Japan | Tanushimaru | 111 | 9 | 4.30 | 3 |
| Italy | Montegiorgio | 110 | 15 | 4.82 | 9 |
| Italy | Rome | 104 | 29 | 4.40 | 11 |
| Greece | Corfu | 83 | 14 | 4.45 | 7 |
| Croatia | Dalmatia | 80 | 9 | 5.18 | 9 |
| Greece | Crete | 66 | 1 | 5.29 | 8 |
| Yugoslavia | Belgrade | 59 | 29 | 5.34 | 12 |
| Mean | | 117 | 24 | 5 | 11 |

It can be seen immediately from Table 30.1 that there is a wide variation in the age-adjusted death rates from all causes (59–186) and from coronary heart disease (1–99). East Finland stands out as appearing to be the unhealthiest place to live, with a particularly high death rate from coronary heart disease. Crete shows an astonishingly low death rate from coronary heart disease, so much so that the quality of these particular data must be in some doubt.

Before the study began Keys, like others, felt that cholesterol and a high-fat diet were the cause of coronary heart disease, based on the pathological descriptions made at the end of the 19th century, and the results of the study were interpreted as supporting this view. The example of East Finland in particular was clearly in keeping with this but what we must remember is that there are many factors that distinguish one country from another that were not measured in this study. Comparing countries can only generate ideas, not conclusions.

The study identified a moderate association between total dietary fat and coronary heart disease mortality, as can be seen in Figure 30.1, the data being taken from Table 30.1. It is important to realise that the fat intake is a population average. In Chapter 22 we looked at a number of later studies that investigated in greater detail the dietary patterns of individuals and their subsequent health risks.

**Figure 30.1  The rate of all causes of death and dietary fat [1].**

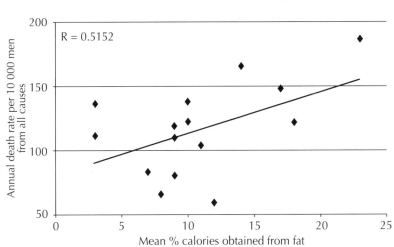

The data are presented as a scattergraph, designed to show the association between two measured variables. In this case the percentage of calories that the population obtains on average from fat is thought, by initial reasoning, to be the moving force, and thus it appears on the *x* (horizontal) axis. The other variable, considered to be the result, appears on the *y* (vertical) axis, which in this scattergraph it is the annual death rate per 10 000 men from all causes, in the locations investigated by Keys and his colleagues [1].

It can be seen that the points are widely scattered. We can also see the trend line. The closer the points are to the line, the more powerful is the association. This is presented mathematically as the correlation coefficient, $R$, a number (a statistic) with a value between $-1$ and $+1$. The closer it is to $+1$ or $-1$, the more powerful the association. If $+$, the trend line will slope upwards from left to right, indicating a positive association; as the proposed moving factor increases, so does the effect, interpreted as causative. If $-$, the association is negative; as the proposed moving factor increases, the effect decreases, interpreted as protective. If $R$ is close to 0, there is no significant association.

In Figure 30.1, the points are not close to the trend line and $R = 0.5152$. The association is therefore weak. We will be looking at more scattergraphs and trend lines in this and later chapters.

Another way to present the result is to square the value of $R$, to create $R^2$. This gives a number between 0 and 1, with no plus or minus. The closer to 1 the stronger the association; the closer to 0 the weaker the association. If we square $R = 0.5152$, then $R^2 = 0.2654$, again indicating a weak association.

Further information from the scattergraph can be obtained by multiplying $R^2$ by 100, and in this case the result is 26.54%. This means that dietary fat might explain 26.54% of the variation of coronary heart disease that we see in the data presented, but only if the association is direct; do not forget the association with radio and television receivers.

If, in the example presented in Figure 30.1, we remove the obvious outlier of East Finland, then analysis of the other points leads to $R$ becoming 0.2691 and $R^2$ 0.0724. This is so close to 0 that there is no association between dietary fat and the all causes of death rate. Only 7% would be explained.

Figure 30.2 shows the association with fat intake, again expressed as the percentage of calories obtained from fat as a population average, and deaths specifically from coronary heart disease. We can immediately see that the data points are much closer to the trend line than in Figure 30.1.

**Figure 30.2 Deaths from coronary heart disease (CHD) and dietary fat [1].**

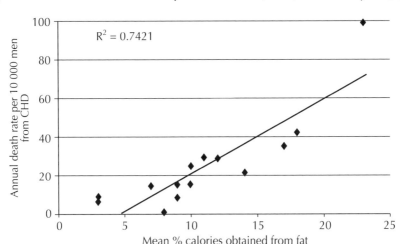

The association is strong but East Finland as an outlier is again very influential. If East Finland is included then $R^2$ is 0.7421. If it is excluded then $R^2$ falls to 0.6934, but this still indicates a significant association. There is something about national diet and in particular the proportion of fat eaten that is somehow associated with death rates from coronary heart disease. But let us not fall into the obvious trap of assuming that this automatically supports the diet–cholesterol–heart hypothesis: the results of studies discussed in Chapter 22 show us that this association does not translate into the experience of individuals within a country.

This brings us to cholesterol in the blood, a major subject of investigation by Keys. The association between dietary fat and serum cholesterol at a population level is shown in Figure 30.3. The association is strong, with $R^2 = 0.7312$ and all points being close to the trend line; East Finland is not a significant outlier. It is easy to appreciate how this study gave great impetus to the diet–cholesterol–heart hypothesis, but again I must emphasise that we are looking at characteristics of countries and regions and not individuals. The association between the population average cholesterol and fat intake might be explained on the basis of common cause rather than cause and effect.

**Figure 30.3 Average population cholesterol and fat intake [1].**

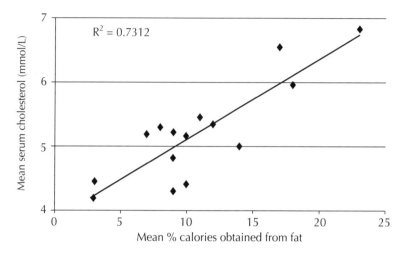

The diet–cholesterol–heart hypothesis is much less convincing when we look at the association between annual death rate from all causes and serum cholesterol in the Seven Countries Study [1]. Figure 30.4 shows a very weak association, with the data points widely scattered around a flat trend line; $R^2$ is close to 0 at 0.0625.

**Figure 30.4 Annual death rate and mean serum cholesterol [1].**

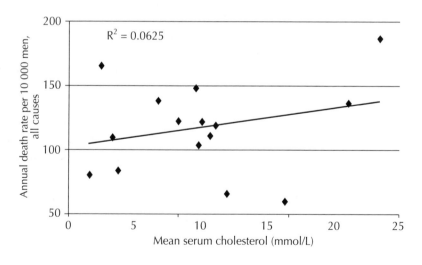

Figure 30.5 shows the association between coronary heart disease death rate and average serum cholesterol. This is much stronger, with $R^2 = 0.6498$. East Finland once again appears to be an outlier but removing it only reduces $R^2$ to 0.5692, still a moderate association. This is in keeping with other studies of working men, as we have seen.

**Figure 30.5 Annual death rate from coronary heart disease (CHD) and mean serum cholesterol [1].**

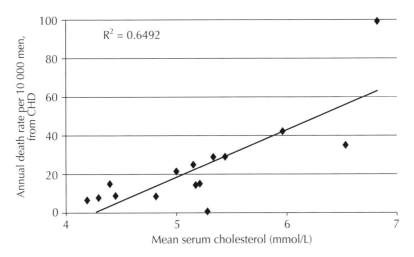

Can we identify a common factor that links dietary fat, serum cholesterol, all causes of death and coronary heart disease, something that might explain the differences between locations in Europe and other countries? We have already considered sunlight to be protective; could it be the factor? We now know that sunlight exposure can explain seasonal variation of disease and it could well control susceptibility to coronary heart disease. We know from our own experience that it controls agriculture and we have seen that it can explain the seasonal variation of cholesterol. Could it explain the geographical variation of cholesterol?

The Seven Countries Study does not provide sunshine data. It does, however, provide accurate geographical locations of its study populations and from these we can obtain latitude measurements. Latitude is a major determinant of the sunlight exposure of a population and the latitude data for the locations of study are shown in Table 30.2.

**Table 30.2 The Seven Countries Study [1]**

| Location | Country | Latitude |
|----------|---------|----------|
| Ushibuka | Japan | 32°9' |
| Tanushimaru | Japan | 33°35' |
| Crete | Greece | 35°01' |
| Corfu | Greece | 39°37' |
| Rome | Italy | 41°48' |
| Dalmatia | Croatia | 43°00' |
| Montegiorgio | Italy | 44°00' |
| Velika Krsna | Yugoslavia | 44°40' |
| Crevalcore | Italy | 44°45' |
| Belgrade | Yugoslavia | 44°48' |
| Zrenjanin | Yugoslavia | 45°30' |
| Slovenia | Slovenia | 46°30' |
| Zutphen | the Netherlands | 52°06' |
| West Finland | Finland | 62°15' |
| East Finland | Finland | 67°30' |

*All degrees north of the equator.*

We are now in a position to investigate possible associations between latitude and the various factors that Keys recorded, but we must remember that associations only produce ideas and not conclusions.

We can see in Figure 30.6 the association between latitude and deaths from all causes. It shows a moderate association, with $R^2 = 0.3494$. The two towns at the lowest latitude were in southern Japan and they had an intermediate mortality rate. There is, however, a trend for the age-standardised mortality rate to increase with distance of residence from the equator, but only in the towns and countries studied. We must remember that there are tropical countries where mortality rates are very high as a result of pestilence, genocide and famine. The suggestion is that at times of relative affluence and social stability, latitude does have an effect on health, but in a way that cannot be concluded from this study alone.

**Figure 30.6  Latitude and all causes of mortality [data from 1].**

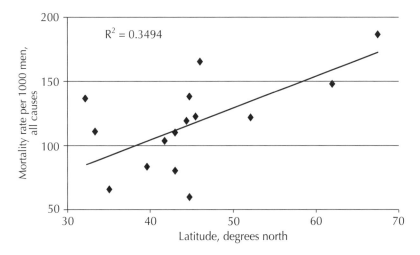

Figure 30.7 shows the association between latitude and mortality rate from coronary heart disease to be much stronger, with $R^2 = 0.7196$. The two southern Japanese towns have a low mortality rate from coronary heart disease; eastern Finland, the area also known as Karelia, has both the most northerly latitude and by far the highest mortality rate. Once again we cannot draw a conclusion about the intermediary mechanism and all we can say is that latitude appears to influence the susceptibility of a population to coronary heart disease.

**Figure 30.7  Latitude and mortality from coronary heart disease (CHD) [data from 1].**

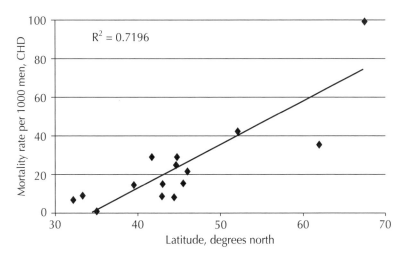

We need to look at the factors that were investigated in the Seven Countries Study, factors that were felt to provide an explanation in accordance with the diet–cholesterol–heart hypothesis. Figure 30.8 shows an extremely strong association between dietary fat intake and latitude.

**Figure 30.8 Latitude and dietary fat intake [data from 1].**

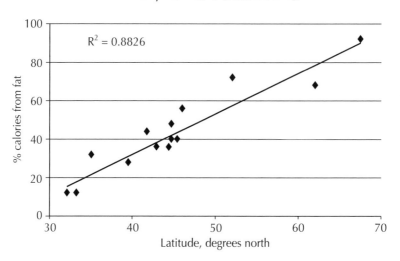

It can be seen that all points are close to the trend line and that $R^2$ =0.8826, which is very close to the maximum of 1. Therefore latitude could be responsible in some way for 88% of the variation of fat intake. There is clearly something about latitude that determines the proportion of calories that the population obtains from fat. Is this purely a matter of tradition and choice of the population, or is it something that results from local agricultural practice, something that is dependent on climate? Could both dietary pattern and death rate from coronary heart disease be related independently to latitude? We will be investigating this further in a later chapter.

We will now look at the geography of cholesterol in more detail. The Seven Countries Study provides data concerning the average serum cholesterol of the men studied in the various locations. The nature of the study meant that the subjects were not always random samples of the population and they did not represent all employment and social groups. For example, those from Rome were railway employees and those from Belgrade were university staff. Keys had to accept this limitation to initiate the study, but the data give us some guide to the characteristics of the various populations.

Figure 30.9 shows the association between average serum cholesterol and latitude. The association is strong, with $R^2$ = 0.6785. The main outliers on the scattergraph are the two Serbian towns of Velika Krsna and Zrenjanin, with cholesterol levels being relatively low for the latitude.

**Figure 30.9  Latitude and serum cholesterol [data from 1].**

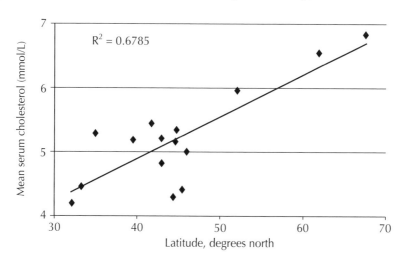

Once again no conclusion can be drawn regarding the cause–effect relationships, as these are merely observations. The starting point for analysis should be that there are no special relationships and that all the factors, mortality rates, dietary fat and serum cholesterol, are independent variables, each of which is associated with latitude in its own right. This is the approach that we must maintain as we move into the next chapters.

A review of the Seven Countries Study was published in 1999, in the form of a lecture on population sciences delivered by Daan Kromhout of the National Institute of Public Health in the Environment in the Netherlands, as a tribute to Ancel Keys [2]. The data he presented are displayed in Figure 30.10.

**Figure 30.10 Twenty-five year coronary heart disease (CHD) mortality related to serum cholesterol [2].**

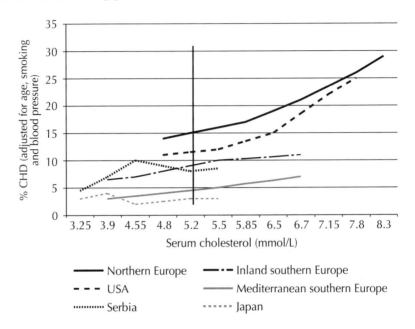

*Adapted with permission from the* European Heart Journal.

Two factors are shown very clearly. First, the population average cholesterol levels are particularly low in Japan and Mediterranean southern Europe, more intermediate in Serbia and inland southern Europe, higher in the USA (railroad workers) and highest of all in northern Europe. Second, it shows that, at a given level of cholesterol, coronary heart disease mortality shows the same pattern, with the lowest level in Japan, followed by Mediterranean southern Europe, then Serbia and inland southern Europe, then the USA, and northern Europe has the highest mortality of all.

This graph allows us to standardise for cholesterol by drawing a vertical line. We can then see that there is a five-fold geographical variation in the age-standardised mortality rate from coronary heart disease with a given serum cholesterol level, in this example 5.2 mmol/L. This variation has obviously nothing to do with serum cholesterol and another explanation must be sought. Kromhout did not bring out this extremely important conclusion in his paper. He discusses diet and its relationship with coronary heart disease in keeping with conventional wisdom but fails to consider any other environmental factors that might be relevant.

Kromhout realised that most of those with coronary heart disease had only small elevations of risk factors but he did not appear to appreciate the significance of this observation. He stated that 'In order to make a large impact in terms of public health, risk factor reduction at the population level is needed' [2]. Perhaps we need more thought.

In the study of Keys [1] and the review by Kromhout [2] there is no mention of latitude and no concept of sunshine as being a possible factor in determining the distribution of disease and local agricultural traditions. We have seen that there is a strong association between serum cholesterol and latitude that would support the hypothesis I have put forward, namely that blood (serum) cholesterol levels are high at times and locations of low levels of sun exposure. Climate has a similar beneficial effect on agriculture as it has on human health.

Having looked at the geography of cholesterol we will now look at the geography of disease.

# PART 6

# THE GEOGRAPHY OF DISEASE

# 31
# BURNLEY, COLNE AND NELSON

One of the major influences on my thinking regarding the environmental factors leading to coronary heart disease came from reading an interesting paper that concerned the locality of east Lancashire, UK, in which I have lived and worked for the past 30 years. The main author was David Barker, Professor of Clinical Epidemiology and Director of the Medical Research Council Environmental Epidemiology Unit at Southampton University, UK. He is a leading epidemiologist whose particular research interest has been the passing of coronary risk from one generation to another by non-genetic processes. As an epidemiologist he is particularly concerned about environmental factors. Although he has assembled a large amount of information for public and professional debate he has not come to a final conclusion and, as far as I am aware, he has not considered that sunlight and stored vitamin D might be important.

Barker used historical records from Burnley and the smaller neighbouring towns of Colne and Nelson, all in east Lancashire [1]. He was able to determine the disease incidence of previous generations and here we can see once again the value of good historical data as a basis for present-day research. He compared the disease profile from the historical records with the experience of the present generation. The sources of information were the 1911 national census, the local government report of England and Wales from 1913 and the local government report of Lancashire from 1914. This process shows the value of detailed local research and access to past quality data collection.

Burnley developed as an important cotton town after the opening of the Leeds and Liverpool canal at the end of the 18th century. The canal passes through Burnley on an impressive high embankment and within the town there remains a collection of 19th century cotton mills congregated around the canal.

Colne, to the north-east of Burnley, changed from its previous rural economy to adapt to the industrial revolution and the opening of the canal. Its industry developed very shortly after that of Burnley, but on a smaller scale.

With the continuing expansion of the cotton industry in the late 19th century after the end of the American civil war, which had reduced the imports of raw cotton into Lancashire, a new location for an industrial community was necessary and Nelson came into being, mid-way between Burnley and Colne. It was a planned town, developing around an east Lancashire railway station that took its name from an adjacent public house called the Nelson Inn, after the victor of the Battle of Trafalgar in 1805. Cotton mills and associated workers' houses were built between 1871 and 1911 to develop the new town of Nelson to a significant size.

Burnley and Colne had by that time a tradition of industrialisation, with the population having perhaps three or even four generations working in the textile mills and other factories. Nelson, on the other hand, acquired its new population mainly from farming communities in nearby Yorkshire. Barker quotes from the 1914 report [1]:

*This fact has an important bearing on the question of infantile mortality, owing to the general good health and habits of cleanliness and thrift characteristic of these immigrants from rural districts.*

We therefore find that Burnley was the first phase of industrial development, Colne the second and Nelson the third. The building of Nelson, as a later phase of development, had an improved standard of the workers' houses, with wider streets providing more space between the houses. Particularly bad health had been associated with the back-to-back style of house, in which there was only a front entrance and the back of the house was physically attached to the back of a similar house. At the end of the 19th century there were 2371 such houses in Burnley and 1000 in Colne, but the improved building standards by that time resulted in only 52 back-to-back houses in Nelson. The newer houses were built around a back alley, a service path between the backyards of adjacent rows of houses.

It is also important to note that Burnley was considered to be a very damp place, with many houses having been built on low-lying marshy land below the high canal embankment in the valley of the rivers Brun and Calder. The low-lying land held not only damp air but also smoke from the factories and domestic chimneys. This older housing of Burnley lies at about 100 metres above sea level. Nelson lies higher, at about 150 metres, and Colne is at about 180 metres above sea level.

The infant mortality report published in 1914 provided specific information about Burnley, Colne and Nelson. In the years leading up to the report, the infant mortality rate in Burnley was 177 deaths per thousand births, in Colne 130 and in Nelson 87 (Table 31.1). This was quite a striking difference in itself. It was also noted that the death rates in Burnley were 73% above average for bronchitis and pneumonia and 105% above average for diarrhoea.

**Table 31.1 Infant mortality rates for 1911–13 from Burnley Colne and Nelson [1]**

|                   | Deaths per 1000 births |
|-------------------|------------------------|
| Burnley           | 177                    |
| Colne             | 130                    |
| Nelson            | 87                     |
| England and Wales | 111                    |

*Adapted with permission from the British Medical Journal Publishing Group.*

After looking at the 1914 local government report for Lancashire, David Barker and his co-author Clive Osmond, senior scientist and medical statistician, decided to undertake a present-day study for comparative purposes [1]. They identified the standardised mortality ratios (SMR) for 1968–78, the England and Wales average being standardised at 100. The SMR for men in Burnley was 121, in Colne 109 and in Nelson 100 (Table 31.2).

**Table 31.2 SMR for ages 55–74 years, both sexes, for 1968–78.**
**CHD = coronary heart disease [1]**

|                   | All causes | CHD | Pneumonia | Bronchitis |
|-------------------|------------|-----|-----------|------------|
| Burnley           | 121        | 120 | 174       | 188        |
| Colne             | 109        | 119 | 125       | 132        |
| Nelson            | 100        | 106 | 108       | 134        |
| England and Wales | 100        | 100 | 100       | 100        |

*Adapted with permission from the British Medical Journal Publishing Group.*

It is interesting to look at the relative mortality rates for these three east Lancashire towns, and it appears that the population of Burnley has a very high burden of illness and premature death. It is also important to remember that this study is dealing with an area and a population of considerable socio-economic deprivation, as shown in Table 31.3.

**Table 31.3 Social profile for 1971, percentage of employed men [1].**
IIIN, non-manual workers; IIIM, manual workers

|             | I | II | IIIN | IIIM | IV | V |
|-------------|---|----|------|------|----|---|
| Burnley     | 3 | 13 | 10   | 45   | 20 | 10 |
| Colne       | 3 | 14 | 10   | 47   | 16 | 11 |
| Nelson      | 2 | 13 | 8    | 48   | 18 | 11 |
| England and |   |    |      |      |    |   |
| Wales       | 5 | 18 | 12   | 38   | 18 | 9 |

*Adapted with permission from the British Medical Journal Publishing Group.*

This study shows how the mortality rate can vary significantly within a short distance, the centres of Burnley, Nelson and Colne being within less than 10 miles of each other. The suggested explanation for the mortality difference in 1914 was that the populations of Colne and Nelson were helped by a higher altitude and better air. The population of Nelson was further helped by the improved housing qualities and also by the 'sturdier and healthier' women, recently agricultural workers. It thus suggested that the health of the mother is of importance to the health of the children. This very important observation, leading to the identification of the 'maternal factor', was made by Professor Barker and is the subject of a later chapter. If we consider the background and good health of the women of Nelson, then perhaps this factor could be a body store of vitamin D, resulting from greater exposure to sunlight.

The most important message from this study is that the variations of mortality rates recorded in Burnley, Colne and Nelson in 1914 could still be identified in 1968–78. The impression is that some environmental factor persists, or perhaps there is a factor being inherited by subsequent generations that is unlikely to be genetically determined.

# 32

# THE GEOGRAPHY OF CORONARY HEART DISEASE IN THE UK

There is a general impression that the populations of the northern parts of the British Isles have poor health as a result of faulty eating. We saw in Chapter 22 that this health profile is true but the presumed reason is false. This information was from the study of three English towns, Ipswich in the south-east, with the lowest standardised death rate from coronary heart disease, Stoke-on-Trent in the midlands, with the intermediate rate, and Wakefield in Yorkshire, with the highest rate. The study showed no dietary explanation for these differences [1].

The reduced life expectancy in the north of the UK is undoubted. The report of the *Health Statistics Quarterly* published in the autumn of 2001 [2] was given wide publicity. It showed that the highest average life expectancy from birth is in Chelsea & Westminster and Kensington, 77.5 years for males and 82.4 years for females. The lowest life expectancy for males is Lanarkshire in Scotland, at 72.1 years. The lowest life expectancy for females is 77.7 years, shared between St Helens & Knowsley and Ayrshire & Arran. However, the variations are not entirely the result of a latitude effect: one of the lowest life expectancies for men, 72.8 years, is in East London and The City, only a short distance from Kensington, which has an average life expectancy of 5 more years. This is a striking variation that requires an explanation, which might have something to do with its high immigrant population and social structure, as we will see later.

In Chapter 30 we noted the relationship between coronary heart disease and latitude, demonstrated in the Seven Countries Study [3], and we can apply this idea to the Three English Towns study that we met in Chapter 22. Figure 32.1 is a scattergraph showing the association between the SMR for these towns and their latitudes. It can be seen that the association is very strong, with $R^2 = 0.9587$.

**Figure 32.1 SMR for coronary heart disease and latitude [1].**

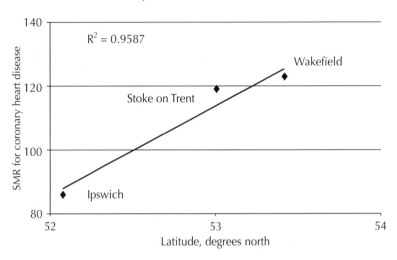

*Adapted with permission from the British Medical Journal Publishing Group.*

Although $R^2$ gives an indication of the strength of an association, the power of this is influenced by the number of points on the scattergraph. The more data points, the greater the power. In, for example, Figure 30.8 there are 13 data points. Two points are necessary to fix the line and so 11 points are present to allow calculation of $R^2$. In statistical language this is referred to as 11 degrees of freedom. In Figure 32.1 there are only three data points and thus only 1 degree of freedom. The power of the association is therefore low.

In the previous chapter we saw that there is a higher incidence of disease and death in Burnley compared with Nelson. I proposed that this is the result of differential levels of sunshine, as a result of housing and altitude characteristics, with a contribution from the inheritance of non-genetic factors from the mother, possibly vitamin D. I suggest that sunshine exposure would explain not just the altitude effect in east Lancashire but also the latitude effect of the three English towns. We need to examine sunshine effects directly.

I obtained annual sunshine data from the Meteorological Office for areas close to the three towns, Sheffield for Wakefield, Stone for Stoke-on-Trent and Wattisham for Ipswich. These data are shown in Table 32.1 together with latitude and SMR for coronary heart disease (CHD).

**Table 32.1 The Three Towns Study [1]**

| Town | SMR CHD | Latitude (degrees north) | Sunshine (hours per year) |
|------|---------|--------------------------|---------------------------|
| Wakefield | 123 | 53.42 | 1259 |
| Stoke | 119 | 53.01 | 1298 |
| Ipswich | 86 | 52.08 | 1591 |

*Adapted with permission from the British Medical Journal Publishing Group.*

The scattergraph derived from the data is displayed in Figure 32.2 and it shows an inverse relationship: the greater the hours of sunshine per annum, the lower the SMR for coronary heart disease. A negative slope of the trend line indicates a protective effect. Once again there is only 1 degree of freedom, but the important finding is that the association is even stronger than for latitude. It can be seen that the three points are on the trend line and $R^2$ is a virtually perfect 0.9999.

**Figure 32.2 SMR for coronary heart disease and hours of sunshine**

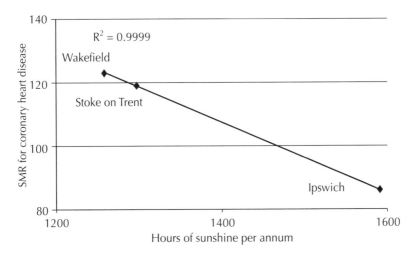

259

To take this a stage further and increase the number of data points on the scattergraph, I looked at the regions of the UK, taking average mortality rates provided by the British Heart Foundation from national statistics [4]. I added hours of sunshine per year obtained by the Manchester Weather Centre from the Meteorological Office. The data can be seen in Table 32.2 and a scattergraph is shown in Figure 32.3. We can see a strong association between the two, with a clear gradient and all points close to the trend line, and $R^2$ is high at 0.7259. This similarly suggests that the latitude effect is a reflection of exposure of the population to sunshine.

**Table 32.2 Hours of sunlight and coronary heart disease mortality in regions of the UK [4].**
CHD = coronary heart disease

| | Average hours of sunshine per annum | Age-standardised mortality rate from CHD per 100 000 |
|---|---|---|
| Wessex | 1623 | 293 |
| South-east Thames | 1613 | 293 |
| South-west Thames | 1583 | 278 |
| South Western | 1582 | 302 |
| East Anglia | 1518 | 289 |
| North-east Thames | 1492 | 300 |
| North-west Thames | 1445 | 293 |
| Oxford | 1435 | 283 |
| Wales | 1405 | 358 |
| Mersey | 1382 | 368 |
| North Western | 1368 | 393 |
| West Midlands | 1357 | 337 |
| Northern | 1347 | 387 |
| Yorkshire | 1339 | 373 |
| Trent | 1329 | 345 |
| Scotland | 1313 | 401 |
| Northern Ireland | 1230 | 443 |

*Crown © 2005, adapted with permission.*

**Figure 32.3 Coronary heart disease (CHD) and sunlight in regions of the UK [4].**

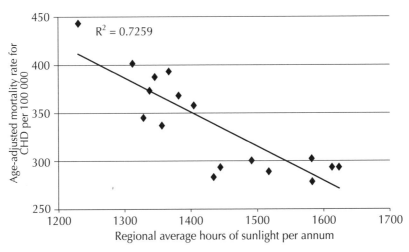

The impressive-looking scattergraph is of only relatively few data points and it cannot be regarded as conclusive, even though it is somewhat encouraging. It is necessary to test the proposal further by increasing the sample size still further. The British Heart Foundation has assembled mortality data for coronary heart disease not only for regions but also for 217 health districts in the UK [4]. I added latitude, based on a grid reference rather than degrees, and generated a scattergraph of mortality against latitude, as shown in Figure 32.4.

**Figure 32.4 The relationship between latitude and coronary heart disease mortality in the UK [4].**

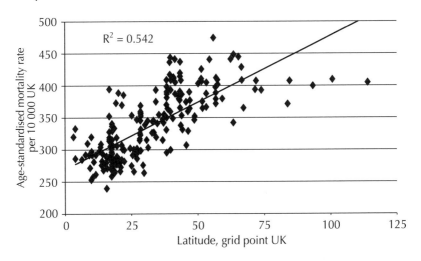

The association is quite strong, with $R^2 = 0.524$, supporting the latitude effect of death from coronary heart disease. It is important to note that, as the number of data points increases, a number of unknown variable factors will be introduced and these might lead to a reduction of $R^2$, but this is offset by the increase of power. We can see that, at a given latitude, there is vertical variation that indicates the presence of factors other than latitude.

In Figure 32.5, I have used data, obtained from the Meteorological Office, of the annual hours of sunshine for a large number of recording stations throughout the UK. I have added the age-standardised mortality rates for coronary heart disease for each locality and created another scattergraph.

**Figure 32.5 The relationship between coronary heart disease (CHD) mortality and sunshine in 217 UK localities [4].**

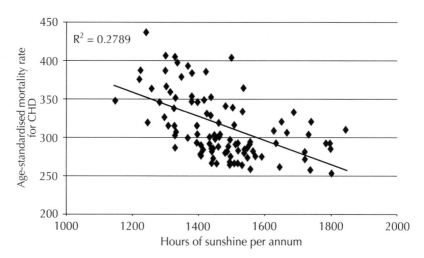

When we use sunshine data in place of latitude we can see a protective effect, with a negative slope. The association is less strong, with $R^2 = 0.2789$. This indicates that, although latitude is a major determinant of mortality rate from coronary heart disease, there is more to the latitude effect than simply the annual hours of sunshine of a wide locality. There appear to be local factors influencing mortality from coronary heart disease.

I would like to draw your attention once again to Lancashire, and to look at four towns of similar size and similar social structure. Burnley, Blackburn, Preston and Blackpool are on the same latitude, little more than 30 miles apart. The air stream is mainly from the west, bringing moist but fairly warm air off the Irish Sea. Burnley is most easterly, lying in the shadow of Pendle Hill, which, although only 500 metres high, exerts a significant effect on the local weather. The local saying is that when you can see Pendle Hill it is going to rain, and when you cannot see it, it is already raining! Blackburn lies more to the west, just among the lower hills rising into the Pennines. Preston lies on flat land on the estuary of the River Ribble. The Fylde, the flat marshy land lying north of the estuary, is now drained and is good agricultural land extending to the coast at Blackpool. The climatic advantages of proximity to the Lancashire coast are obvious to all who live there; Blackpool has been the traditional holiday and retirement destination of people from Lancashire towns.

The annual hours of sunshine of each of these towns are shown in Table 32.3 along with the respective SMR for coronary heart disease.

**Table 32.3 Sunshine and mortality in four Lancashire towns. CHD = coronary heart disease [4]**

|  | Average hours of sunshine per annum | Age-standardised mortality rate from CHD per 100 000 |
|---|---|---|
| Burnley | 1196.9 | 414.2 |
| Blackburn | 1281.3 | 407.6 |
| Preston | 1476.4 | 392.0 |
| Blackpool | 1522.4 | 378.9 |

*Crown © 2005, adapted with permission.*

It can be seen that Blackpool has the lowest SMR and Burnley the highest; the annual hours of sunshine are the opposite. Plotting these as a scattergraph, Figure 32.6 shows an extremely strong association, with $R^2 = 0.9495$. It appears, therefore, that for comparable towns on the same latitude, cloud cover reducing sunlight penetration to ground level is associated with an increased mortality from at least coronary heart disease.

**Figure 32.6 Sunshine and mortality from coronary heart disease (CHD) in four Lancashire towns [4].**

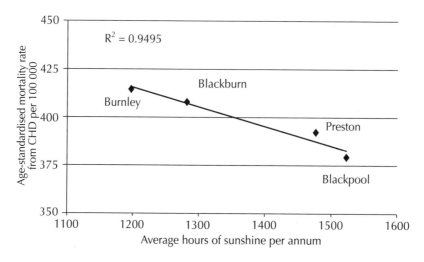

Although the national overview has some advantages, there is a need to look at some localities in more detail. For example, the more detailed analysis of the four Lancashire towns has provided some interesting information. And we have already noted the remarkable difference in life expectancy between Kensington and nearby East London.

Blackburn in Lancashire, where I work, is the centre of a population of about 250 000, with an age-standardised mortality rate above the national average. Looking in more detail, we find that the population of the inner parts of the town has an SMR of 144 compared with villages of the Ribble Valley, only about 10 miles away, where the SMR is 95. Such local differences are likely to have local rather than climatic explanations. We saw that in the 18th century the rural villages surrounding Manchester had approximately half the mortality of the inner city, and I suggested that the explanation might have been atmospheric pollution in the city, thus reducing sunlight penetration. Similarly we noted the higher mortality rates in Burnley in 1914 compared with Colne and Nelson; although there were specific explanations for the low mortality in Nelson, these did not apply to Colne. We noted that the housing in Burnley was low-lying; it would trap damp and polluted air so that sunlight penetration would be very low.

In Blackburn and other cities today there is little atmospheric pollution, but nevertheless I suggest that there is insufficient exposure of the population to sunlight. The streets are narrow and the houses are small but, of greatest importance, is that they have no gardens. This is in contrast to the Ribble Valley villages and it is an important factor in the increased susceptibility of the inner city population to premature death. We have seen that people who have gardens have higher blood vitamin D levels than those who do not, and also lower cholesterol levels. The important factor is the opportunities available to a population for leisure in the open air.

We can also see the increased burden of illness in the northern parts of the UK when we examine data for influenza. There was a minor epidemic of influenza in the UK in January 2000 and it caused a great deal of pressure on hospital beds. Figure 32.7 shows the general practice consultation rates for influenza and influenza-like illness in the second week in January 2000.

**Figure 32.7  General practitioner (GP) consultation rates for influenza in the second week in January 2000 [5].**

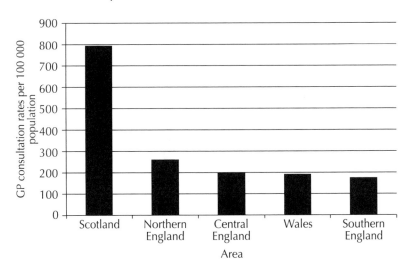

*Crown © 2005, adapted with permission.*

It is important to note the north–south gradient. Scotland showed a spectacular burden of illness, as judged from the data provided by the Public Health Laboratory Service, based on returns by the Royal College of General Practitioners [5]. We have already looked at the increased rates of illness, in particular respiratory illness, in the winter, and this could well be an effect of vitamin D insufficiency. The particularly high incidence of influenza in Scotland could be a result of particularly low vitamin D levels.

The point is that it is not just coronary heart disease that shows geographical variation within the UK, as the influenza epidemic indicates. There is a more fundamental aspect of health and susceptibility to disease. We can also see it with variant Creutzfeldt–Jakob disease (vCJD) [6]. We can see in Figure 32.8 that there is a relatively high incidence in northern England and Scotland. There might be specific explanations in respect of specific diseases such as vCJD, but the overall pattern and susceptibility of the northern populations must not be forgotten.

**Figure 32.8  Incidence of vCJD by place of residence in 1991 [6].**

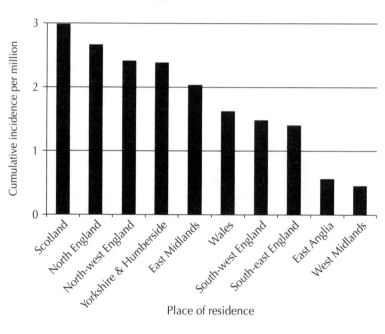

© 2001, adapted from The Lancet with permission from Elsevier.

Table 32.4 looks at the bigger picture and shows age-standardised mortality rates for a wide range of fatal diseases in the UK. We can see quite clearly that there is an increased mortality in northern areas from coronary heart disease, stroke, bronchitis and cancer. There is something that increases the susceptibility of northern populations to early death and I propose that it is a relative lack of sunlight exposure and thereby insufficiency of vitamin D.

**Table 32.4  Age-standardised mortality rates for 2000 in the UK [7].**
CHD = coronary heart disease

|  | CHD | Stroke | Bronchitis | Cancer | All causes |
|---|---|---|---|---|---|
| Males |  |  |  |  |  |
| North East | 240 | 88 | 56 | 300 | 1002 |
| North West | 235 | 84 | 54 | 279 | 982 |
| Yorkshire & Humber | 225 | 80 | 51 | 258 | 912 |
| East Midlands | 199 | 73 | 47 | 236 | 862 |
| West Midlands | 211 | 79 | 44 | 249 | 904 |
| East Anglia | 181 | 62 | 39 | 230 | 797 |
| London | 193 | 71 | 48 | 252 | 890 |
| South East | 172 | 66 | 37 | 231 | 791 |
| South West | 182 | 67 | 36 | 225 | 784 |
| England | 201 | 73 | 45 | 248 | 870 |
| Wales | 226 | 77 | 46 | 260 | 921 |
| Scotland | 238 | 92 | 54 | 298 | 1044 |
| Northern Ireland | 226 | 76 | 43 | 259 | 924 |
| UK | 207 | 75 | 45 | 254 | 892 |
| Females |  |  |  |  |  |
| North East | 200 | 137 | 55 | 275 | 1095 |
| North West | 200 | 138 | 53 | 260 | 1090 |
| Yorkshire & Humber | 183 | 129 | 47 | 248 | 1005 |
| East Midlands | 171 | 133 | 36 | 237 | 1000 |
| West Midlands | 175 | 134 | 38 | 234 | 1002 |
| East Anglia | 149 | 118 | 31 | 230 | 939 |
| London | 152 | 111 | 39 | 235 | 963 |
| South East | 144 | 119 | 30 | 228 | 917 |
| South West | 153 | 122 | 26 | 218 | 893 |
| England | 167 | 126 | 38 | 238 | 981 |
| Wales | 191 | 136 | 45 | 251 | 1039 |
| Scotland | 212 | 155 | 54 | 277 | 1121 |
| Northern Ireland | 201 | 130 | 36 | 235 | 1019 |
| UK | 173 | 129 | 40 | 243 | 999 |

*Crown © 2001, adapted with permission.*

The data also indicate an east–west gradient. The population of the East Midlands has more favourable mortality rates than that of the West Midlands. East Anglia has a similar advantage over London. The climate of the UK has not just a north–south gradient but, more accurately, a north-west to south-east gradient, characterised by wetness to dryness, the result of different amounts of cloud cover that brings rain as well as reducing the penetration of ultraviolet light to ground level.

The geography of coronary heart disease in the UK leads us to understand that place of residence is a determinant of health. The studies from Burnley, Colne and Nelson suggest that it is not just location of residence that is important but also place of birth, and it is necessary to look at the effect of migration. Does an individual take with him or her the health profile determined by place of birth, or does he or she acquire the health profile of the new location of residence?

This was investigated by the Regional Heart Study, working from the departments of clinical epidemiology and general practice at the Royal Free Hospital School of Medicine, London, UK. In this study 7735 middle-aged men were followed up for 6.5 years [8]. The geographical gradient of poor health from the south to the north of the UK was confirmed and the authors concluded [8]:

*Regardless of where they were born, men examined in Scotland experienced the highest IHD [ischaemic/coronary heart disease] risk, while those examined in the South of England had the lowest.*

In other words, an acquired local environmental factor, and I propose sunlight, is more important than inherited factors, either genetic or non-genetic. The data can be seen in Table 32.5.

**Table 32.5  Risk of major coronary event by zone of residence and migration status in 7735 middle-aged men with a 6.5-year follow-up [8].**
CHD = coronary heart disease

| | Risk of CHD event per 1000 men per year | | | | |
| --- | --- | --- | --- | --- | --- |
| | South | Midlands & Wales | North | Scotland | All zones |
| All men | 4.7 | 8.0 | 8.4 | 9.9 | 7.4 |
| Non-migrants | 6.3 | 8.6 | 9.3 | 10.6 | 8.7 |
| Internal migrants | 4.1 | 7.8 | 7.6 | 9.0 | 6.7 |
| International migrants | 2.5 | 5.6 | 7.5 | 14.7 | 5.8 |

© 1989, adapted from The Lancet with permission from Elsevier.

It is particularly noticeable that migrants into the south have a slightly lower coronary risk rate than those born in the south but certainly a lower risk than those in other locations. By far the highest risk are migrants from overseas who settle in Scotland. The overall impression is that the location of residence (columns) show greater conformity than location of birth (rows) and explains most of the risk.

We will need to look at factors other than sunshine exposure to explain the influences other than latitude. We have identified altitude and cloud cover in Lancashire and we have considered patterns of housing. But can the geographic and latitude influences on health be identified in other countries? We will need to look at Europe in more detail, and also North America, where we are likely to find accurate data.

# 33
# THE GEOGRAPHY OF CORONARY HEART DISEASE IN EUROPE

We have already touched upon this subject in Chapter 30, with the analysis of data from the Seven Countries Study [1]. The data were opportunistic and it is a tribute to Ancel Keys that he achieved so much. But the studies were not national: they were the result of the motivation of individuals who could only achieve what was possible for the clinical situations in which they found themselves. The Rome population sample was of railway workers; the Belgrade sample was university staff; other groups were agricultural workers. Although the study was extremely valuable, better sampling of the population would be necessary for greater understanding.

I think that it is likely that the inception of the Seven Countries Study inspired the World Health Organization (WHO) to gather data on disease that was not obviously microbial in causation. International epidemiology had previously been concerned mainly with infectious disease but, during the past 30 years in particular, WHO has gathered an impressive amount of data on non-infectious disease, assembled into annual reports. This has enabled the development of studies of the geography of coronary heart and other diseases, in Europe and elsewhere.

There remains the problem of the diagnostic criteria of a disease and whether they are really the same from one country to another. Death rate rather than disease incidence is the most exact measurement, and has been used extensively, but it still does not solve the problem of the accuracy of the stated cause of death. Medical communication between countries has improved, and English has become the major medical language of many countries for which English is by no means the mother tongue. This in itself is likely to improve accuracy.

I extracted relevant information from the WHO annual review of 1986 [2], specifically mortality rates for coronary heart disease, which are recorded within each nation using the International Classification of Disease (ICD). To test further the hypothesis that sunlight exposure has a major protective effect against coronary heart disease, I not only took the coronary heart disease rates for the nations concerned but also determined the latitude of those countries. This immediately presented a problem: how do we define the latitude of a country that might be, as with Japan, 1000 miles from north to south? I took the main population centre of each of the nations and determined its latitude. I obtained the sunshine data for the UK from the Manchester Weather Centre but such data were not available on an international basis. I had to use latitude as an approximation for sunshine in Europe, and the limitations of this will become obvious.

The results are shown in Table 33.1. It can be seen that the highest death rates from coronary heart disease are in northern European countries, led by Scotland, Northern Ireland, Sweden, Eire, Finland, England and Wales. The southern European countries of Spain, Portugal, Greece and France have much lower levels. Hong Kong and Japan, lying significantly closer to the equator, have the lowest levels of all.

Figure 33.1 uses the data from Table 33.1, and shows the association between age-standardised death rates from coronary heart disease and latitude. There is a moderately strong association, with $R = 0.7459$ and $R^2 = 0.5699$, which means that 57% of the variation of death rate from myocardial infarction could be explained by latitude alone. But what of the remainder? If we look at the data points above the trend line, at high latitude levels we find the countries with the highest death rates, namely Scotland, Northern Ireland, England & Wales and Sweden. These countries are close to the Atlantic Ocean and have appreciable cloud cover. We could investigate this further if the data were available, but that appears not to be the case. However, I suggest that cloud cover reducing sunlight penetration is a factor that can be added to latitude to explain susceptibility to coronary heart disease. We have seen a good example of this in the four Lancashire towns (see Chapter 32, Table 32.3).

**Table 33.1  Death rates from coronary heart disease and latitude in European and other countries [2]**

| | Age-standardised death rate for males from myocardial infarction | Latitude, degrees north |
|---|---|---|
| Scotland | 275.5 | 56 |
| Northern Ireland | 243.6 | 55 |
| Sweden | 242.4 | 58 |
| Eire | 217.9 | 53 |
| Finland | 217.3 | 61 |
| Norway | 213.7 | 60 |
| England & Wales | 200.9 | 52 |
| Czechoslovakia | 191.5 | 49 |
| Hungary | 171.5 | 47 |
| Iceland | 146.2 | 64 |
| Malta | 141.3 | 36 |
| the Netherlands | 140.9 | 52 |
| Austria | 133.5 | 48 |
| Poland | 116.5 | 52 |
| Canada | 115.1 | 47 |
| Greece | 110.2 | 39 |
| Israel | 97.0 | 33 |
| Yugoslavia | 90.7 | 43 |
| Portugal | 88.9 | 39 |
| Spain | 80.0 | 40 |
| France | 68.5 | 47 |
| Romania | 62.8 | 44 |
| Hong Kong | 34.2 | 23 |
| Japan | 29.7 | 35 |

**Figure 33.1 Mortality rate from myocardial infarction (MI) and latitude [2].**

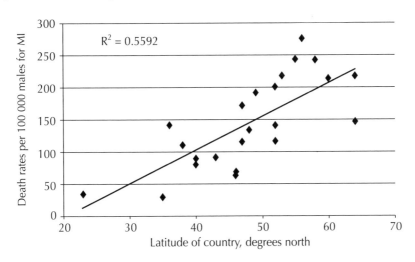

Europe in 1985 was not the same as Europe today. Since then the Soviet Union has ceased to exist, bringing independence to a significant number of countries. 1986 saw the beginning of perestroika, followed by openness of information. We now have access to reliable health data from eastern Europe and we can see that the health profile of many of these countries is very bad. Figure 33.2 shows age-standardised death rates for coronary heart disease for 1995–98; these new data were brought to my attention by a recent paper from a Swiss group [3]. The constituent countries of the UK are not identified separately and we can see that many previous Soviet nations have high age-standardised death rates, but otherwise the variations in death rates are similar to 1985.

**Figure 33.2 Age-standardised death rates for coronary heart disease, 1995–98 [3].**

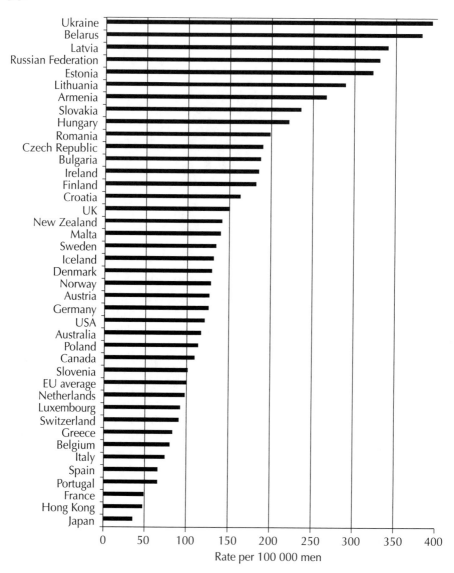

*Adapted with permission from the British Medical Journal Publishing Group.*

We can see in Figure 33.3 that once again there is an association between death rates from coronary heart disease and latitude. But there is a vertical scatter along a specific latitude. For example, if we look at latitude 50° north we can see a range of death rates from coronary heart disease. Luxembourg is the lowest, at 92.3, Germany has a rate of 125.8, the Czech Republic 190, and then Ukraine has an exceptionally high male death rate from coronary heart disease, at 393.8 per 100 000 per annum.

**Figure 33.3 Latitude and death rates from coronary heart disease [3].**

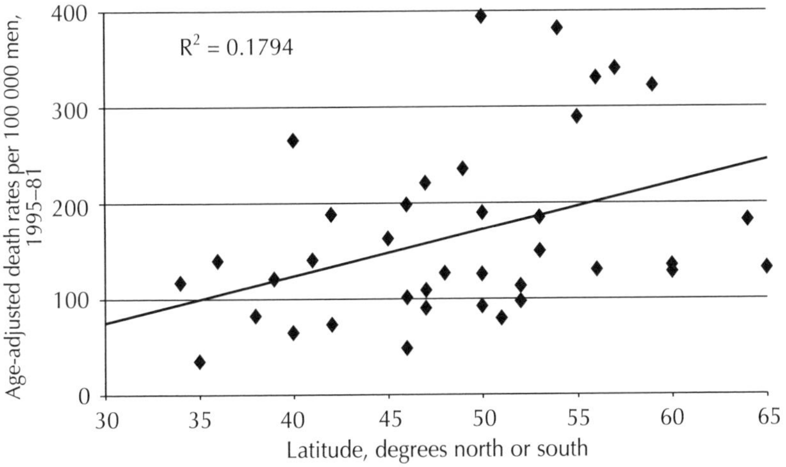

*Adapted with permission from the British Medical Journal Publishing Group.*

It is also interesting to look at the top end of the trend line of Figure 33.3, shown in more detail in Figure 33.4. We can see above the line a cluster of eastern European countries with relatively high death rates from coronary heart disease. Then we see below the line a cluster of western European countries with relatively low death rates. The difference is dramatic and indicates that in Europe there is not only a north–south gradient but also an east–west gradient.

**Figure 33.4 Latitude and death rates from coronary heart disease [3].**

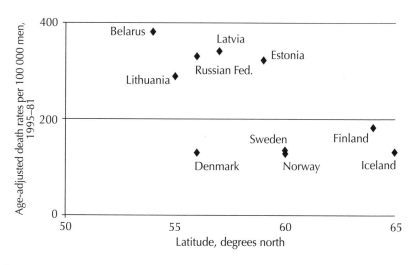

*Adapted with permission from the British Medical Journal Publishing Group.*

We do not really know a great deal about countries such as Ukraine and Belarus. We cannot be certain of their diagnostic processes or accuracy and perhaps there is over-reporting of deaths from coronary heart disease. It is easy to attribute the death of an individual to 'heart attack', as obviously the heart stops beating, but this might not be an accurate cause of death. There is probably inadequate medical intervention in poor former Soviet countries but, despite these reservations, we cannot ignore the data and we must try to learn something from it. We have seen the Leningrad paradox, in Chapter 23, that the severe social and dietary deprivations of the years of the Second World War are thought to be responsible for current high coronary death rates; perhaps the same is true for other eastern European countries. We hope that the death rates in the eastern European nations will improve in the future, with improvements in economic development, but let us not pretend that food shortages are somehow a good thing and that food surpluses automatically lead to poorer health.

I have also drawn attention to the atmospheric pollution of the UK, and London in particular, that came to an end only from the late 1950s onwards. I have mentioned in Chapter 3 that the Clean Air Act was a major public health initiative, and in a later chapter we will be looking in more detail at the relationship between atmospheric pollution and coronary heart disease. For now I would like to raise the possibility that atmospheric pollution in the major population centres of eastern European countries is likely to interact with latitude and cloud cover to reduce sunlight penetration to ground level. There may of course be other population factors, such as cigarette smoking and housing characteristics, but we will also be looking at these topics in more detail.

Martin Bobak qualified in medicine at the Charles University in Prague, Czech Republic, and with Professor Michael Marmot he has been leading the east–west research group at the London School of Hygiene and Tropical Medicine, UK. A recent review stated in reference to the east–west mortality divide [4]:

> *The reasons for these differences in mortality are not clear and data currently available permit only speculation. Determinants of the mortality gap between eastern and western Europe are probably related to the contrast in their social environments and may be similar to those underlying the social gradients mortality within countries.*

Another aspect of the geography of disease in Europe came to light in early 2005, in a Europe-wide study of antibiotic use, published in *The Lancet* [5]. There was a three-fold variation between the country with the highest antibiotic use, France, and the country with the lowest, the Netherlands. The data refer to outpatient antibiotic use only and are expressed as the defined daily dose measurement unit used by WHO. Figure 33.5 shows the details.

It is quite remarkable that the countries with the highest antibiotic use tend to be in the south of Europe and those with the lowest use tend to be in the north. The southern European countries also show a much wider seasonal variation than those in the north, with higher prescribing in the winter months. The comparison between the UK and Greece is illuminating, as shown in Figure 33.6, and it poses more questions than answers.

**Figure 33.5 Antibiotic use in European countries [5].**

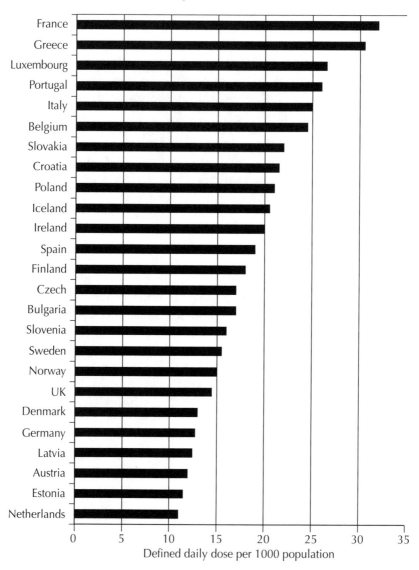

Defined daily dose per 1000 population

*© 2005, adapted from The Lancet with permission from Elsevier.*

**Figure 33.6 Seasonal variation of antibiotic use [5].**

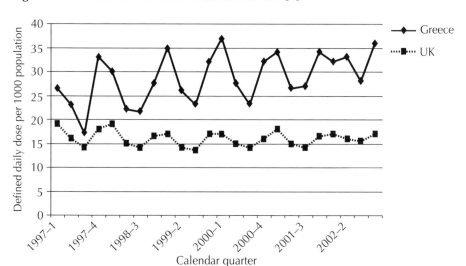

We cannot escape the possibility that the greater use of antibiotics in Mediterranean countries might be responsible for the better health of their populations. This, of course, assumes that the illness behaviour of the population and the behaviour of the doctors is the same throughout Europe, and there are reasons to believe that this is not the case. Are Mediterranean people more inclined to visit the doctor with minor illness? Is the population more demanding of antibiotics and other medications? Do Mediterranean doctors have a lower threshold for prescribing? It is likely that these suggestions are correct and that prescribing of medications other than antibiotics is higher in southern European. It is less likely that there is a greater illness burden in southern Europe that is counteracted by a widespread prescription of highly active antibiotics.

The concern about behavioural issues brings us to the important topic of social influences on life expectancy in general and the incidence of coronary heart disease in particular. But first we must look west across the Atlantic for further clues from the geography of coronary heart disease.

# 34
# THE GEOGRAPHY OF CORONARY HEART DISEASE IN THE USA

Geographical variation in the incidence of coronary heart disease in the USA has been noted for several years [1]. There is a definite pattern, with higher mortality rates in the inner cities compared with rural locations, similar to the pattern Thomas Percival observed in Manchester, England, in the late 18th century. The recognition of a pattern in Europe based on latitude provoked international interest, and led to similar investigations being undertaken in the USA.

The results were that latitude in the USA proved to have a very poor correlation with death rates from coronary heart disease. Instead, rather surprisingly, longitude seemed to be a better predictor [2]. The mortality rates were high on the east coast of the USA, gradually decreasing across the USA to the west and finally rising again on the west coast. We can see this in Figure 34.1. The data were obtained from more than 3000 counties in the USA, looking at deaths from both coronary heart disease and cerebrovascular disease. The interesting thing is that the graph looks like an inverse of the land profile of the USA, shown in Figure 34.2.

**Figure 34.1 Mortality rates for coronary heart disease and cerebrovascular disease in men in the USA [2].**

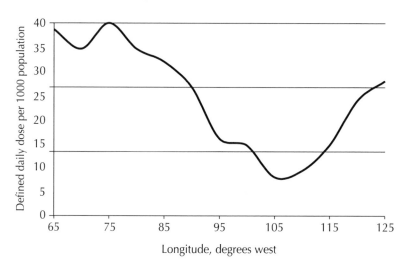

**Figure 34.2 Land mass profile of the USA.**

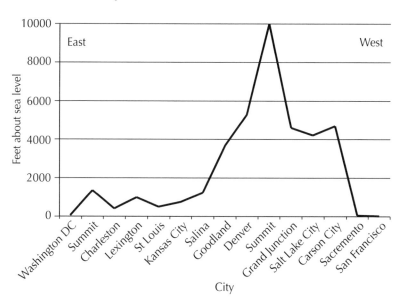

The authors performed a regression analysis of coronary heart disease rates in the 3000 locations against longitude. They found that in men there was a very strong association, with $R^2 = 0.7903$. The explanation for this phenomenon was not immediately obvious but it became clear that people living at high altitudes were somehow protected against death from coronary heart disease and stroke. A further study supported the suggestion of a decreased mortality from cardiovascular disease in people living at high altitudes [3].

A slightly earlier but less extensive study had been undertaken in New Mexico, a state in which a significant proportion of the population lives at a high altitude [4]. For the purpose of the study, the counties of the state were divided into five groups, based on altitude, the lowest being 914–1219 and the highest more than 2133 metres above sea level. The association between age-standardised death rates per 100 000 men with altitude of residence can be seen in Figure 34.3.

**Figure 34.3 Coronary heart disease (CHD) mortality and altitude of residence in New Mexico [4].**

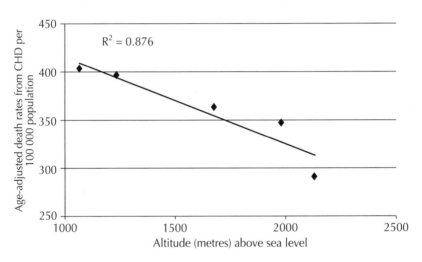

The association is very strong, with $R^2 = 0.876$. New Mexico was chosen for this study because of the range of altitude and also because it eliminated the possibility of ethnic variation influencing the longitude effect. The population of New Mexico is almost exclusively white, with only about 2% black. Slightly more than 90% of the population is white and the rest is Native American.

This study was purely observational, but with such studies there usually follows an attempt to explain the phenomenon identified in terms of existing scientific knowledge and conforming to conventional wisdom, no matter how fragile the arguments might become. In this case the authors proposed that the low oxygen concentrations of the rarefied atmosphere at high altitude would stimulate the growth of additional blood vessels within the heart muscle, improving its blood supply. This was clearly very speculative. No mention was made that the rarefied atmosphere would allow greater sunlight penetration to ground level and that this might be protective. This would conform with the experience of the Swiss, who developed heliotherapy centres at high altitude. It would also conform with the benefits of living in Nelson rather than Burnley in Lancashire, UK, early in the 20th century, where the thicker smoke-polluted and damp air in a lower lying location would prevent the penetration of sunlight, leading to higher levels of disease.

So we can see that geography describes the distribution of disease and gives us a major clue regarding the explanation of its cause. Living relatively close to the equator and living at high altitudes have one thing in common: they both result in high exposure of an individual to ultraviolet light. We should also remember that the heliotherapy of tuberculosis in Switzerland was organised to maximise ultraviolet light exposure.

This provides extremely persuasive evidence implicating sunshine as a protective mechanism against coronary heart disease and perhaps other diseases, but we must remain mindful of the fact that, whereas rickets is directly caused by vitamin D deficiency, we cannot regard vitamin D deficiency as being the direct cause of coronary heart disease. Vitamin D can only be a powerful defence factor and the cause of the disease has yet to emerge.

# 35

# THE NORTHERN IRELAND PARADOX

In Chapter 13 we looked at the geography of disease by comparing Belfast with Toulouse. We found significantly higher age-standardised rates in Belfast for coronary heart disease in particular (4.3 times that in Toulouse) but also for stroke (2.1), other cardiovascular diseases (1.4), cancer (1.3) and 'all causes' (1.8). The risks shown applied to men aged between 55 and 64 years, and the details can be seen in Table 13.1.

This was given as an example of the geographical variation of disease, without an attempt at explanation. However, the health disadvantages of living in Belfast require an explanation if public health action is to be taken, and the explanation must be robust. It has generally been based on victim-blaming: it is the fault of the people of Northern Ireland that they smoke too much, drink too much alcohol and eat the wrong foods. Before accepting such a conclusion, based on the diet–cholesterol–heart hypothesis underpinned by puritanical thinking, we need to examine the facts.

The data presented are from the MONICA study [1]. The study provides more details about the populations, in particular looking at the usual risk factors for coronary heart disease. These can be seen in Table 35.1; the data include only men.

**Table 35.1  Risk factor profiles for men from Belfast and Toulouse [1].**
HDL = high-density lipoprotein; BP = blood pressure; BMI = body mass index

| | Age 45–54 years | | Age 55–64 years | |
| --- | --- | --- | --- | --- |
| | **Belfast** | **Toulouse** | **Belfast** | **Toulouse** |
| Diabetes, % | 2.6 | 7.2 | 3.5 | 10.9 |
| Hypertension, % | 20.6 | 27.5 | 33.5 | 49 |
| Cigarette smoking, % | 32.2 | 35.3 | 22.9 | 36.2 |
| Total cholesterol, mmol/L | 6.19 | 5.94 | 6.12 | 5.98 |
| HDL cholesterol, mmol/L | 1.22 | 1.39 | 1.28 | 1.34 |
| BP, mean mm Hg | 101.3 | 102.1 | 103.8 | 106.7 |
| BMI, kg/m$^2$ | 26.3 | 26.0 | 26.7 | 26.4 |
| Probability of CHD | 0.016 | 0.015 | 0.042 | 0.041 |

*Adapted from the* QMJ *with permission from Oxford University Press.*

If we look at this carefully, we can see that it is not the background characteristics that make the people of Belfast more susceptible to coronary heart disease. Diabetes is perhaps surprisingly more than twice as common in Toulouse and so is hypertension (high blood pressure). A greater proportion of the population of Toulouse smokes and blood pressure (BP) is slightly higher. The body mass index (BMI) is calculated as weight in kilograms divided by body surface area, a height–weight index; the average is similar for the two populations. We can see that total serum cholesterol is higher in Belfast, but we now know that this is a latitude effect. The other advantage of the population of Toulouse is a higher high-density lipoprotein (HDL) cholesterol level.

Overall, however, there is little to separate the two populations and they have the same overall risk factors for developing coronary heart disease. The risks are amalgamated into a risk score, shown on the bottom line of Table 35.1, indicating the probability of developing coronary heart disease. The score is based on age, cigarette smoking, serum total cholesterol, systolic blood pressure and body mass index. The scores for Belfast and Toulouse are identical, indicating that the different mortality rates cannot be explained on existing understanding. Note that it does not involve diabetes: a score doing so would give the population of Belfast a distinct risk advantage.

Why is there such a difference between the predictions shown in Table 35.1 and the observations that we have seen in Table 13.1? There is clearly a major factor that is not yet recognised. The original authors inevitably looked at diet for an explanation but, as is shown in Table 35.2, no obvious explanation appeared.

**Table 35.2 Nutrient intake in Belfast and Toulouse, average per day (men aged 45–64 years) [1]**

|  | Belfast | Toulouse |
|---|---|---|
| Total energy, kcal | 2340 | 2295 |
| Protein, g | 82.8 | 96.8 |
| Fat, g | 99.8 | 92.3 |
| Carbohydrate, g | 270 | 235 |
| Cholesterol, g | 319 | 479 |
| Alcohol, g | 12.1 | 21.7 |
| Sugar, g | 104 | 79.1 |
| Starch, g | 151 | 143 |
| Fibre, g | 21.1 | 19.5 |

*Adapted from the QMJ with permission from Oxford University Press.*

In particular, dietary excesses of protein, fat and cholesterol could not explain the great excess of mortality in Belfast. The population of Toulouse consumed more tomatoes per head than that of Belfast, but there was no obvious food that might have been damaging and, as the authors expressed [1]:

*Neither the classic risk factor scores nor the similarity in major nutrient intake adequately explain the large differences in IHD [ischaemic/ coronary heart disease] and other causes of mortality between the centres.*

So this is what we might call the Northern Ireland paradox: a population with an extremely high incidence of coronary heart disease that does not demonstrate the risk factors or dietary indiscretions that would be expected from the diet–cholesterol–heart hypothesis.

The MONICA study referred to above was fairly small. The mortality data applied to the total populations of the cities but the risk factor profiles were based on samples of 366 people in Belfast and 400 in Toulouse. The dietary assessments were based on 80 and 40 men, respectively.

This publication was followed in 1998 by the PRIME study, also appearing in the *Quarterly Journal of Medicine* [2]. The purpose of this study was to explore further the Northern Ireland paradox, to try to explain 'the several-fold differences in risk of coronary heart disease between France and Northern Ireland'. The study investigated much larger population samples, 2748 men in Belfast and 2610 in Toulouse. The pattern of coronary heart disease is shown in Table 35.3.

**Table 35.3  Coronary heart disease in Belfast and Toulouse (men aged 45–64 years) [2]**

|  | Belfast | Toulouse |
|---|---|---|
| Myocardial infarction (MI) (% of total population) | 6.1 | 1.1 |
| Angina (% of total population) | 7.1 | 1.5 |
| Other coronary heart disease (% of total population) | 1.2 | 0.5 |
| MI rate men aged 35–64 years (per 100 000 population) | 781 | 240 |

*Adapted from the QMJ with permission from Oxford University Press.*

We see once again the extraordinarily high rate of coronary heart disease in men living in Belfast compared with those living in Toulouse; the incidence of myocardial infarction is three times higher. The study looked at the background risk indicators to attempt to find an explanation, and these are shown in Table 35.4.

**Table 35.4  Risk indicators for coronary heart disease in men in Belfast and Toulouse [2]**

|  | Belfast | Toulouse |
|---|---|---|
| Diabetes, % | 1.6 | 8.9 |
| Hypertension, % | 17.2 | 24.7 |
| Cigarette smoking, % | 24.6 | 20 |
| Total cholesterol, mmol/L | 5.9 | 5.51 |
| HDL cholesterol, mmol/L | 1.19 | 1.24 |
| Triglyceride, mmol/L | 2 | 1.49 |
| Fibrinogen, g/L | 3.64 | 3.15 |
| BP, mean mm Hg | 107.8 | 103.1 |
| BMI, kg/m$^2$ | 26.3 | 26.0 |
| Probability of CHD | 0.022 | 0.016 |

*Adapted from the QMJ with permission from Oxford University Press.*

Here we draw a blank. The various risk indicators, excluding diabetes (which is very powerful), show only a very marginally increased risk for the men of Belfast. The prediction of coronary heart disease thus falls very far short of the observed three-fold difference in disease incidence. The conclusion of the study is that 'The levels of the classical risk factors found in this study … cannot explain the large differences in the incidence of IHD [CHD] which exist' [2].

I emphasise that the classical risk factors are based mainly on the diet–cholesterol–heart hypothesis, which is clearly untenable but on which public health policies continue to be based. The authors of this study did not suggest a latitude effect, a climatic factor or differential rates of sunshine exposure.

Let us not forget that the MONICA study showed increased death rates in Belfast not only from cardiovascular disease but also from 'all causes', including cancer. There is clearly some fundamental aspect of health that is disordered in Northern Ireland and the evidence is strong that this is lack of sunlight and thereby vitamin D.

# 36
# THE FRENCH PARADOX AND THE EFFECT OF ALCOHOL

Conventional wisdom based on the diet–cholesterol–heart hypothesis is that a diet high in animal fat is the cause of coronary heart disease, mediated by an excess of cholesterol in the blood with consequent deposition of cholesterol in the coronary and other arteries. We have seen that this hypothesis has come up against several uncomfortable and undisputed observations. The Northern Ireland paradox is one of these, but there is also the better-known French paradox.

In France a high animal fat diet is considered the norm, and we have seen this in the previous chapter. This discordance with the diet–cholesterol–heart hypothesis led to the identification of the 'French paradox', reviewed in 1992 by Renaud and de Lorgeril of the Nutrition and Vascular Pathophysiology Research Unit, Bron Cedex, France [1]. The phenomenon of a diet high in animal fat with a low incidence of coronary heart disease is not confined to France, thus it is sometimes called the Mediterranean paradox.

Gerona, on the Mediterranean coast of northern Spain, is a place where the incidence of myocardial infarction is low but there is a high incidence of cardiovascular risk factors [2]. An investigation was undertaken by the Lipid and Cardiovascular Epidemiology Unit in Barcelona, Spain, looking at the population of Gerona. The group studied 2004 inhabitants aged between 25 and 74 years and found the coronary risk factors to be as shown in Table 36.1.

**Table 36.1  Characteristics of the population of Gerona, Spain [2]**

|                      | Men  | Women |
| -------------------- | ---- | ----- |
| Cholesterol, mean mmol/L | 5.72 | 5.66 |
| Hypertension, %      | 38.3 | 35.2 |
| Cigarette smoking, % | 29.6 | 17.0 |
| BMI, kg/m$^2$        | 26.0 | 26.0 |
| Definite angina, %   | 3.0  | 3.9 |

We can see the corresponding distribution of serum cholesterol in Figure 36.1, and it shows that more than 50% of the population sample from Gerona has a serum cholesterol higher than the 5.2 mmol/L, now recommended as the threshold for 'treatment'.

**Figure 36.1  Distribution of serum cholesterol in Gerona, Spain (population aged 25–74 years) [2].**

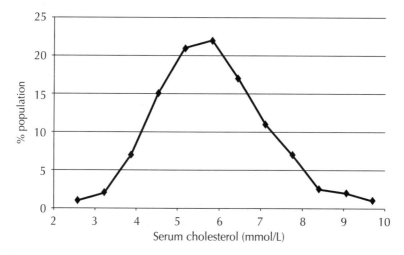

We therefore might identify this as the Gerona paradox, to add to the French paradox; it casts further doubt on the validity of the traditional view of causation of coronary heart disease.

A paradox, or anomaly, means that data do not fit in with expectations of the popular hypothesis. Either the original hypothesis must be rejected or the paradox must be explained away by a subordinate hypothesis. There is a great reluctance to reject the diet–cholesterol–heart hypothesis as there is so much vested interest in research and medical establishments, research grants and the nutrition industry. The tendency is for subordinate hypotheses to be generated.

A recent review by Professor Jean Ferrières of the Department of Epidemiology, University School of Medicine, Toulouse, France, published in the specialist journal *Heart*, made no acknowledgement that the French paradox might invalidate the diet–heart hypothesis [3]. He summarised a large number of subordinate hypotheses that might allow the French paradox to be incorporated into the major hypothesis without disrupting conventional wisdom. The most popular of these is that the low coronary heart disease mortality in France is the result of a high consumption of red wine that somehow more than compensates for the high cholesterol diet. In Table 35.2, we have seen that the population of Toulouse consumes a greater average intake of alcohol than the population of Belfast and that, of course, fuelled suggestions that alcohol, or specifically red wine, might be protective. At present there is a crisis among the wine producers of France as the per capita alcohol consumption has fallen by 50% [4]. This is the result of public health initiatives. Based on the general explanation of the French paradox, that wine is protective against coronary heart disease, and the diet–cholesterol–heart hypothesis, we should expect to see a significant increase in deaths from coronary heart disease in France. We have not done so far. If it does not happen then it could be called the second French paradox or, more simply, invalidation of the postulated health benefit of red wine.

Once again, we have an attempt to explain away a paradox by special reasoning and this has been accepted without significant supportive evidence. Red wine is being scrutinised to find a chemical property that might possibly and logically be cardioprotective, but protective against what? What is the nature of the disease? The scrutiny that we have applied indicates that coronary heart disease cannot be the result of faulty diet. We must observe the reasoning of Paracelsus, that coronary heart disease is a specific disease and we must look for a specific cause.

The red wine subordinate hypothesis has generated further research to identify components of red wine that might have a beneficial effect on cardiovascular physiology. However, this misses the point that we are really looking at a Mediterranean paradox; the expression French paradox should be abandoned. Furthermore, the Mediterranean area exerts an effect that goes well beyond cardiovascular disease; it is of benefit to health in general, including cancer, as we have already seen.

Medicine is so often driven by evangelism rather than reason and this has led to the red wine story reaching what can only be called silly proportions. For example, in a UK hospital red wine is offered on wards to patients who have survived a heart attack [4] but without supportive evidence of benefit [5]. It shows how vulnerable clinical medicine can be to fashion, especially when promoted by a passionate supporter. Of course the alcohol industry itself is powerful and sees an opportunity in the medical use of red wine.

There are voices of caution, those who believe that there should be restraint in the medical use of alcohol [6]. They have pointed out that the US Bureau of Alcohol, Tobacco and Firearms has approved new wine labels that advise patients to consult their family doctor about 'the health effects of wine consumption'.

There have been reports of the relationship between alcohol and mortality being U-shaped, as illustrated in Figure 36.2. The study shown was undertaken by Michael Marmot and his colleagues at the London School of Hygiene and Tropical Medicine, UK [7].

**Figure 36.2 Ten-year mortality related to alcohol consumption [7].**
CHD = coronary heart disease

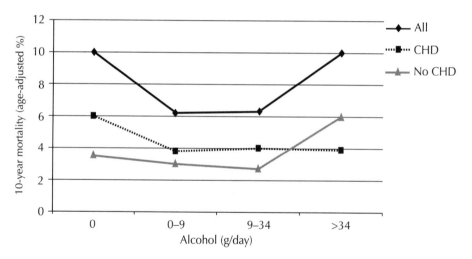

© 1981, adapted from The Lancet with permission from Elsevier.

The lowest mortality was observed among those who drank some alcohol, with a higher mortality among those who drank none. Not surprisingly those who drink large amounts of alcohol had the highest mortality, but not from coronary heart disease. These findings can be interpreted as showing that a little alcohol is beneficial but there is no obvious or plausible explanation of why this should be. Alcohol is not known to contain specific vitamins or essential trace elements, but the possibility of benefit from alcohol cannot be discounted.

On the other hand, members of the Church of the Latter Day Saints, Seventh Day Adventists and other Christian religious groups drink no alcohol and have an extremely good health profile, well above average [8]. Priests of the Church of the Latter Day Saints, mainly in the state of Utah in the USA, have the best health in that country, with an SMR of only 35, against the national average of 100. But it is not just in this church that religious practice appears to be of major importance regarding population health. Susan Lutgendorf and her colleagues from the University of Iowa, USA, conducted a detailed study of the long-term effects of religious worship, which showed a remarkably beneficial effect, illustrated in Figure 36.3 [9]. This was a very detailed sociological prospective study of 557 people, followed up for 6 years; the frequency of religious attendance was one of many parameters measured.

**Figure 36.3 Religious participation and mortality [9].**

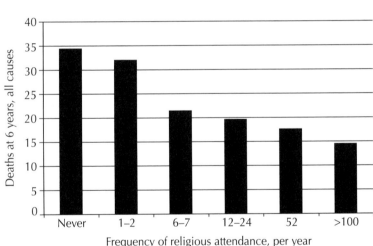

*Adapted from Health Psychology with permission from the American Psychological Association.*

The 6-year mortality of those with no religious attendance was twice that of those who attended twice per week or more. Here is perhaps a great opportunity for preventive medicine, but also a great challenge.

The mechanism linking religious devotion with good health is far from clear. Perhaps it is the result of divine intervention acting with an ecumenical perspective, but we must also look at explanations from aspects of human behaviour. People who devote themselves to religion tend to lead lives without risk and with minimal misbehaviour. They usually avoid 'sins of the flesh' and pleasures such as cigarettes and alcohol. Lutgendorf and colleagues [9] went on to look at the relationship between religious attendance and inflammatory markers in the blood, choosing interleukin-6 (IL-6). They found that the lowest level of IL-6 was found in those with the most frequent attendance, indicating a low level of inflammatory activity.

As those who practise religious worship tend to drink very little if any alcohol, it has been questioned whether the alleged benefit from a small amount of alcohol is real or an observation for which a different interpretation would be appropriate. The alternative interpretation, with some objective foundation, is that many people drink no alcohol because they are ill, and this illness could be responsible for their higher mortality, not the absence of alcohol.

Katherine Bradley and Joseph Merrill of the departments of Medicine and Health Science at the University of Washington, USA, writing in a commentary in *The Lancet*, drew attention to the fact that all the evidence regarding a possible beneficial effect of alcohol on the heart has been based on simple uncontrolled observations. There are no intervention studies to see whether alcohol is of benefit, but of course such a clinical experiment would be impossible to implement. A study of 22 071 USA male physicians reported the following conclusion: 'Light-to-moderate alcohol consumption reduces the overall risk of stroke … in men' [10]. This illustrates a careless use of language: it was an observational study and not an intervention study. The word 'reduces' is not appropriate; it should read: 'Light-to-moderate alcohol consumption is associated with a lower risk of stroke in men'. The benefit of a small amount of alcohol has not always been identified but the disadvantage of a large amount is clear [11].

We must therefore use judgement in our advice to patients, by which I mean giving advice without conclusive evidence. Personal prejudices come into play and different doctors will have different opinions. My view is that if the advice to drink red wine is based on the so-called French paradox, and that would appear to be the case, then there is an inherent fault and the advice is baseless. If people wish to drink wine or any other alcoholic beverage for pleasure rather than a sense of duty, then they should do so, while accepting that a large amount can, and indeed does, cause serious illness.

But let us return to the French paradox. When we compare France with Northern Ireland, for example, we are looking at geography as well as national characteristics. The PRIME study [12] provides much more information than just the comparison between Belfast and Toulouse [13], it also provides information about the populations of Lille and Strasbourg. We have seen that a great deal of information can be obtained by looking at patterns within countries. Investigations in the UK and USA have demonstrated differences in mortality that can be explained on the basis of physical geography; differential exposure to sunlight seems to hold the key to understanding. Might the same be true in France?

Toulouse is in the south of France, Strasbourg in the centre, close to the border with Germany, and Lille is in the north. Table 36.2 gives their geographical characteristics.

**Table 36.2 Characteristics of three cities in France**

|  | Latitude, degrees north | Altitude, metres above sea level |
| --- | --- | --- |
| Lille | 50° 40′ | 48 |
| Strasbourg | 49° 15′ | 154 |
| Toulouse | 43° 25′ | 152 |

Table 36.3 gives details of the mortality patterns of the three cities and, once again, we can see a relationship with latitude, with the highest death rate in Lille in the north, the lowest in Toulouse in the south and an intermediate level in Strasbourg.

**Table 36.3 Coronary heart disease in France, deaths per 100 population per annum [12]**

|  | Lille | Strasbourg | Toulouse |
| --- | --- | --- | --- |
| Myocardial infarction | 2.1 | 1.8 | 1.1 |
| Angina | 3.6 | 2.9 | 1.5 |
| Other coronary heart disease | 1.3 | 0.2 | 0.4 |

*Adapted from the* QMJ *with permission from Oxford University Press.*

Figure 36.4 shows this in graphical form and we can see a strong association, with $R^2 = 0.9899$ being almost the maximum, but must acknowledge that the sample size of three is the very minimum.

**Figure 36.4 Latitude and deaths from myocardial infarction in France [12].**

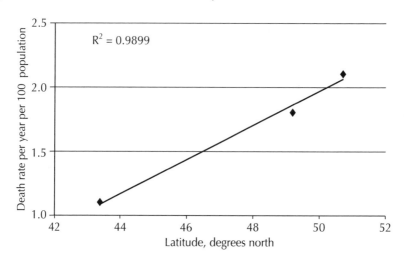

Adapted from the QMJ with permission from Oxford University Press.

Once again we can see from Table 36.4 that classical risk factors provide no explanation for the increased incidence of coronary heart disease in the centre and north of France. Most lifestyle indicators, for example cigarette smoking, are similar for all three cities. Toulouse in the south has the lowest average serum cholesterol level, as we might now expect.

**Table 36.4 Risk factor profiles for Belfast and Toulouse [12]**

|  | Lille | Strasbourg | Toulouse |
|---|---|---|---|
| Diabetes, % | 12.6 | 9.3 | 8.9 |
| Hypertension, % | 25.8 | 23.4 | 24.7 |
| Cigarette smoking, % | 19.9 | 19.5 | 20.0 |
| Total cholesterol, mmol/L | 5.7 | 5.8 | 5.5 |
| HDL cholesterol, mmol/L | 1.4 | 1.3 | 1.2 |
| Triglyceride, mmol/L | 1.6 | 1.7 | 1.5 |
| Fibrinogen, g/L | 3.2 | 3.2 | 3.2 |
| BP, mean mm Hg | 112.8 | 111.0 | 103.1 |
| BMI, kg/m$^2$ | 26.5 | 27.4 | 26.3 |
| Probability of CHD | 0.023 | 0.021 | 0.016 |

Adapted from the QMJ with permission from Oxford University Press.

The French paradox is not specifically French: it is an expression of the general latitude effect of mortality in Europe. If we acknowledge this and recognise the importance of sunlight as a unifying factor of susceptibility to disease, then the paradox ceases to exist: it is something that is only to be expected. We do not require subordinate hypotheses, such as the supposed red wine effect; we just need to reject the underlying diet–cholesterol–heart hypothesis. The French paradox simply indicates the protective effect of the Mediterranean sun and vitamin D. It is unfortunate that the epidemiological investigations did not include blood levels of vitamin D of the populations studies. Such investigations will only take place if a supporting hypothesis has been developed and that is not the case at the present time. It is possible that there are blood samples from previous studies that are stored frozen, awaiting further testing in the future. Perhaps such testing will be for vitamin D levels, as calcidiol.

We clearly need to take a fresh look at the French, or Mediterranean, paradox. To try to bring together health issues, food, alcohol and climate, it might be useful to investigate the agricultural patterns within Europe.

# 37
# THE GEOGRAPHY OF
# AGRICULTURE IN EUROPE

Minerva presents a weekly column on the last page of the *British Medical Journal*, in which she gives brief comments on and reviews of the world medical press. A recent statement was as follows [1]:

> *Japanese eat very little fat, while people in Mexico eat lots. Both groups suffer fewer heart attacks than the British or Americans. Africans drink very little red wine, while the Italians drink large volumes of the stuff – both of these groups too have fewer heart attacks. An epidemiological conclusion might be that you should eat and drink what you like: speaking English seems to be what kills you.*

I would endorse the advice that we should eat and drink what we like, but we should control the quantity. Changing our language cannot be expected to help, it is one of those factors that must be regarded as an indicator rather than a cause. It is the location in which we live that determines both the English language we speak and early death. Minerva was issuing a warning about jumping to dietary conclusions, and we have seen that the diet–cholesterol–heart hypothesis does not have a strong foundation. Once again the association between speaking English and having a life span that, by present-day European standards, is not very long cannot be assumed to be a simple cause–effect relationship but must be linked by some common cause.

Let us remember the two foundations of the diet–cholesterol–heart hypothesis. The first was the observation of cholesterol in the atherosclerotic lesions of the coronary and other arteries. It was assumed that it was a prime mover of disease and no-one really questioned its role, no-one, that is, until fairly recently. We will be dealing with this in a later chapter.

The other foundation was the work of Ancel Keys, with the Seven Countries Study [2]; he noted an association between the average animal fat intake of a population and mortality rate from coronary heart disease. We saw this in Figure 30.2, and also in Figure 30.1, which showed an association with all causes of death, an observation that suggests a more fundamental factor relating to health. But on the basis of observation alone and without the support of intervention studies, Keys became a strong proponent of the 'healthy low fat' diet. In fact he helped his wife produce a recipe book!

We have seen that the associations demonstrated by Keys are an effect of latitude. The relationship between diet, latitude and coronary heart disease is generally explained by the traditional model. There is an assumed direct relationship between these factors: climate, acting particularly through sunshine, influences local diet, which in turn influences serum cholesterol and thereby influences the risk of development of coronary heart disease. This, the diet–cholesterol–heart hypothesis, is shown in Figure 37.1.

**Figure 37.1 A model of the relationships between climate, diet and coronary heart disease.**

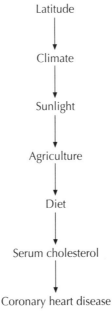

Latitude

↓

Climate

↓

Sunlight

↓

Agriculture

↓

Diet

↓

Serum cholesterol

↓

Coronary heart disease

The second model is the one that I propose, and it can be seen in Figure 37.2. Sunlight protects against coronary heart disease directly and thereby has an important role in maintaining good health. Sunshine also has an effect on local agriculture and thus on diet. Sunshine has a direct influence on serum cholesterol, as we have seen in earlier chapters.

**Figure 37.2 An alternative model of the relationships between climate, diet and coronary heart disease.**

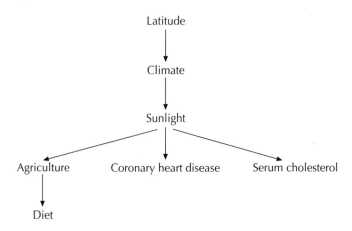

We can see the close associations between agriculture and diet with coronary heart disease and serum cholesterol. It is thus easy to see why the three have been linked together to form the diet–cholesterol–heart hypothesis. I propose that this is an incorrect interpretation and that the true interpretation is as shown in Figure 37.2. Sunshine has the three separate effects mentioned; it acts directly and favourably on human metabolism and not via a dietary intermediary mechanism.

Let us look at some evidence to support such an assertion, in particular evidence concerning agriculture. We can obtain health and mortality data from the WHO yearbooks [3]. We can obtain data concerning agriculture from *Eurostat*, a monthly publication of the European Union (EU), although, of course, the latter data apply only to Europe [4].

Several foods have been linked with coronary heart disease but, with the exception of oily fish, the associations are far from convincing. Dairy products and animal fats have been proposed as damaging; olive oil and wine have been proposed as protective. We can see the production of these in Table 37.1, which shows the agricultural production of various crops in countries of the EU.

Table 37.1 Agricultural production in the EU [3,4]. h = hectares; t = tonnes

| | Beef 1000 h 2002 | Sheep 1000 h 2002 | Milk 1000 t 2002 | Barley 1000 t 2001–02 | Wheat 1000 t 2001–02 | Seed oil 1000 t 2000–01 | Veg. oils 1000 t 1999–2000 | Wine 1000 hl 2001–02 | Death rate from CHD | Population 000s |
|---|---|---|---|---|---|---|---|---|---|---|
| Finland | 1012 | 67 | 2532 | 1786 | 489 | 72 | 85 | 96 | 217 | 5183 |
| Sweden | 1576 | 427 | 3274 | 1642 | 2345 | 129 | 98 | 241 | 242 | 8835 |
| Denmark | 1740 | 92 | 4590 | 3966 | 4664 | 292 | 193 | | 190 | 1700 |
| UK | 10 381 | 24 888 | 14 912 | 6700 | 11 564 | 1172 | 855 | 1392 | 200.5 | 59 200 |
| Ireland | 6333 | 4829 | 5230 | 1277 | 769 | 13 | 1103 | 124 | 218 | 3883 |
| the Netherlands | 3780 | 1300 | 10 795 | 387 | 991 | | 1183 | | 141 | 15 892 |
| Belgium | 2758 | 146 | 3160 | 369 | 1457 | 29 | 657 | 407 | 140 | 10 200 |
| Luxembourg | 190 | 8 | 271 | 54 | 54 | | | 250 | 104 | 439 |
| Germany | 13 732 | 2145 | 27 904 | 13 434 | 22 708 | 3798 | 2899 | 14 770 | 159 | 82 425 |
| Austria | 2067 | 304 | 3316 | 1012 | 1462 | 229 | 119 | 2988 | 133.5 | 8151 |
| France | 19 777 | 9127 | 26 029 | 9799 | 30 189 | 5626 | 1254 | 55 072 | 68.5 | 60 424 |
| Spain | 6478 | 23 813 | 7521 | 6245 | 3342 | 6057 | 1846 | 32 091 | 80 | 40 217 |
| Portugal | 1395 | 3457 | 2235 | 13 | 51 | 396 | 243 | 11 984 | 89 | 10 524 |
| Italy | 6695 | 8138 | 11 467 | 1126 | 2789 | 4219 | 1368 | 34 877 | 98 | 58 057 |
| Greece | 573 | 8932 | 1903 | 249 | 401 | 2927 | 591 | 1903 | 110 | 10 648 |

**Table 37.2 Agricultural production in the EU per million population [3,4]. h = hectares; t = tonnes**

| | Beef 1000 h 2002 | Sheep 1000 h 2002 | Milk 1000 t 2002 | Barley 1000 t 2001–02 | Wheat 1000 t 2001–02 | Seed oil 1000 t 2000–01 | Veg. oils 1000 t 1999–2000 | Wine 1000 hl 2001–02 | Death rate from CHD | Population 000s |
|---|---|---|---|---|---|---|---|---|---|---|
| Finland | 195 | 13 | 489 | 345 | 94 | 14 | 16 | 19 | 217 | 5183 |
| Sweden | 178 | 48 | 371 | 186 | 265 | 15 | 11 | 27 | 242 | 8835 |
| Denmark | 1024 | 54 | 2700 | 2333 | 2744 | 172 | 114 | | 190 | 1700 |
| UK | 175 | 420 | 252 | 113 | 195 | 20 | 14 | 24 | 200.5 | 59 200 |
| Ireland | 1631 | 1244 | 1347 | 329 | 198 | 3 | 284 | 32 | 218 | 3883 |
| the Netherlands | 238 | 82 | 679 | 24 | 62 | | 74 | | 141 | 15 892 |
| Belgium | 270 | 14 | 310 | 36 | 143 | 3 | 64 | 40 | 140 | 10 200 |
| Luxembourg | 433 | 18 | 617 | 123 | 123 | | | 569 | 104 | 439 |
| Germany | 167 | 26 | 339 | 163 | 275 | 46 | 35 | 179 | 159 | 82 425 |
| Austria | 254 | 37 | 407 | 124 | 179 | 28 | 15 | 367 | 133.5 | 8151 |
| France | 327 | 151 | 431 | 162 | 500 | 93 | 21 | 911 | 68.5 | 60 424 |
| Spain | 161 | 592 | 187 | 155 | 83 | 151 | 46 | 798 | 80 | 40 217 |
| Portugal | 133 | 328 | 212 | 1 | 5 | 38 | 23 | 1139 | 89 | 10 524 |
| Italy | 115 | 140 | 198 | 19 | 48 | 73 | 24 | 601 | 98 | 58 057 |
| Greece | 54 | 839 | 179 | 23 | 38 | 275 | 56 | 179 | 110 | 10 648 |

302

Of course some countries are large and some are small. Some export agricultural products and some import. Table 37.2 shows the same data but, in an attempt to introduce comparability, I have related the production to head of population for each of the countries. In this table we can see the enormous productivity of agriculture in Ireland and Denmark in relation to their small populations.

Ireland's agriculture is based on beef, sheep and milk production. All these require grass and a great deal of water. Ireland has both of these: the climate prohibits the growth of most foods on a large scale but water is readily available through almost constant rainfall. Denmark has a high production of cereals: wheat and barley. For these to reach maturity, dryness and sunshine are necessary on a scale not available in Ireland.

Whereas Ireland and Denmark are agricultural nations, the UK is largely industrial. However, the production of beef, sheep, milk, barley and wheat are high in absolute terms (Table 37.1), once again reflecting the climate. We shall be looking at the regional productions shortly.

Sheep can survive with little water and sheep grazing is a feature of all countries. Although Ireland is most productive, there is no association between sheep and coronary heart disease deaths. The $R^2$ is only 0.0019 (Figure 37.3).

**Figure 37.3 Sheep production and coronary heart disease (CHD) in the EU.**

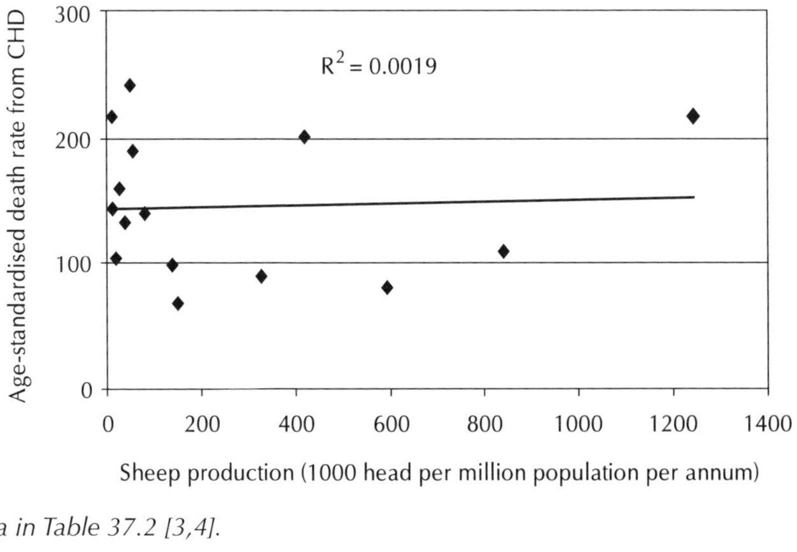

Sheep production (1000 head per million population per annum)

*Data in Table 37.2 [3,4].*

Beef production is also widespread with no overall association with coronary heart disease. Figure 37.4 and Table 37.2 show the very high productivity per capita of beef in Ireland, seemingly associated with a high death rate from coronary heart disease, but the overall picture including other countries in the regression analysis leads to the conclusion that there is no cause–effect relationship between the two.

**Figure 37.4  Beef production and coronary heart disease (CHD) in the EU.**

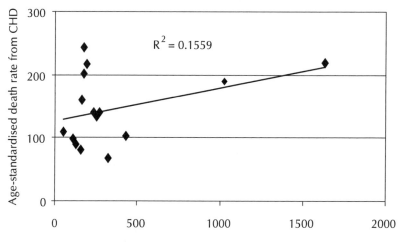

Beef production (1000 head per million population per annum)

*Data in Table 37.2 [3,4].*

Milk production is similar to that of beef, and only Ireland and Denmark, with high coronary heart disease incidences, have particularly high productivity (Figure 37.5). Despite advice to avoid dairy products, there is no association to suggest that milk production might cause high mortality from coronary heart disease: I would suggest that climate is responsible for both.

**Figure 37.5  Milk production and coronary heart disease (CHD) in the EU.**

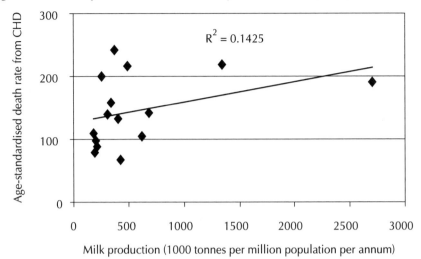

*Data in Table 37.2 [3,4].*

Barley production similarly shows no significant association with coronary heart disease (Figure 37.6). Barley production is extraordinarily high in Denmark, whose population has just above average risk of death from coronary heart disease.

**Figure 37.6  Barley production and coronary heart disease (CHD) in the EU.**

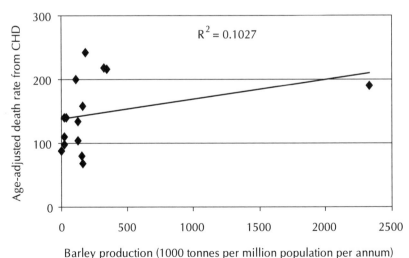

*Data in Table 37.2 [3,4].*

The production of wheat requires much more sunlight than other cereals and it will not mature without plenty of sun in July and August. If the rainfall is too great, wheat cannot be harvested and will rot in the fields, as happened in the UK in the summer of 2004. The grey skies of the British Isles do not enable the harvesting of wheat to the same extent as the clear blue skies of southern and central Europe. However, wheat contributes so much to our diet that its production occurs all over Europe. France produces the most wheat, and Denmark has by far the highest productivity per capita. There is no association between wheat production and death from coronary heart disease (Figure 37.7), the poor association shown by $R^2 = 0.0549$.

**Figure 37.7 Wheat production and coronary heart disease (CHD) in the EU.**

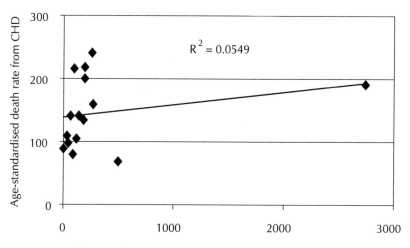

*Data in Table 37.2 [3,4].*

Although vegetable oils are generally thought to be good for us, containing polyunsaturated fats, Figure 37.8 shows no association between their production and coronary heart disease deaths. What can be seen is the particularly high productivity in Ireland, a country where the population has a high mortality from coronary heart disease, indicating lack of protection.

**Figure 37.8 Vegetable oil production and coronary heart disease (CHD) in the EU.**

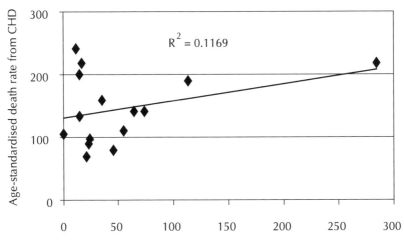

Data in Table 37.2 [3,4].

Seed oils include olive oil and grape seed oil. Spain, Greece, Italy France and Germany are the highest producers of seed oil, although olive oil is not produced in Germany; the production of that country refers to grape seed oil. Greece has the highest production per capita of mainly olive oil. There is a negative association of seed oil production with deaths from coronary heart disease, shown in Figure 37.9, but only with an $R^2$ of 0.1182. Those countries producing seed oils have lower mortality rates from coronary heart disease. My interpretation is that a climate with adequate sunshine to allow the production of olive oil gives the local population a significant health advantage.

**Figure 37.9 Seed oil production and coronary heart disease (CHD) in the EU.**

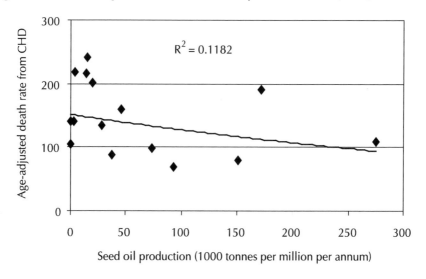

*Data in Table 37.2 [3,4].*

And finally wine. Those countries that produce little or no wine have high mortality rates from coronary heart disease; those that produce large amounts of wine have lower mortality rates. There is a strong negative association, with $R^2 = 0.6866$, shown in Figure 37.10.

**Figure 37.10 Wine production and coronary heart disease (CHD) in the EU.**

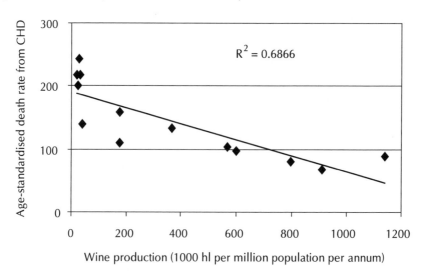

*Data in Table 37.2 [3,4].*

It is of course understandable that people jump to the conclusion that the wine is responsible for a low mortality rate from coronary heart disease. However, my alternative interpretation is that a climate with adequate sunshine to allow the production of wine also protects the population against coronary heart disease and a number of other conditions. Wine production and sunshine are inseparable; Galileo is reputed to have said 'Wine is sunshine held together by water'.

It is difficult to imagine the production of olives and grapes under grey skies with little sun. We have looked at the photosynthesis of vitamin D in humans; photosynthesis in plants involves the input of sunlight energy to produce complex energy-rich carbohydrates and fats. In respect of vines, sugars produced in the leaves are transported to the grapes; the synthesis of sugars is totally dependent on sunlight energy and not air temperature. Grapes can be produced in quite mountainous regions with cold winters and relatively cool but very sunny summers. For adequate sugar synthesis, a long growing season is necessary, hence the limitation of altitude for large-scale production.

Olive trees photosynthesise fatty acids that are stored in the fruit, and once again a large input of sunlight energy is essential, plus a long growing season. Olive oil production is not compatible with a location that has grey skies for most of the year. Even though there might be no winter frosts, as in the coastal areas of most of the UK, the high latitude, with inclination of the sun, means that there is insufficient sunlight energy at ground level to allow the synthesis of olive oil.

I hope that I have been able to demonstrate that the connection between olive oil, wine and human health is the climate that favours all of them. The so-called Mediterranean diet is a myth. In Spain and Portugal it is fish; in France it is meat and wine; in Italy it is pasta; in Greece it is olive oil. The common factor is the sunlight energy at ground level, and this cannot be put on the dinner table. In the same way that living in the UK, and therefore speaking English, is bad for health, living on the Mediterranean coast, and therefore speaking the local language and eating the local food, is good for health.

France is a large country with about four times the land area of England and a similar population. We have seen that the French population health varies, with the highest mortality rate from coronary heart disease occurring in the north. Agriculture differs throughout France: although champagne is produced in the north, red wines are produced only in the south and that is where olive trees grow. Puglia in the south of Italy is a vast agricultural production area, now that the swamps have been drained. In the UK we also see that agriculture is more productive in the south.

Table 37.3 shows the agricultural production of the UK regions. Of course we see no olive oil production and there is just a tiny production of wine in the south-east. An important finding is so little wheat production in the north of England. We can see that, as in Europe as a whole, where wheat is produced the death rate from myocardial infarction is relatively low. Also, where there is a predominant production of grass, death rates are relatively high.

**Table 37.3 Agricultural production in the UK (1000 ha in production). Death rates from myocardial infarction (MI; deaths per 100 000 males per year) [4,5]**

|  | Olive | Vine | Wheat | Barley | Grass | MI death |
|---|---|---|---|---|---|---|
| South-east | 0 | 1 | 492 | 262 | 446 | 293 |
| South-west | 0 | 0 | 194 | 219 | 979 | 302 |
| East Anglia | 0 | 0 | 343 | 204 | 105 | 289 |
| East Midlands | 0 | 0 | 389 | 188 | 324 | 337 |
| West Midlands | 0 | 0 | 143 | 137 | 428 | 345 |
| Yorkshire | 0 | 0 | 231 | 196 | 431 | 373 |
| North | 0 | 0 | 61 | 93 | 736 | 387 |
| North-west | 0 | 0 | 19 | 45 | 300 | 393 |
| Wales | 0 | 0 | 11 | 51 | 1395 | 358 |
| Scotland | 0 | 0 | 104 | 387 | 4691 | 401 |
| Northern Ireland | 0 | 0 | 5 | 45 | 766 | 443 |

*Crown © 2005, adapted with permission.*

So we see again the connection between agriculture and coronary heart disease, the link being sunlight energy rather than diet.

There is more to location than just the physical geography of the land. As early as the late 18th century we could already see that people living in the inner cities had a worse health profile than those living in rural environments. We need to explore these factors in more detail. How do people live their lives and what influences might this have on their health?

# PART 7

# THE SOCIOLOGY OF DISEASE

# 38
# SOCIO-ECONOMIC DEPRIVATION
# AND DISEASE

I have already mentioned that at one time it was felt quite confidently that a heart attack was the prerogative of the hard-working businessman, but it ultimately became clear that this was not the case. The social distribution of coronary heart disease and other conditions required a more structured and objective analysis.

It is worth reminding ourselves of the Registrar General's social classification in the UK, which is based upon employment: social class one, professional and executive; social class two, semi-professional and managerial; social class three, clerical and skilled workers; social class four, semi-skilled workers; social class five, unskilled workers and unemployed. Whatever the deficiencies of this classification, it has been used in the UK for many years and provides valuable insights into society. It allows a certain measurement of advantage and disadvantage based on a variety of social factors, with a reliable but not absolute correlation with disposable income. It might have led to UK being seen as a class-ridden society. Other countries have been slow to develop a social classification, but when they have done so it has been shown that social differences exist and are identical to those in the UK.

The first time that I came across details of the social dimensions of disease and death was a publication by Peter Townsend, at the time Professor of Sociology at the University of Essex, UK, and later co-author of the Black Report that I have referred to earlier (see Chapter 21) [1]. The text of a lecture by Townsend was published in *The Lancet* in 1974

[2], the year of the restructuring of the National Health Service (NHS) with a new emphasis on the integration of general practice and hospital medicine but, most importantly, with public health physicians having a pivotal role in planning and service development.

It is important to note that Townsend was not concerned with coronary heart disease itself but with the overall relationship between health and social issues. We must not forget this when we consider later data that concentrated on coronary heart disease, about which so much data have been generated but about which such a puzzle remains.

Townsend demonstrated the disturbing fact that, whereas the survival of the privileged groups improved during the years 1930–63, in relative terms the survival of groups 3 and 4 did not change and that of social group 5 deteriorated (Figure 38.1). This is called the widening social gap. In absolute terms, the health of all groups improved but that of the socio-economically privileged improved most of all.

**Figure 38.1 Standardised mortality ratios (SMR) by social class [2].**

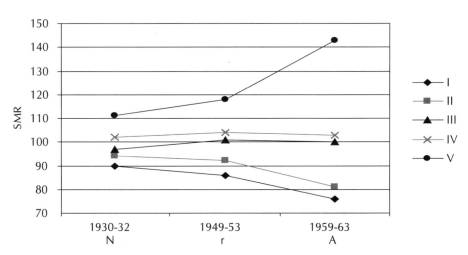

His challenge to the new NHS was to tackle these social inequalities, but this has not been easy; the causes of the inequalities cannot readily be explained. Furthermore, at about the same time, Thomas McKeown, former Professor of Social Medicine at the University of Birmingham, UK, indicated that the major improvements in the health of the public were the result of civil engineering rather than medical achievements [3]. I am sure that he was correct in this assertion when applied to the 19th and early 20th centuries but I feel that he underestimated the importance of clean air. Most commentators felt that he failed to acknowledge medical contributions in the latter half of the 20th century.

Anders Forsdahl, from the Institute of Community Health, University of Tromsø, Norway, [4] was aware of the variations in mortality from coronary heart disease in Norway. He linked a high mortality to poor living conditions in childhood, drawing attention to the long lead-time (incubation period) of coronary heart disease, and also acknowledging a social gradient in a nation other than the UK. David Barker, from the University of Southampton, UK, showed the same thing in the UK, a strong relationship between infant mortality rate and coronary heart disease in adults [5].

In 1984, Michael (now Sir Michael) Marmot and his colleagues from the London School of Hygiene and Tropical Medicine, UK, reported the result of the follow-up of 17 530 civil servants participating in the Whitehall Study [6]. The 10-year mortality from coronary heart disease can be seen in Figure 38.2, categorised according to the civil service employment scale: administrative, professional/executive, clerical and other. This has some similarity to the first four social classes of the Registrar General of the UK.

**Figure 38.2  Age-adjusted mortality from coronary heart disease [6].**

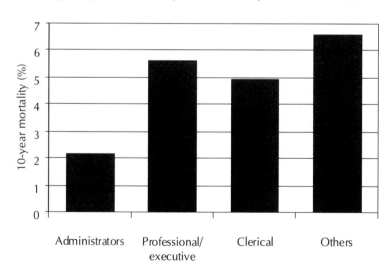

*Adapted from* The Lancet. *Copyright © 1984, with permission from Elsevier.*

We can see a clear gradient, with the lowest mortality from coronary heart disease being associated with positions at the top of the organisation, representing people with the highest educational achievement and income. To quote the authors [6]:

*For every cause of death except genito-urinary diseases ... the two lower grades have higher mortality risks than the two higher grades. For nearly every cause there is a step-wise relation between grade and mortality.*

It is possible or even likely that the earliest recognition of coronary heart disease in the upper social groups was not just because of their better access to medical care but because the disease first emerged in these groups. It was soon to become dominant in those who were less privileged.

Before we start to look for specific explanations concerning the social class differences of coronary heart disease, it is important to recognise that the same social gradient exists for a number of other conditions, as shown in Figure 38.3, again from data from the Whitehall study [6].

**Figure 38.3 Age-adjusted mortality at 10 years [6].**

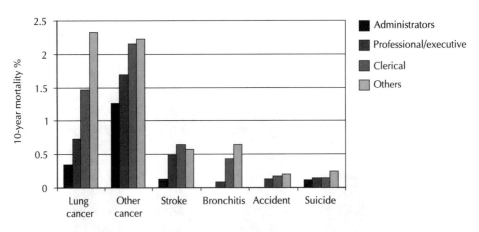

*© 1984, adapted from* The Lancet *with permission from Elsevier.*

The administrators have an obvious and significant health advantage across a wide range of causes of death. The authors comment 'a large part of the differences in mortality remains unexplained' [6]. That is still the case 20 years later. In a further publication in 1986, Marmot & McDowall [7] reported that the social difference was widening; although there were overall health improvements, they were greater in those with socio-economic privileges.

The social gradient of coronary heart disease has also been identified in Sweden [8]. Although there was no official social description in what was thought to be an egalitarian society, it was of course possible to define the population according to occupation. The groups, as in the UK, were unskilled manual, skilled manual, foremen, intermediate and professional/ executive. It was found that that the mortality rate from coronary heart disease in the unskilled group was twice that in the professional/executive group (Figure 38.4).

**Figure 38.4 Mortality and occupational classes (men) in Sweden [8].**
CHD = coronary heart disease.

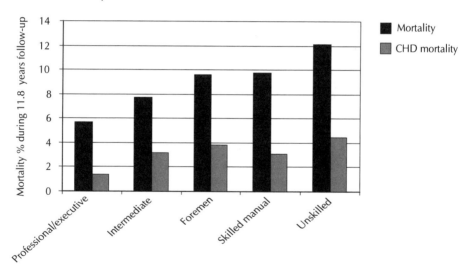

*Adapted with permission from the British Medical Journal Publishing Group.*

Social differences in health have been explained in the UK mainly (but incompletely) on the basis of cigarette smoking, but this would not be an explanation in Sweden. Fifty-four per cent of the unskilled workers smoked, not dissimilar to 47.5% of the professional/executive workers.

But it is not just death, including coronary deaths, that is related to social conditions. Long-term illness also shows a social gradient, in both Britain and in Sweden, as shown in Figure 38.5 [9]. Differences between the social groups are less in the Swedish population than in that of England and Wales, but the social gradient still exists. There is something that helps the health of the socio-economically privileged other than specific factors that relate to coronary heart disease.

**Figure 38.5  Relative prevalence of long-term illness by social class in 1981 [9].**

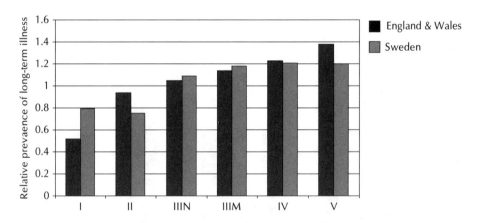

A study of the various employment groups of the NHS was undertaken by R. Balarajan, Professor of Epidemiology and Public Health Medicine at the University of Surrey, UK [10]. This showed the same pattern during the years 1979–83: mortality rates from all causes were lowest in those with the highest educational achievement and income, in particular the doctors and dentists. The results of the study can be seen in Figure 38.6. Deaths from coronary heart disease were twice as high in hospital porters as in doctors, and lung cancer deaths were more than five times higher.

**Figure 38.6  All causes of mortality in the NHS by occupational group [10].**

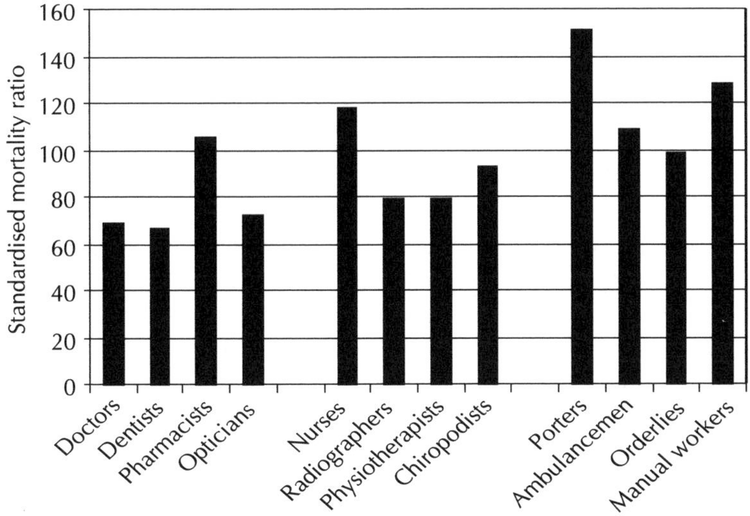

*Adapted with permission from the British Medical Journal Publishing Group.*

The association between socio-economic status and coronary heart disease has also been demonstrated in Finland [11]. The age-adjusted rate in the lowest socio-economic third was 44% higher than in the most privileged third. This was independent of known factors such as smoking, cholesterol levels, etc.

Further information was added by the UK Office of National Statistics (ONS) in February 2005 [12]. This study assembled data for more than 8500 local authority wards in the UK, recording age at death, levels of illness and measures of income and socio-economic deprivation. It reported both age of death according to social class and the years of ill-health, providing expressions of life expectancy and, of more importance, healthy life expectancy. We have already seen, in Chapter 1, the compression of morbidity, that life expectancy and healthy life expectancy have become virtually the same. Raymond Tallis, Professor of Geriatric Medicine at the University of Manchester, UK, regards the pursuit of this as the prime purpose of medicine [13].

The UK ONS tells us that a man living in a prosperous location would be expected to live on average until the age of 77.4 years and have a healthy life expectancy of 66.2 years. He would have on average 11.2 years of ill-health. A man living in one of the least prosperous locations would be expected to live on average to 71.4 years and have a healthy life expectancy of only 49.4 years. He would have on average 17 years less healthy life than the man living in the prosperous location. For women, the corresponding difference is 16.8 years.

The link between socio-economic deprivation and poor health is unclear. The assumption that it is the result of behavioural indiscretions such as cigarette smoking is supported by observations that in the UK smoking shows a social gradient, being much more common in the socio-economically deprived. For example, an NHS press release on 1999 indicated cigarette smoking in 21% of men and 18% of women in the highest income quintile, compared with 42% of men and 37% of women in the lowest income quintile [14]. But this is not the case in other countries, such as Sweden and Finland, where smoking is more uniform but a social gradient of health is still evident. And, as in Finland, there is objective evidence of a social gradient of health in the UK, leading Peter Phillimore of the University of Newcastle, UK and colleagues (including Peter Townsend) to suggest re-emphasising 'the case for linking mortality patterns with material conditions rather than individual behaviour' [15]. This early voice against victim blaming appears to have gone unheeded.

There is a suggestion that the behaviour of doctors rather than behaviour of patients might have a bearing on unfavourable outcome [16]. This conclusion, based on research undertaken in Scotland, was that:

*Socio-economically deprived patients are thought to be more likely to develop coronary heart disease but are less likely to be investigated and offered surgery once it has developed. Such patients may be further disadvantaged by having to wait longer for surgery because of it being given lower priority.*

This is an example of the inverse care law, first described by Julian Tudor Hart, a general practitioner working in South Wales [17]. It indicates that those who are most in need of health care are least likely to receive it. In respect of the social gradient of illness, it is the healthier middle classes who tend to be at the front of the queue for treatment. I have already mentioned the view of Thomas McKeown [3], that clinical medicine has little relevance to the health of the population. If this assertion were true, then a place in the queue would be of no consequence, but in practice clinical medicine does have a role to play in the treatment of disease, and access to treatment is important.

However, although access to treatment is of importance, it appears that the biology of coronary heart disease is the main determinant of the higher mortality in the socio-economically deprived. Furthermore, it is not just the long-term aspects of disease and mortality but some aspects of the short-term manifestation of coronary heart disease that show increased severity in the socio-economically deprived. An interesting finding from Scotland indicates that the death rate following a first myocardial infarction is higher in the socio-economically deprived. This is particularly noticeable in those below the age of 65 years and it applies to deaths before arrival in hospital and also during stay in hospital [18]. This is shown in Figure 38.7.

**Figure 38.7 Mortality at 30 days following myocardial infarction at < 65 years of age [18].**

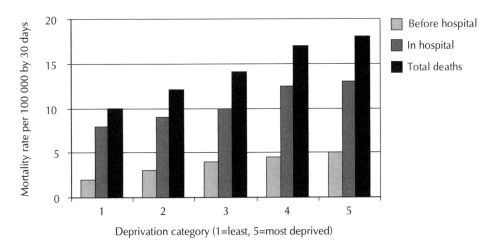

*Adapted with permission from the British Medical Journal Publishing Group.*

The authors were unable to offer an explanation for their finding and research into possible mechanisms was not part of the study. An explanation could only have been speculative, but the total absence of a possible explanation was disguised by the statement 'How socioeconomic deprivation increases these risks is probably multifaceted', a rather meaningless comment.

This finding from Scotland has also been shown in a report from London, in a study from the Newham General Hospital [19], where 1417 patients were divided into four groups according to socio-economic deprivation. The short-term mortality at 30 days was higher, at 18%, in the most deprived class, compared with 12% in the least deprived. The difference had disappeared at 3 years (Table 38.1). New coronary events at 30 days were 21% in the most deprived and 15% in least deprived groups. As the difference diminished over 3 years, in this instance the socio-economic deprivation factor, whatever it is, acts over a short time-scale.

**Table 38.1  Coronary events, including death after myocardial infarction [19]**

| | Socio-economic deprivation group | | | |
| --- | --- | --- | --- | --- |
| | 1 (least) | 2 | 3 | 4 (most) |
| Coronary events, % | | | | |
| 30 days | 15 | 17 | 17 | 21 |
| 6 months | 25 | 26 | 27 | 30 |
| 1 year | 30 | 35 | 30 | 36 |
| 3 years | 42 | 50 | 44 | 47 |
| Death, % | | | | |
| 30 days | 12 | 13 | 14 | 18 |
| 6 months | 16 | 19 | 18 | 21 |
| 1 year | 19 | 24 | 20 | 23 |
| 3 years | 28 | 35 | 31 | 28 |

*Adapted with permission from the British Medical Journal Publishing Group.*

It will be noted that the terminology has changed. The five population groups are not described as social classes but by degree of socio-economic deprivation. This is important, drawing attention to both the social aspects of life and income, rather than occupation.

I would also emphasise again that, although these studies have looked at coronary heart disease in some detail, a greater burden of illness is a general feature of the socio-economically deprived. Another study from Scotland looked at a group of the population (a cohort) all born in 1920. By the end of 1974, 33 208 men and 37 157 women were still alive. They were investigated in 1997, and at that time 44% of the least deprived men had died compared with 77% of the most deprived. The corresponding figures for women were 30% and 50%, shown in Figure 38.8 [20].

**Figure 38.8  Percentage mortality between the ages of 54 and 77 years [20].**

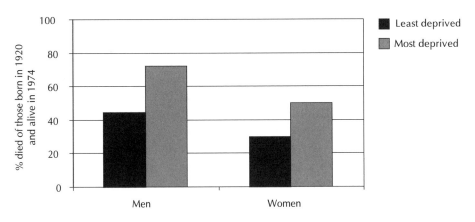

*Adapted with permission from the British Medical Journal Publishing Group.*

There is thus something about being socio-economically privileged that gives an enormous health advantage and it has a wide range of clinical expressions. This socio-economic gradient is more pronounced in the north-west of England than in the south-east, as demonstrated in the 2001 Report of the Chief Medical Officer of the Department of Health [21], shown in Figure 38.9.

**Figure 38.9  Death rates relating to social class groups [21].**

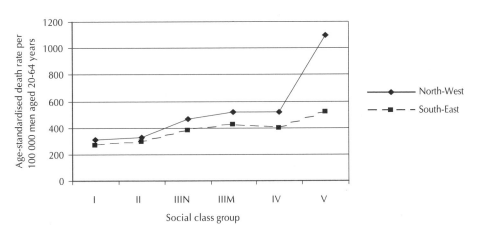

*Crown © 2001, adapted with permission.*

I have already indicated the possibility that the geographical variations of mortality rates in the UK, Europe and USA might be explained on the basis of differential rates of sunlight exposure. Could insufficient sunlight exposure be the cause of the social variation of mortality within the UK and its particular impact in the north of England?

'Poverty is a greater predictor of heart disease than risk factors such as smoking, obesity, stress, or blood cholesterol concentrations' [22]. This is stated in a report by Dennis Raphael of the Department of Public Health Sciences at the University of Toronto, Canada [22]. But why is this? What is the mechanism that links poverty and heart disease? Is it really poverty, when people living in many countries of the world have very low rates of coronary heart disease despite living in much greater poverty than the poorest of Canada and the industrialised world?

There would appear to be a general and fundamental factor relating social class and susceptibility to disease in temperate climates. As mentioned earlier, the single social factor that correlates most powerfully with life expectancy is eating an evening meal with the family while sitting around a table. Clearly this in itself is no guarantee of a long life but it is an indicator of certain unclear social factors that convey a very great advantage.

The data presented concerning the social distribution of heart disease in this country should cause great concern and the answers are not clear. There has been a tendency towards victim blaming, that is socio-economically deprived people who have a high mortality rate from heart disease are considered to be victims of their own unhealthy lifestyles. It is their own fault, and indeed lifestylism has become very much part of the whole paradigm of coronary heart disease. Not only do the working classes eat the wrong foods but they also take too little exercise. It interesting to recall the comments of William Heberden from 1801 [23]:

*The poor, who have little care of preserving their lives beyond getting their daily bread, make a very large part of mankind. Their prejudices are strong, and not easily overcome by reason.*

It is too easy to take a middle-class moral high ground and wrongly regard the poor as architects of their own health disadvantages. Take, for example, cigarette smoking. The Chief Medical Officer gives data in the 2001 report [21] that smoking is more common in the socio-economically deprived of the UK, and we can see this in Figure 38.10.

**Figure 38.10  Cigarette smoking and social class group [21.**

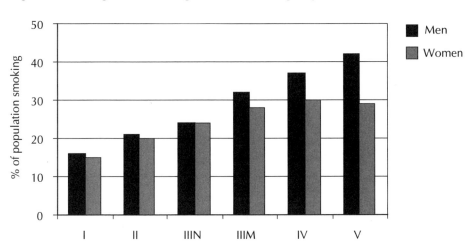

*Crown © 2001, adapted with permission.*

But it is not quite as simple as this. Much of the data that we have seen have been standardised for smoking but the social class gradient remains. We all know that cigarette smoking causes lung cancer, a subject that we will revisit in a later chapter. For now, let us note the uncomfortable fact from Denmark that social class has a strong effect on the risk of developing lung cancer and the reason is completely unknown [24]. This was demonstrated in a study of 4931 men followed up for nearly 20 years, during which 144 men developed lung cancer and 135 died as a result. It was noted that, for a given number of cigarettes smoked over a long period of time, the risk of developing lung cancer was three times higher for the men of the most deprived social group compared with those who were least deprived. Full adjustments were made for factors such as the form of smoking, amount smoked, whether or not inhalation took place, number of 'pack years' and age. The incidence curves are shown in Figure 38.11.

**Figure 38.11  Incidence of lung cancer in smokers by social class [24].**

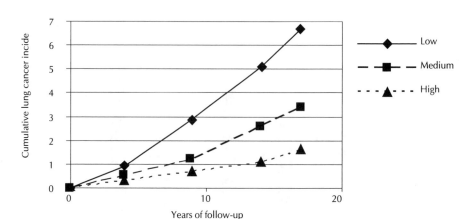

Lung cancer is therefore a further example of the wide range of illness showing a social gradient. The possible influence of sunlight and vitamin D will be reviewed later.

Scotland has a long history of good-quality clinical research. In an earlier chapter, I drew attention to the excellent book *To Improve the Evidence of Medicine. The 18th Century British Origins of a Critical Approach* [25]. The author, Professor Ulrich Tröhler of the University of Freiburg, Germany, commented on the extraordinary contribution of Scottish physicians to the development of structured data collection and statistical analysis, a tradition that continues to the present day. Many of the papers on socio-economic deprivation that I have reviewed have originated in Scottish hospitals and universities. General practice has also made an important contribution, and again because of structured data collection.

A study of 307 741 patients from 53 general practices in Scotland revealed that 2186 adults developed heart failure [26] (Table 38.2). Today the major cause is coronary heart disease, in a late stage of which the heart muscle becomes irreversibly damaged. The study showed that [26]:

*Compared with affluent patients, socioeconomically deprived patients were 44% more likely to develop heart failure but 23% less likely to see their general practitioner on an on-going basis.*

**Table 38.2 Heart failure in Scotland. GP, general practitioner [26]**

| Deprivation category | Number | Prevalence per 1000 pop. | Annual GP contacts | Mean survival (years) |
|---|---|---|---|---|
| 1 (least) | 70 761 | 6.4 | 2.6 | 3.5 |
| 2 | 66 633 | 7.4 | 2.7 | 4.4 |
| 3 | 93 258 | 7.5 | 2.4 | 3.8 |
| 4 | 34 627 | 7.5 | 2.3 | 2.8 |
| 5 (most) | 28 633 | 7.2 | 2 | 2.8 |

*Adapted with permission from the British Medical Journal Publishing Group.*

Here we have more evidence of the socio-economic gradient of disease and another example of the inverse care law. It is reassuring to note that prescribing of medications did not differ between the socio-economic groups.

The model presented in this book is that the social gradient of disease is mediated by insufficient exposure to the sun by the socio-economically deprived. We need to appreciate that this is a feature of the population but also that the various diseases are more likely to occur in the absence of sunshine and vitamin D. Heart failure is an example of this; we have seen that it is more likely to occur in the socio-economically deprived. There is also evidence from Germany that heart failure is associated with vitamin D insufficiency, with low levels of calcidiol because of a shortage of vitamin D from the diet or the sun, and low levels of calcitriol, the active metabolite [27]. The authors also indicate that vitamin D is necessary for heart function and that heart muscle cells have vitamin D receptors (VDRs). Figure 38.12 demonstrates the low levels of serum calcidiol in patients with congestive heart failure compared with controls and Figure 38.13 shows similar findings for calcitriol.

**Figure 38.12 Vitamin D as calcidiol and congestive heart failure (CHF) [27].**

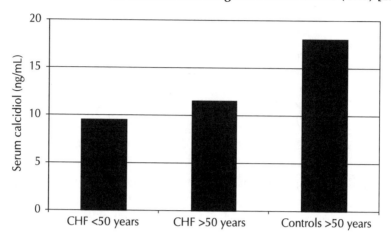

**Figure 38.13 Vitamin D as calcitriol and congestive heart failure (CHF) [27].**

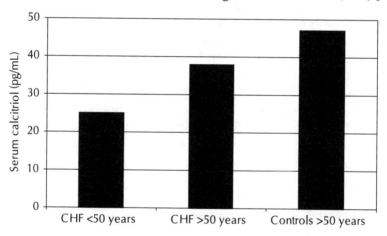

A report from Liverpool, UK, has indicated a social gradient for diabetes [28]. Of the total population of 176 682 in South Sefton, 2585 were known to have diabetes. The study was not able to give a socio-economic score to each person and so they were grouped by place of residence. The prevalence of diabetes obtained from disease registers was mapped on to the geography of this part of north Liverpool using the electoral wards. Each of these had a socio-economic profile and a Townsend score of deprivation. The analysis can be seen in Figure 38.14.

**Figure 38.14 Socio-economic deprivation and prevalence of diabetes [28].**

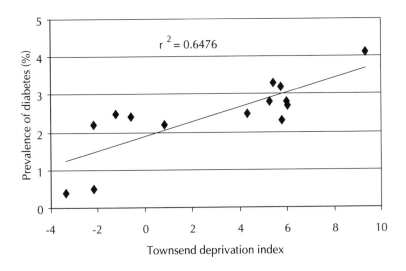

Adapted from the QMJ with permission from the Oxford University Press.

The crude data show a ten-fold greater prevalence of diabetes (Type 2) in the most deprived communities compared with the least deprived. The association is very strong, with $R^2 = 0.6476$. Once again we have no immediate explanation for this observation and the authors did not speculate. However, we need to put the association of socio-economic deprivation with diabetes into the general context that we have already seen. I have suggested that the social gradient of disease might be mediated by inadequate sunlight exposure, and in a later chapter we will look at the associations between diabetes and vitamin D insufficiency.

It is now time to look at other aspects of socio-economic deprivation, to see whether we can find clues regarding the nature of the factor that causes the ill-health that we have seen.

Whenever we look at a variable that has a relationship with coronary heart disease, we find that there is also almost certainly a relationship with social class. An example of this is exercise; we have been told over recent years that exercise is good for us and protects us against heart disease. Observational studies indicate that people who exercise have a relatively low rate of coronary heart disease and a longer life, but it is too easy to jump to the conclusion that exercise is beneficial and cardio-protective. In reality, it is the middle classes who dominate jogging and gyms, and there is a clear social gradient of leisure exercise [29], shown in Figure 38.15.

**Figure 38.15 Physical activity in leisure time by social group [29].**

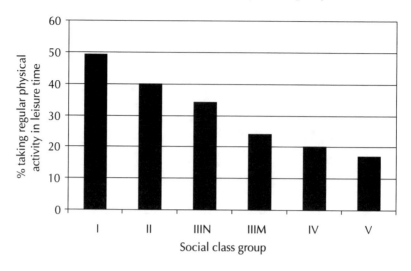

The socio-economically deprived spend a disproportionate time watching the television, an indoor activity, and this has been demonstrated in a study by the Henley Centre for Social Research, London, UK [30]. It was found that 'The poorest spend around 11 hours a week more than the richest watching TV'. The report also suggested that:

> *A cultural underclass might be developing as those on low incomes are restricted to the cheaper entertainment of television while those on higher incomes take advantage of other leisure activities.*

The television is thus seen as the antithesis of leisure activities that might involve exercise with or without outdoor exposure to the sun. Television viewing as a major leisure activity has associations with a number of factors that indicate poor health. In particular there is currently concern regarding childhood obesity and whether lack of physical activity might be as much a cause as over-nutrition. This was the subject of a recent study from New Zealand [31]. A study of 100 unselected individuals born in Dunedin indicated that adolescents in the top quartile of watching television (more than 3 hours per day), compared with those in the lowest quartile (less than 1 hour per day), are more likely to smoke, be overweight, be unfit and have a high cholesterol or high blood pressure (Figure 38.16). These factors could be mediated by a lack of exercise and also lack of outdoor activity with a consequent lack of exposure to the sun.

**Figure 38.16 Television viewing and health in children and adolescents [31].**

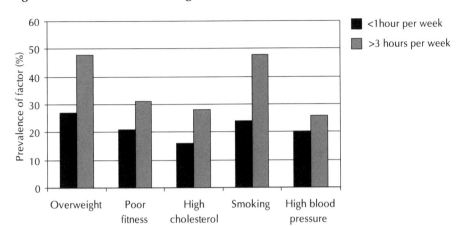

© 2004, adapted from The Lancet with permission from Elsevier.

Working-time compared with leisure-time physical activity has not been investigated. It would generally be greater in social classes four and five and we need to know if it is an advantage in those groups. Observational studies need to be stratified or standardised to a given socio-economic group, but this is not usually the case. There is not very much to be gained by comparing a golf-playing business executive with an unemployed labourer who has no recreational physical activity.

Observations of exercise and other variables can only lead to the generation of ideas, suggestions and hypotheses. The hypothesis must be tested by intervention and that means randomly assigning people to exercise programmes, keeping everything else unchanged. It is difficult to achieve this in the human world. Where it has been attempted, the results can only be regarded as disappointing, and there is a lack of consistent and convincing evidence that exercise is of benefit in protection against cardiovascular disease. If individual people feel that exercise is a good thing, then I would be the last to discourage them, but I would not wish to impose it in the form of compulsory medicine.

There seems to be something rather absolute about social class and its relationship with coronary heart disease. The variables associated with social class do not seem to be adequately powerful to explain the very major differences. Diet and exercise do not appear to hold the answer but the differences of health in relation to social class are striking and an explanation must be sought.

For example, if we look at the geography of disease in East Lancashire, UK, we find that the standardised mortality ratio (SMR) in the Ribble Valley is 98 but it is 148 in the inner city parts of Blackburn and Accrington [32]. The risk of dying from coronary heart disease at a given age is 50% higher in Blackburn than in, for example, the villages of the Ribble Valley. This is, once again, as Thomas Percival described in Manchester and the surrounding villages in 1770 [33].

The inner city parts of Blackburn are characterised by traditional terraced housing and, until their recent demolition, high-rise flats built in the 1960s. The Ribble Valley, in contrast, is almost entirely a rural environment with many villages, a predominantly middle-class population and most houses have a garden. Could housing have an influence of health?

We have already looked at gardens and found that people who have gardens have on average lower cholesterol and higher vitamin D levels in the blood (see Chapter 26). Could this be the key? Could the social class differences of mortality from coronary heart and other diseases be explained by housing that provides different levels of sun exposure? This first came into my mind about 15 years ago when, one Saturday afternoon in the summer, I was asked to visit a sick person at home, in a terraced house in Blackburn. It was a beautiful day and when I received the telephone call I had just finished lunch in my garden in the Ribble Valley. The illness of the individual is not relevant to the present subject, but I was struck by the fact that the family members were sitting inside the house watching the television. An elderly neighbour was sitting in the sun on his chair at his front door but otherwise the street was empty. So here we had a family that was denied sun exposure because there was no garden, nowhere to sit peacefully outside and no park readily available. Here was a lifestyle so different from my own that I felt it could well play a part in the differential risk of death from coronary heart and other diseases. But it was not a chosen lifestyle; it was the inevitable result of a lack of education, relative poverty and low socio-economic privilege.

The family was poor and did not possess a car. Whereas I could easily drive to the sea-side, the hills of the forest of Bowland, the Yorkshire Dales or the Lake District, in order to enjoy a walk in the open air and sunshine, this opportunity did not appear to be available to the family I had just met. The convenience of a car must not be underestimated. Similarly, I can take holidays abroad in winter and summer, but this was something else that the family could not afford. Many such families do not take holidays at all. It is my assertion that the social class gradient of coronary heart disease in the UK, and probably also in Sweden, is because of the differential rate of exposure to sunshine, the low levels of sunshine exposure of the socio-economically deprived.

Much of the work on the socio-economic epidemiology of health in the UK has been undertaken by Sir Michael Marmot, and we have seen some examples of his work. He has recently brought much of his evidence together in a book entitled *The Status Syndrome* [34]. I must emphasise the word evidence; observations are facts. There might inevitably be a statistical error when testing samples, but most observational research in recent years has been of a very high standard. We can rely to a major extent on it being robust, and this book has displayed much of the evidence in figures and tables. But then the observation must be explained; this process is what might be called common sense, often based on conventional wisdom. Regarding coronary heart disease in particular, conventional wisdom is usually something to do with diet, especially fat. The other major conventional wisdom, which I have already touched upon, is the mind, the psychological explanation. This is the basis of Marmot's explanation of the social gradients of disease, as expressed in his book.

Marmot suggests a psychological explanation and it sounds very plausible [34]. People who are relatively poor and underprivileged, even if wealthy by international standards, have no social standing or status in this country and in their larger community. He states that this leads directly to ill-health and premature death.

There are undoubtedly links between behaviour and disease or death. The relationship between the development of sexually transmitted disease and a large number of sexual partners is an obvious example. The observation that men are almost three times more likely than women to die as the result of a road traffic accident is also a result of behaviour. But disease is different. Scientific philosophy since the time of Paracelsus tells us that a specific disease has a specific cause and this is a model that has proven to be powerful in our understanding of disease. The teaching of Paracelsus is ignored by those such as Marmot who suggest a direct effect of psychological and behavioural factors on the development of disease and premature death: an intervening mechanism is never identified. As shown in Figure 38.17, there must be an intervening mechanism when we are dealing with disease.

**Figure 38.17  Mechanism of disease.**

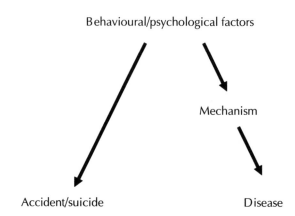

Behavioural/psychological factors

Mechanism

Accident/suicide                    Disease

I therefore reject the direct link but I propose that psychological and behavioural factors influence the susceptibility to disease.

It is interesting to reflect on whether obesity is a disease or a behavioural characteristic. Most people believe that it is the latter, and thereby under the control of the individual; were it a disease, it would be mainly outside individual control, as with most other diseases. The behavioural causation of obesity is considered to explain its higher prevalence in socio-economically deprived groups, as shown in Figure 38.18 with data taken from a report commissioned by the UK Department of Health and Medical Research Council (MRC) [35].

**Figure 38.18 Prevalence of obesity by socio-economic group and age [35].**

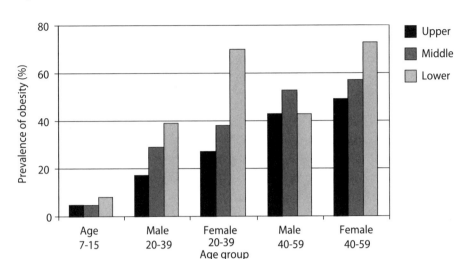

In young adults the prevalence of obesity in the lower socio-economic groups is twice that in the upper. The difference becomes less marked in middle age and disappears in men. It has been suggested that women in the lower social groups have such low feelings of self-worth that they cease to take a pride in their appearance, compared with women in the higher social groups who are forever striving to look slim and youthful. This has no evidence base: it is conjecture arising from a middle-class viewpoint and I am unaware of any research on this important topic. It is, however, an example of how a health characteristic that is not a disease might be directly behavioural.

It is interesting to consider illness rather than disease incidence in various social groups in more detail. Figure 38.19 shows national data taken from the UK census of 2001 [36]. It indicates the social gradient of health that has already been identified among the employment groups. It also indicates an exceptionally higher perception of ill-health among those who have never worked or who have been unemployed for a long time.

**Figure 38.19 Self-reported ill-health by social class in Great Britain [36].**

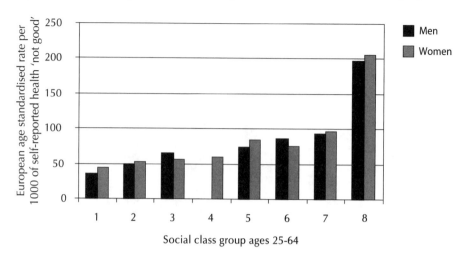

Social class group ages 25-64

*Adapted with permission from the British Medical Journal Publishing Group.*

The definition of the social groups are: social group 1, higher managerial and professional occupations; social group 2, lower managerial and professional occupations; social group 3, intermediate occupations; social group 4, small employers and own account workers; social group 5, lower supervisory and technical occupations; social group 6, semi-routine occupations; social group 7, routine occupations; social group 8, long-term unemployed and never worked. I suggest that the long-term unemployed have a lack of self-worth from which they have a perception of ill-health, but that they also have an increased susceptibility to disease and premature death by virtue of low levels of sunshine exposure and therefore of vitamin D.

There are several reasons for this, and the most important is housing, which will inevitably be in undesirable locations with no outdoor leisure opportunity. The houses will not usually have gardens and, if they do, the garden is likely to be untended and unused. There is unlikely to be a usable local park, and the local environment is likely to be violent and unlikely to encourage outdoor leisure. Compared with children of socio-economically privileged families, children in these areas are more likely to die as a result of accident or violence. The location will probably be inner city with run-down local amenities and no opportunity for upward mobility. The lifestyle will probably continue from generation to generation and the biological inheritance will be detrimental to health. The families will not have the money to develop outdoor leisure pursuits and life is likely to be focused on the television. There will be no money for a car and no safe place to keep one; opportunities to travel and reach the countryside will be few, and the motivation to do so will be absent. Clothing and general demeanour will not enable blending into a social environment outside the home, and there will be no money for holidays in the sun. The little money that might be available for leisure is likely to be spent on television and cigarettes, perhaps on illicit drugs, all items that Aldous Huxley indicated provide the 'artificial paradises' that are avidly sought by those who live such lives [37]:

> Most men and women lead lives at the worst so painful, at the best so monotonous, poor, and limited, that their urge to escape, the longing to transcend themselves if only for a few moments, is and always has been one of the principal appetites of the soul.

It is possible that, in the past 50 years since Huxley wrote this book, 'most' might have diminished to 'many'. I hope so. But there remains this 'many' and these are the people who have been left outside the health improvements that we have seen. It is this group that represents the challenge to health policy and for which victim-blaming is unhelpful and incorrect. I therefore agree totally with the observations and initial interpretation of Michael Marmot in his book *Status Syndrome* [34]. I part with him in his contention that the link with disease is direct and effectively psychological: I believe that it is mediated by lack of sunshine and consequent vitamin D insufficiency.

# 39

# TWO ALBANIAN PARADOXES

The social distribution of coronary heart disease in the UK indicates that the socio-economically disadvantaged members of the population are at a much greater risk compared with the affluent. We have seen the same thing in other countries of northern Europe.

In Albania, however, there are two paradoxes. The first is this: why is it that Albania, the poorest country in Europe, with the most socio-economically disadvantaged population, has a particularly low incidence of coronary heart disease?

Perhaps the main indicator of the low socio-economic status of the population of Albania is the high infant mortality rate, as shown in Figure 39.1.

**Figure 39.1  Infant mortality in European countries [1].**

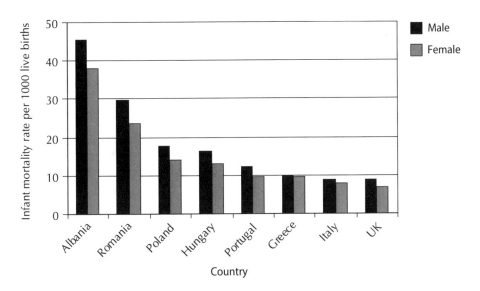

The infant mortality rate of a nation is strongly related to its socio-economic development, and it is lowest in the most economically advanced countries. In this group of countries we can see that the lowest infant mortality rate is in the UK, which is the fourth largest economy in the world and has the highest income per head of population in the group. Albania is at the opposite end of the spectrum: it has the highest infant mortality rate and the lowest income per capita. It can also be seen that infant mortality rates are higher in the eastern European countries, Hungary, Poland and Romania, compared with their western European counterparts. This is likely to be the result of the economic suppression of the communist era.

But when we look at mortality rates from coronary heart disease, we see a very different picture and Albania has one of the lowest mortality rates, comparable with Italy, Greece and Portugal. This is shown in Figure 38.2.

**Figure 39.2  Coronary heart disease mortality rates in European countries [1].**

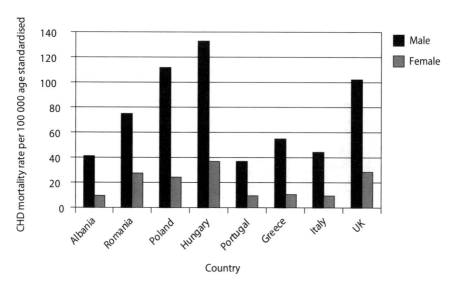

© *1997, adapted from* The Lancet *with permission from Elsevier.*

If we compare Albania with the other former Eastern Bloc countries, we can see that, despite the fact that it is poorer, it has the lowest mortality rate from coronary heart disease. The authors of the paper recognised that the Albanian paradox indicates that low socio-economic status cannot have a direct effect on coronary heart disease [1]. The observation is, however, entirely in keeping with the French, or Mediterranean, paradox, in other words it demonstrates a latitude effect.

The authors also realised that the common feature between Albania, Italy, Greece and Portugal could not be the so-called Mediterranean diet. The population of Albania eats significantly less than those of the other Mediterranean countries. Details of wine consumption in Albania are not available but it is thought to be the lowest in Europe. This is the second Albanian paradox: the population of a European country with one of the lowest death rates from coronary heart disease has the lowest consumption of wine. So much for the protective effect of red wine as a universal panacea. The authors suggest the protective effect not of a Mediterranean diet but of a Mediterranean lifestyle, without specifying what this means. No doubt it means living on or close to the Mediterranean coast.

In relation to other observations that we have reviewed, the obvious reason for the low mortality rate from coronary heart disease in Albania is its low latitude, low level of cloud cover and high exposure of the population to the sun. Insufficient exposure to sunlight might be a characteristic of the socio-economically deprived of northern Europe, but not of Mediterranean Europe. Similar to the poor of India, a warm dry climate and employment that, if it is available, is mainly outdoor agricultural, will result in plenty of time for the population to benefit from exposure to the sun.

There is another piece of information in the study of Arjan Gjonça, of the Department of Social Policy and Administration, London School of Economics and Political Science, and Martin Bobak, of the International Centre for Health and Society, University College London, UK [1]. They also displayed the geographical distribution of mortality from coronary heart disease within Albania using 1978 data. It was clear that the mortality rates were lowest in the southern parts of the country and highest in the northern parts. The authors stated [1]:

*There is a striking north–south gradient, with mortality in the north-eastern districts being almost twice higher than in the south-western districts. This mortality pattern has been stable over time; it was already present in the 1950s, when the earliest data are available, and is identical today.*

They also presented a map showing that the districts in which the mortality rates from coronary heart disease are lowest are those in which olives are cultivated. This conforms with Europe as a whole and I suggest that these are the locations of maximum sunlight energy available at ground level.

The Albanian paradoxes indicate that poor people in Europe can have a low incidence of coronary heart disease irrespective of what they eat or drink, as long as they have high exposure to the sun. The contrast with Leningrad/St Petersburg is obvious. From an international perspective, poverty itself does not predispose to coronary heart disease, but insufficient exposure to sunlight does.

# 40

# THE GREEK PARADOX: SMOKING AND CORONARY HEART DISEASE

In 1980 an editorial of the *British Medical Journal* stated: 'Cigarette smoking doubles the mortality from coronary heart disease but the mechanism is unknown' [1]. It seems strange that the way in which cigarette smoking affects the heart remains unknown 25 years later; but we all know that smoking is bad for us and it kills.

We have seen that the mortality rate from coronary heart disease is very low in the populations of the Mediterranean countries. This can be seen in previous chapters, in Figure 33.2 and also in Figures 37.3 and 39.2.

The Greek paradox is this: why is it that the people of Greece, who enjoy one of the lowest mortality rates from coronary heart disease and one of the highest life expectancies in Europe, smoke the most cigarettes per head of population?

The answer to the Greek paradox is becoming clear. Greece enjoys a location in the most southerly part of Europe, in a location where the olive can grow to maturity, indicating a very high level of sunshine energy at ground level, and where outdoor leisure is comfortable. It is this that promotes good health, and appears to protect against both coronary heart disease and other effects of cigarette smoking, such as lung cancer, as we will see later. The Greek paradox, like the French, Albanian, Leningrad, west of Scotland and Northern Ireland paradoxes, disappears if we change the model of the development of coronary heart disease. We need to look at cigarette smoking in more detail, noting the relative frequency within Europe, as shown in Table 40.1 from data provided by the European Union (EU) through its 2002 edition of Eurostat.

**Table 40.1 Cigarette smoking by country in Europe [2]**

|  | % of adult population who smoke |
| --- | --- |
| Greece | 44.9 |
| France | 38.3 |
| Denmark | 38.2 |
| Austria | 37.8 |
| Spain | 37.3 |
| Belgium | 37.2 |
| UK | 34.9 |
| Germany | 33.8 |
| Luxembourg | 33.7 |
| Ireland | 32.3 |
| the Netherlands | 31.4 |
| Finland | 30.1 |
| Portugal | 28.1 |
| Italy | 26.9 |
| Sweden | 22.1 |

We can see that Greece is at the top of the list and France second. We can add to this table data on death rates from coronary heart disease, also obtained from Eurostat, and look at the association between national smoking characteristics and coronary heart disease death rates. The association can be seen in Figure 40.1, presented as a scattergraph, which reveals another conundrum.

**Figure 40.1 Smoking and coronary heart disease (CHD) deaths in European countries [2].**

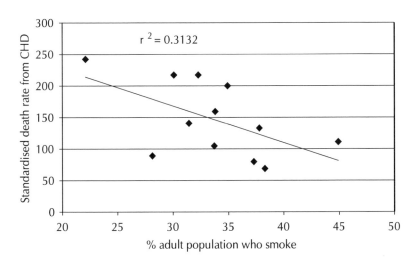

We can see that $R^2 = 0.3132$, a moderately strong association, but the association is negative. The greater the percentage of smokers in the adult population of the country, the lower the death rate from coronary heart disease. This is hardly to be expected: surely something is wrong. It is an extension of the Greek paradox and we might call it the European smoking paradox. I would not regard the negative association displayed in Figure 40.1 as indicating that smoking is in some way protective or otherwise beneficial: I suggest that there is a climatic factor, namely sunshine, that protects the populations of southern Europe against the damaging effects of cigarette smoking.

We are all taught that smoking kills and that cigarette smoking is bad for us. We have seen in Chapter 38 that smoking is much more dangerous for people who are socio-economically deprived (Figure 38.11, data from Denmark). It would therefore appear that there is something about the danger of cigarette smoking that is not quite straightforward.

We can also see from the Greek paradox that cigarette smoking is not as dangerous to the population of Greece as it is to those who live in northern Europe. In fact this observation was made by Ancel Keys in his 1980 publication *The Seven Countries Study* [3], which has provided us with a great deal of information so far. His observations on the relationship between cigarette smoking and coronary heart disease can be seen in Figure 40.2.

**Figure 40.2  Smoking and risk of coronary heard disease (CHD) by location in Europe [3].**

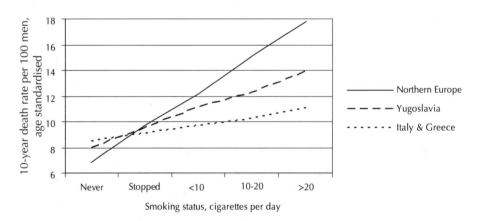

This figure represents what is effectively a set of three dose–response curves for cigarette smoking. It shows a typical toxic effect in that the higher the consumption of cigarettes, the greater the incidence of coronary heart disease, but the interesting observation is that the response depends on the location of residence in Europe. The response line is fairly flat in the south of Europe and there the risk of coronary heart disease for heavy smokers is only slightly greater than for those who do not smoke. In the north of Europe, those who smoke heavily (more than 20 per day) have a risk of coronary heart disease about 250% higher than those who do not smoke. There is some other factor present, something that is protective to those in the south of Europe or something that increases susceptibility to coronary heart disease in the north of Europe. Could it be sunlight?

This is an appropriate moment to stop and consider the relationship between cigarette smoking and coronary heart disease. We have seen that in the north of Europe it is for the socio-economically underprivileged that smoking is particularly dangerous. We now know that sunlight insufficiency is likely to be the major factor influencing the health of those who live in the north of Europe.

It is important to remember the importance of poverty and socio-economic deprivation in relationship to any assessment of coronary heart disease. We can see that coronary heart disease is more common in people who smoke, as is shown in Figure 40.2, and that this is likely to be a social class effect. We must also remember that, for a given level of cigarette smoking, a person who is socio-economically deprived is about three times more likely to develop lung cancer than someone who is affluent. Figure 40.3 reminds us of the social distribution of cigarette smoking in the UK (see Chapter 38) [4].

**Figure 40.3 Cigarette smoking and social class group [4].**

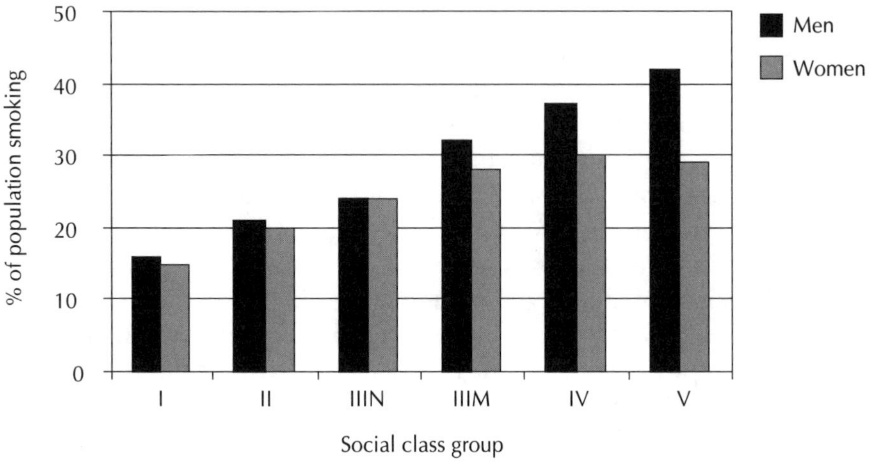

*Crown © 2001, adapted with permission.*

It is generally considered that cigarette smoke contains several toxins and nicotine, a cardiac and neurological stimulant, is the most well-known. Tars are thought to cause cancer of the lung. It is assumed that there is a chemical that has a direct toxic effect on the endothelium, the lining of the arteries, but no such toxin has been identified. The mechanism of the relationship between cigarette smoking and coronary heart disease is by no means clear. In general terms, we have seen that an association cannot always be interpreted in terms of a direct cause–effect relationship and other interpretations must be considered, especially if a well-defined causative mechanism is not obvious.

An interesting and informative analysis of the relationship between cigarette smoking and disease was undertaken by Robert West, of the Department of Epidemiology at the University of Wales College of Medicine, Cardiff, UK. He noted fundamental differences in the relationships of smoking with coronary heart disease and lung cancer [5] and we must examine them here.

If we are to look at the influence of cigarette smoking on lung cancer, coronary heart disease and life expectancy, it is important to look at just one social class in order to avoid confounding variables as much as possible. The data to enable this are provided in the monumental study by Doll and Hill into the smoking habits of doctors and the long-term outcome [6]. Sir Richard Doll (1912–2005) was one of the leading British epidemiologists of the 20th century, becoming Regius Professor of Medicine at Oxford University, UK. He worked alongside Sir Austin Bradford Hill (1897–1991), a brilliant statistician in the UK MRC.

Cigarette smoking is not an all-or-nothing activity and a toxic effect would be expected to increase as the dose or exposure increases. Doll and Hill grouped the study population of doctors into non-smokers, light smokers, medium smokers and heavy smokers. Looking at death rates from lung cancer within these groups, we can see in Figure 40.4 that, with increasing age, the mortality from lung cancer increases, as we would expect. We can also see that the mortality rate is extremely low in non-smokers, overall 0.07 per 1000 per annum. This represents only three deaths in the study sample of 5272 non-smokers out of a total of 31 208 men and women enrolled in the study. The death rate gradually increases with light, medium and heavy smoking. This pattern conforms to a direct effect of cigarette smoking, causing lung cancer with an increasing frequency with more cigarettes smoked.

**Figure 40.4 Mortality from lung cancer by age and smoking status (doctors) [6].**

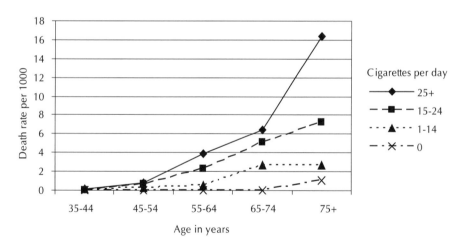

*Adapted with permission from the British Medical Journal Publishing Group.*

The relationship between cigarette smoking and coronary heart disease is very different. Table 40.2 shows the overall mortality rates from coronary heart disease, these data being from the paper by Robert West but originally extracted from that of Doll and Hill.

**Table 40.2  Deaths from coronary heart disease [5]**

| Cigarettes per day | Percentage of all causes of death | |
| --- | --- | --- |
| | **Men** | **Women** |
| Nil | 30.6 | 15.3 |
| 1–14 | 32.6 | 14.2 |
| 15–24 | 29.3 | 21.9 |
| 25+ | 28.5 | 16.9 |

The risk of death from coronary heart disease for someone who smokes heavily, 25 or more cigarettes per day, is approximately the same as someone who has never smoked, very different from the risks of death from lung cancer.

More detail is given in Figure 40.5, which looks at the death rates in each age group in relation to cigarette smoking, comparable with the data presentation of Figure 40.3. The shapes of the curves are very important.

**Figure 40.5  Mortality from myocardial infarction by age and smoking status (doctors) [7].**

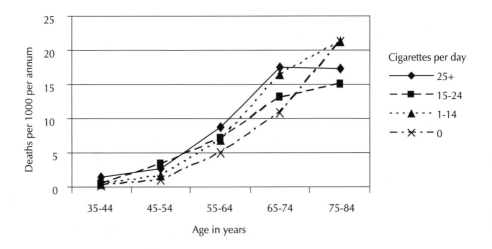

Whereas the curves for lung cancer shown in Figure 40.3 diverge very obviously, there is no divergence of the curves for coronary heart disease and they are all the same shape. Whereas the relationship between cigarette smoking and lung cancer indicates a clear cause–effect relationship, the relationship with coronary heart disease indicates something different.

What we can see is that, within the age group 55–64 years, twice as many heavy smokers have died from coronary heart disease than non-smokers. Furthermore, we can see that a given death rate from coronary heart disease, of say 8 per 1000 per annum, occurs in heavy smokers about 10 years earlier than in non-smokers. In other words, cigarette smoking has an accelerating rather than a causative effect on coronary heart disease. This is the point that was made by West: cigarette smoking causes earlier deaths rather than more deaths. We must always remember that we are all mortal; it is the age at death that is important, not the fact that we die.

What might be the nature of this acceleration? It has long been assumed that cigarette smoke contains a chemical substance that causes coronary heart disease, but such a hypothesis has received no substantiation despite much research. It is now known that cigarette smoke contains more than 4000 identified chemicals and 400–500 gases but none of these has been identified as causing coronary heart disease [7].

The Greek paradox indicates that the relationship between cigarette smoking and coronary heart disease is not direct. The Greek or Mediterranean experience indicates that cigarette smoking cannot be the cause of coronary heart disease: it can hardly be the cause in one country but not in another. A cause is a cause irrespective of location, accepting that there might be local factors providing relative protection or susceptibility.

Cigarette smoking is therefore another factor that influences the development of coronary heart disease but that cannot be the cause. Perhaps the high level of sunshine in Greece is protective against whatever it is about cigarette smoking that causes an acceleration of coronary heart disease. Cigarette smoking has its most obvious effect on the respiratory tract, in its relationship with bronchitis and lung cancer. Could the relationship between cigarette smoking and the heart be mediated by respiratory disease, with protection by sunlight and vitamin D?

The relationship between respiratory disease, coronary heart disease and geography needs to explored further.

# 41

# RESPIRATORY DISEASE AND CORONARY HEART DISEASE

We noted in Chapter 7 that both respiratory disease and coronary heart disease have something in common, a seasonal variation, with an increased frequency in the winter. We know from personal experience and common knowledge that chest problems are more common in the winter but an association with coronary heart disease is not immediately obvious.

In Chapter 31, we looked at three Lancashire mill towns, Burnley, Colne and Nelson, noting excessive mortality rates of the population in 1917 and 60 years later. A close association between respiratory disease and subsequent coronary heart disease was highlighted, suggesting that the two are linked in terms of causation. The interpretation could be that respiratory disease leads to coronary heart disease or that the two have a common cause or a common susceptibility factor.

A study from Finland investigated the association between chronic bronchitis and the subsequent development of coronary heart disease in a 13-year follow-up of 19 444 men and women living in North Karelia and Kuopio [1]. The subjects of the study were grouped according to whether or not they smoked, and the results of the study are outlined in Figure 41.1. Chronic bronchitis was defined in the traditional way, as cough with phlegm (sputum) on most days or nights for 3 months every year.

**Figure 41.1  Chronic bronchitis and coronary heart disease (CHD) in Finland [1].**

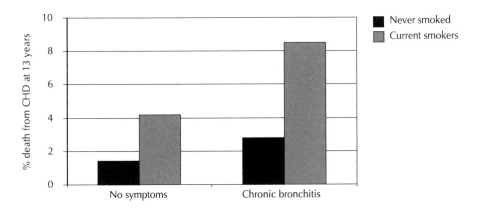

We can see that death from coronary heart disease was more common in those with chronic bronchitis compared with those with no respiratory symptoms. This was true for those who smoked (8.49% versus 4.22%) and those who did not smoke (2.77% versus 1.41%). The death rate from coronary heart disease is very obviously the greatest for those who smoke and have chronic bronchitis.

We have noted in the previous chapter that there is an association between cigarette smoking and coronary heart disease. The data suggest that the link between the two is not direct but that cigarette smoking has an accelerating effect on the development of coronary heart disease.

Cigarette smoking leads to chronic lung disease. In the Finland study, chronic bronchitis was more common in those who smoked than in those who did not smoke, and more noticeable in men than in women, as shown in Figure 41.2.

**Figure 41.2 Prevalence of chronic bronchitis in east Finland [1].**

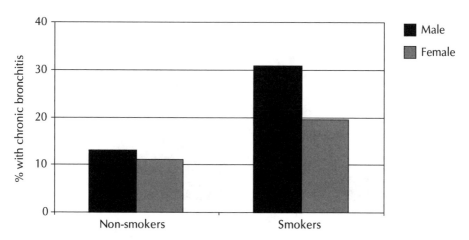

Chronic bronchitis has sometimes been known in Europe as the British Disease because of its high prevalence in the UK. Clinical medicine in this country now tends to use the term chronic obstructive pulmonary disease (COPD), emphasising the presence of small airway obstruction causing wheezing and being at least partially reversible by medical intervention.

In the UK we have a high prevalence of chronic lung disease and also of coronary heart disease. Is this association a coincidence? The study from Finland suggests the relationship might be cause–effect, but is the association widespread?

We can turn to the World Health Organization (WHO) for a source of information [2]. There are data on chronic lung disease in addition to the heart disease data that we have already used. However, there is a nomenclature problem with chronic lung disease, which can be seen not only in national use but also individual use. A patient might receive a diagnostic label of chronic bronchitis from one doctor, COPD from another and asthma from another. There is an overlap between them all and it is probably best to group them together for the purpose of investigating the relationship with coronary heart disease.

The data shown in Table 41.1 indicate that populations in the UK, and Scotland in particular, have a surprisingly low death rate from respiratory disease, but we must remember that the term British disease was applied in the early parts of the 20th century. Things will have changed quite dramatically following smoke control legislation in the 1950s and the data shown are from 1992.

**Table 41.1  Death rates from chronic respiratory disease per 100 000 males [2]**

| | |
|---|---|
| Ukraine | 74.9 |
| Hungary | 63.9 |
| Denmark | 58.5 |
| Belarus | 52.2 |
| Lithuania | 46.2 |
| Italy | 46.0 |
| Russia | 41.5 |
| Belgium | 39.6 |
| Germany | 35.6 |
| Switzerland | 34.6 |
| Luxembourg | 34.2 |
| Finland | 31.2 |
| Czech | 30.3 |
| Poland | 28.4 |
| the Netherlands | 25.8 |
| Austria | 25.2 |
| Slovenia | 24.4 |
| Latvia | 24.3 |
| Sweden | 21.4 |
| England & Wales | 21.2 |
| Estonia | 20.6 |
| Norway | 20.6 |
| Portugal | 17.2 |
| Northern Ireland | 16.7 |
| Ireland | 16.6 |
| France | 15.7 |
| Bulgaria | 15.6 |
| Spain | 13.1 |
| Scotland | 12.5 |
| Albania | 12.1 |
| Malta | 10.2 |
| Greece | 4.8 |

We can see some wide variations that are difficult to explain. The exceptionally low level in Greece (4.8) contrasts with a surprisingly high level in near-by Italy (46). Can we explain this 10-fold difference? It might something to do with the nomenclature of disease on death certificates rather than the true incidence of disease. Lithuania has a mortality rate from chronic respiratory disease twice that of neighbouring Latvia and Estonia. The data were collected by WHO from returns from the countries concerned and imperfections are inevitable. However, they are the best available.

We can add to this table the mortality rates for coronary heart disease that we encountered in Figure 33.2. This enables us to produce another scattergraph, looking at the association with respiratory disease, as shown in Figure 41.3.

**Figure 41.3 Deaths from chronic respiratory disease and coronary heat disease (CHD) [2].**

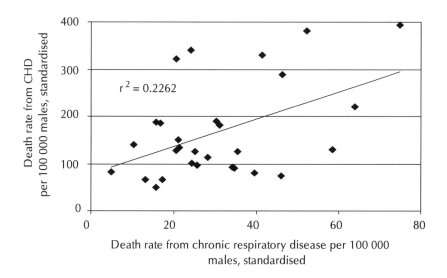

It can be seen that there is a modest relationship between respiratory disease and coronary heart disease, with $R^2=0.2262$. As with the Finland study, this could be interpreted as chronic or recurrent respiratory infections having a causative role in the development of coronary heart disease. We are now perhaps getting closer to the cause of coronary heart disease.

However, we must consider the possibility that the association between chronic respiratory disease and coronary heart disease is one of common causation or common susceptibility. I have mentioned at some length that insufficiency of sunlight and vitamin D might be a common susceptibility factor; this could be the case for the association between coronary heart disease and chronic respiratory disease. If so, then they might show a similar association with latitude, and we can test this using a scattergraph of deaths from chronic respiratory disease against latitude. The mortality data can be seen in Table 41.1 and the scattergraph including latitude in Figure 41.4.

**Figure 41.4 Deaths from chronic respiratory disease and latitude [2].**

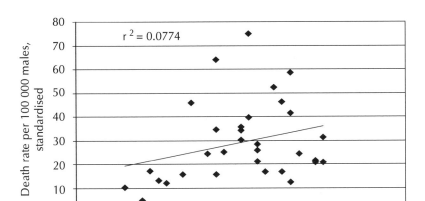

There is no association, the $R^2$ being only 0.0774. There are some obvious outliers, with high mortality rates from chronic respiratory disease associated with relatively low latitudes. These are the former Eastern Bloc countries Ukraine, Hungary and Belarus. But Denmark and Italy have particularly high mortality rates from chronic respiratory disease in association with latitude. It appears that latitude does not provide a common causative link between respiratory disease and coronary heart disease; the model of chronic respiratory disease being the precursor of coronary heart disease is thus stronger.

Other studies have demonstrated a link between chronic respiratory disease and subsequent death from coronary heart disease. One study from Glasgow indicated that the risk was 2.53 higher than the population average, after correction for social class [3]. There is a social class gradient for chronic respiratory disease. The morbidity ratio for those in social classes 1 and 2 is 63, and for social classes 4 and 5 it is twice as high at 131, the population average being, of course, 100 [4].

If chronic or recurrent respiratory disease is the precursor of coronary heart disease, then we can possibly see a mechanism whereby cigarette smoking accelerates the development of coronary heart disease: through respiratory disease. We have already seen an example in the Finland study of chronic bronchitis being more common in those who smoke [1]. There is also evidence that cigarette smoking is a major risk factor for respiratory infections. In a study from the US National Center for Infectious diseases in Atlanta, Georgia, 58% of patients found to have invasive infection with *Pneumococcus* (a common respiratory pathogenic bacterium) were current smokers, compared with 24% of a control population [5]. These patients did not have any recognisable immunodeficiency.

The message from this study is that cigarette smoking encourages infection that invades through the respiratory tract, supporting the mechanism of causation of coronary heart disease via respiratory infection. This brings us back to the question: what sort of disease is coronary heart disease? The next chapter will look at evidence that it might be inflammatory, rather than dietary.

# 42
# INFLAMMATION AND CORONARY HEART DISEASE

It has long been assumed by most people that coronary heart disease, in keeping with associated atherosclerotic disease affecting the brain and the legs, is in some way a degenerative disease. This implies that it is either because of wearing out under continual use (such as arthritis of the hips and knees) or an inevitable accompaniment of getting older. The diet–cholesterol–heart hypothesis implies that there is a steady accumulation of cholesterol in the walls of the arteries, starting in young adult life and continuing inevitably towards death. The higher the dietary cholesterol and the higher the blood cholesterol, the earlier the end-point of death is likely to be reached. We have already noted the weakness of the diet–cholesterol–heart hypothesis in respect of both diet and blood level of cholesterol.

One of the problems with the ready acceptance of the diet–cholesterol–heart hypothesis by the medical, scientific and lay populations has been that it has stifled alternative thinking and research into the causation of coronary heart disease. In particular, and until very recently, there has been neglect of an old observation that inflammatory cells can be seen by microscopy of atheromatous plaques. This initially led to the suggestion that the process might be inflammatory and, after being forgotten in the shadow of cholesterol, the idea has been resurrected in recent years. The evidence that the pathology of coronary heart disease is clearly linked to an inflammatory process comes as a great surprise to many people and it has not yet been absorbed into current medical thinking. Douglas Mann of the Houston Veterans Administration Medical Center, Texas, wrote in an editorial for *The Lancet* in 1999 [1]:

*Although clinicians have recognised the importance of inflammatory mediators in the pathogenesis of heart disease for well over 200 years, clinicians and scientists have taken nearly as many years to focus on the basic biological mechanisms by which inflammatory mediators contribute to the pathogenesis of cardiac disease states.*

It was in the late 1980s that renewed interest in the inflammatory processes in atheromatous plaques appeared. The key cell identified by microscopy is the macrophage, the English translation of which is 'big eater'. The macrophages in tissues are derived from monocytes in blood. Their function is generally to clean up inflamed tissues, consuming tissue debris through the process of phagocytosis. Macrophages are present in unstable atheromatous plaques, which might rupture and lead to surface thrombosis, with subsequent clinical events. An interesting and important study to demonstrate these processes was undertaken using carotid artery atheromatous tissue obtained at surgery [2].

There are two general ways by which inflammation can be detected. The first is histological evidence, looking for inflammatory cells by microscopy of biopsy tissue. This is not generally applicable for the living patient with coronary heart disease because of the inaccessibility of biopsy tissue for histological examination. Even surgical removal of arterial tissue would not usually be appropriate. Autopsy material is available but this limits the opportunities for detailed study because of the interruption of inflammatory processes when a patient dies.

The second method of detecting inflammation is to look for inflammatory markers in the blood. One is the erythrocyte sedimentation rate (ESR), a measure of the speed at which the red blood cells settle to the bottom of a tube of blood to which an anticoagulant has been added. Inflammatory proteins tend to cause the red cells to clump together into larger particles that settle more quickly. ESR is non-specific regarding diagnosis but it is widely used in clinical medicine to help identify or follow the progress of an inflammatory condition. It is not particularly sensitive and has not been useful for coronary heart disease.

Another inflammatory marker is the C-reactive protein (CRP), which appears in blood in response to inflammatory processes in a number of conditions. It is more sensitive than ESR in that it is more likely to be elevated in a patient with inflammatory disease. It can be measured in the blood and the concentration is usually less than 10 mg/L. It can rise to 300 mg/L or more in patients with, for example, severe pneumonia.

A study of the relationship between CRP and coronary syndromes was undertaken in Rome, Italy [3]. The resulting observation was that CRP is elevated in most patients with newly presenting angina and in all patients admitted to hospital because of pre-existing unstable angina or myocardial infarction. The authors commented that in patients with angina, another expression of coronary heart disease, the blood levels of the markers of heart muscle damage (troponin T and creatine kinase) were normal. They concluded that the CRP increase was not the result of the coronary heart disease but linked to its cause. They also noted that, in patients with angina, the outcome was much worse in those with an elevated CRP, regarding early myocardial infarction, the need for emergency surgery and death, as shown in Figure 42.1.

**Figure 42.1 Cardiac events following admission with unstable angina [3].**

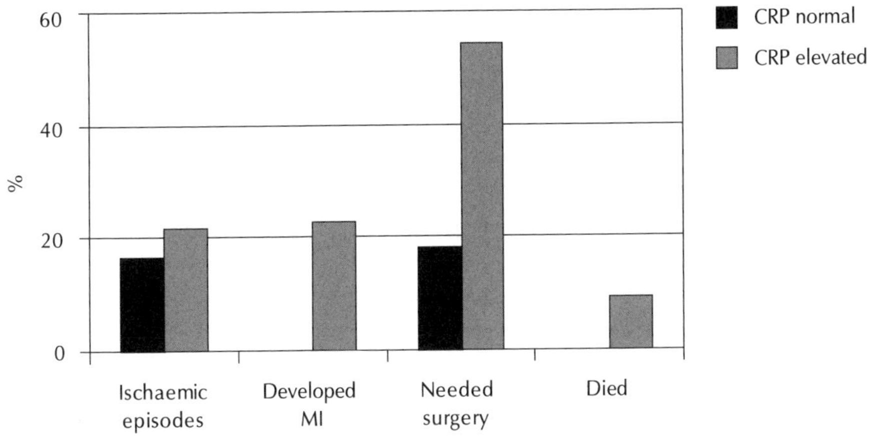

CRP has also been associated with coronary heart disease in a long-term community setting. This was a population study in south-west London, UK, based around St George's Hospital Medical School [4]. The study population of 388 men aged 50–69 years was divided into five groups based on blood levels of CRP; 1.6% of those in the lowest quintile of CRP had a history of coronary heart disease, compared with 32% of those in the highest quintile. The full details are shown in Figure 42.2.

**Figure 42.2 CRP quintiles and coronary heart disease (men aged 50–69 years) [4].**

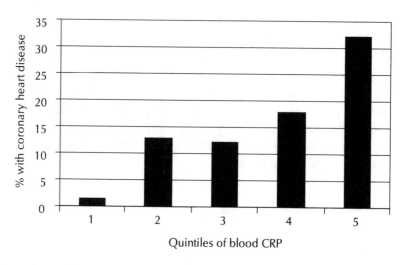

Adapted with permission from the British Medical Journal Publishing Group.

This study identified other relationships with CRP and we will revisit it later. It does, however, confirm a strong association between CRP and coronary heart disease, suggesting that it is mediated by an inflammatory process.

The south-west London study was retrospective, looking at historical coronary heart disease in the study population. A larger and prospective study of coronary events in relation to blood CRP was undertaken by the European Concerted Action on Thrombosis and Disabilities Angina Pectoris Study Group (ECAT) [5]. This looked at 2121 out-patients with angina from 15 European centres, grouped on recruitment into quintiles on the basis of blood CRP. The occurrence of new coronary events in the highest quintile of CRP during the follow-up period of 2 years was three times higher than in the lowest quintile. This is shown in Figure 42.3, the risk of coronary events in the quintiles being age-standardised and relative to a standard score of one in the lowest quintile.

**Figure 42.3 Quintiles of CRP and 2-year coronary events [5].**

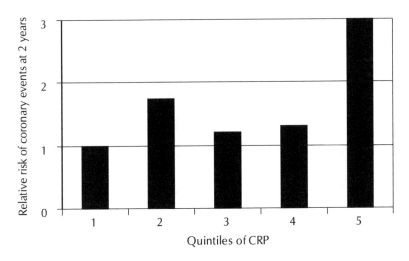

This shows once again that the occurrence of acute coronary events is predicted by the blood level of CRP, suggesting that there is an inflammatory process preceding the clinical expressions of coronary heart disease.

It has been demonstrated in a study from Germany that, the more extensive the coronary heart disease, the higher the CRP [6]. The extent of the disease was assessed regarding whether one, two or three of the major coronary arteries showed evidence of disease on coronary angiography. The results, shown in Figure 42.4, indicated that, the more arteries affected, the more severe the disease and the higher the CRP level in the blood. This again indicates the role of inflammation in the causation of coronary heart disease.

**Figure 42.4  CRP and severity of coronary heart disease [6].**

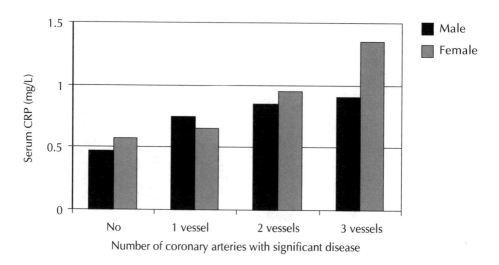

There has been a suggestion that the inflammation might be a secondary process confined to atheromatous plaques, leading them to rupture and cause acute coronary events, including sudden death. However, a study from Rome and Milan indicates that the inflammatory process is widespread within the coronary arteries in patients with angina, and is not confined to the culprit coronary artery stenosis [7].

Another interesting study from Germany, from the University of Ulm, looked at the relationship between alcohol intake and CRP [8]. Those subjects with a moderate intake of alcohol had a lower CRP level than those who drank either little or no alcohol or a great deal of alcohol (Figure 42.5).

**Figure 42.5 CRP and alcohol consumption [8].**

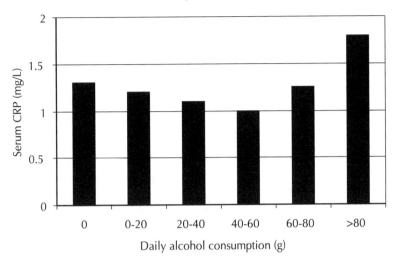

This is the same as the U-shaped curve of alcohol and coronary heart disease. The authors suggested that alcohol might have a direct effect on the inflammatory process, thus providing protection against coronary heart disease. It not possible to reach a conclusion regarding these findings and a number of different interpretations can be applied. It is likely that the CRP levels represent associated diseases rather than being a response to alcohol.

An elevated CRP is associated with coronary heart disease and precedes its clinical manifestations; the higher the CRP, the more extensive the disease and the worse the outcome. These observations suggest that an inflammatory process is very important in the development of coronary heart disease but this is generally not considered in clinical practice. Whereas in other diseases in which inflammation is a major factor, for example ulcerative colitis, the main objective of treatment is to suppress inflammation, this is not the objective in the management of patients with acute coronary syndromes. The identification of inflammation has not really made any impact on the general understanding of the causation of coronary heart disease.

CRP is a more powerful predictor of coronary heart disease than cholesterol, as has been demonstrated by a group from Harvard, who looked at stroke as well as coronary heart disease [9]. A comparison of serum CRP and cholesterol for predicting coronary heart disease is shown in Figure 42.6, and CRP is clearly superior.

**Figure 42.6  Cholesterol and CRP as predictors of coronary heart disease (CHD) [9].**

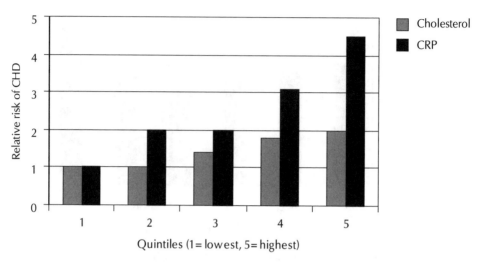

Similarly, CRP is superior to cholesterol in predicting stroke, specifically ischaemic stroke (interruption of blood supply) rather than haemorrhagic stroke. This is shown in Figure 42.7.

**Figure 42.7  Cholesterol and CRP as predictors of ischaemic stroke [9].**

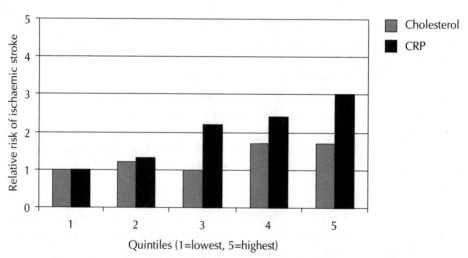

These and other similar observations have led the Honolulu Heart Program group to suggest that 'Atherosclerosis could have origins more closely linked with inflammation than with other processes' [10]. This comment acknowledges the weakness of the diet–cholesterol–heart hypothesis, whose adherents have generally ignored the importance of inflammation in the development of coronary heart disease.

This brings us to what must be a close relationship between cholesterol and CRP. The Harvard group have developed this further, investigating 14 916 middle-aged men who were not known to have coronary heart disease [11]. The risk of myocardial infarction increases with increasing serum cholesterol, especially if the CRP is elevated. Similarly, the risk of myocardial infarction increases with increasing serum CRP, but especially if the cholesterol is elevated. The results can be seen in Figure 42.8, a three-dimensional bar chart. The subjects are divided into three groups on the basis of CRP and cholesterol.

**Figure 42.8 Relative risk of myocardial infarction (MI) with cholesterol and CRP [11].**

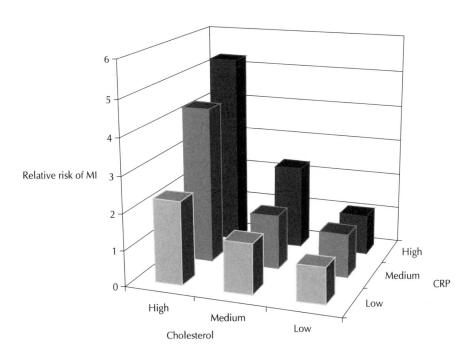

*Adapted from* Circulation *with permission from Lippincott, Williams and Watkins.*

The risk of myocardial infarction is lowest in those with the lowest CRP and cholesterol, and highest in those with the highest CRP and cholesterol. Cholesterol and CRP are clearly working together, synergistically. It appears that both might have a role in the causation of coronary heart disease. CRP is clearly part of the inflammatory process; could this be the case with cholesterol? Are they both telling us the same thing? We will look at this possibility in the next chapter, but first we must deal with a further dimension of inflammation and coronary heart disease.

Inflammatory processes are by no means straightforward and can be difficult to understand. New research information is being generated continually. A very good review of CRP and its relationship with coronary heart disease appeared in the *Quarterly Journal of Medicine* in 2003, authored by Hirschfield and Professor Mark Pepys from the Royal Free Hospital Medical School, London, UK [12].

In the same journal in the previous year, another group from the Royal London Hospital had looked at the involvement of vitamin D in the inflammatory process [13]. As this is clearly relevant to the main theme of this book, I will briefly review the paper, although its content is highly technical.

The mechanisms of the inflammatory process are not entirely understood but it would appear to involve tissue enzymes called metaloproteinases (MMPs) that control remodelling of the blood vessel wall and other tissues during and after inflammatory disruption. This is an important part of the restoration of normal structure and function following any inflammatory disease. Vitamin D (in its most active form, calcitriol) modulates tissue MMP and thus influences recovery from inflammation. We have previously encountered VDRs and these can also be found in the walls of arteries. This is further evidence that vitamin D is important in the inflammatory process generally and in the atherosclerotic process in particular.

We have looked at the history, geography and sociology of coronary heart disease, and we will shortly be looking at its ethnic dimension. For now I will mention that the South Asian ethnic population of the UK has an extraordinarily high incidence of coronary heart disease and the group from the Royal London Hospital felt that this might be a result of vitamin D insufficiency. The study of Timms *et al.* [13] was to investigate in more detail the inflammatory process of atherosclerosis and coronary heart disease, and they studied the Bangladeshi population living in Tower Hamlets, London. They found, as might be expected, a high incidence of vitamin D insufficiency in this population and it was associated with unusually high levels of circulating MMP9 and CRP. The study also confirmed that people with mutations of VDR are at particular risk of vitamin D deficiency when receiving only low exposure to sunlight. We have already seen that such people are at risk of developing tuberculosis.

The conclusion was that the tissue damage in coronary heart disease, and in particular the plaque rupture that might lead to sudden death or acute coronary event, is at least in part because of a lack of MMP in the tissues, and that this in turn is the result of an insufficiency of vitamin D.

We will now review briefly the relationship between cholesterol and inflammation and then we will look in more detail at the ethnicity of coronary heart disease.

# 43
# CHOLESTEROL AND INFLAMMATION

I have tried to emphasize the importance of not assuming a cause–effect relationship when two factors are found to occur more frequently than would be expected by chance. There is rather more caution in science today, but a century ago that was not always the case. Following the observations of Virchow, it was readily assumed that the cholesterol he had identified in diseased arterial tissue was driving the disease process; this assumption has continued to the present as part of the diet–cholesterol–heart hypothesis and it has been questioned by very few people.

We saw in Chapter 24 that two particular studies, MRFIT and Whitehall [1,2], have shown in young and middle-aged men a relationship between a high blood cholesterol concentration and subsequent development of coronary heart disease. This has been a very powerful influence on scientific and popular opinion, reinforcing the conventional wisdom that cholesterol in the blood is causing the disease.

Temporal relationships require more thought and attention. During the MRFIT and Whitehall studies, there was no way of knowing whether or not the participants of the study had coronary heart disease. They certainly had no clinical manifestations of the disease at the time of recruitment, but the general thinking is that coronary heart disease has a latent period of a minimum of about 20 years. As most people who experience myocardial infarction are above the age of 70, it must be assumed that the disease is commonly established although latent by the age of 50 years.

The elevated blood cholesterol levels in the MRFIT and Whitehall studies were shown to predict the clinical manifestations of coronary heart disease, sudden death, angina or myocardial infarction. The long latent interval of subclinical disease (what is called an incubation period in acute viral infections) means that most of those in the study probably had the disease in a subclinical form. The high blood cholesterol levels were therefore not necessarily preceding coronary heart disease, and it is possible that the high blood cholesterol levels were reflecting an active but latent disease process.

We have seen in the previous chapter that active inflammation, as shown by an elevated CRP, is a powerful predictor of coronary events and a poor outcome. Is it possible that elevated blood cholesterol is simply telling us the same thing? We have also seen the elderly paradox, which indicates quite clearly that, in elderly people, high cholesterol is an advantage regarding all causes of mortality. This immediately suggests that cholesterol might have an overall protective role.

We have also seen, as illustrated in Figure 24.6, that, before the epidemic of coronary heart disease in western Europe, members of the well-researched family in the Netherlands with familial hypercholesterolaemia had a health advantage [3]. They had, between 1800 and 1869, an SMR of 40 in female members of the family and 70 in males. They were starting to lose this advantage between 1870 and 1900, when the SMR was 80 for women and 90 for men. When the coronary heart disease epidemic was emerging between 1901 and 1929, the SMR had risen to well above the population average, to 150 in women and 180 in men.

There is thus no question that the genetic mutation became a disadvantage during the epidemic of coronary heart disease, but its health advantage in the absence of coronary heart disease suggests that cholesterol might then have a protective role. The health advantage of the family with hypercholesterolaemia was particularly obvious at a time when most deaths were caused by infectious diseases, suggesting that cholesterol might have a role in protection against acute infections.

Coronary heart and other atherosclerotic diseases are very common causes of illness and death in western countries. If they were the result of cholesterol, then this would indicate an evolutionary disaster: why should the body be programmed to synthesise a substance that we are told is so harmful? The fact that coronary heart disease has been an epidemic indicates that it is not genetically determined, but the family from the Netherlands was clearly at more than average risk.

Evolutionary survival is the result of genetic advantages; if the body produces cholesterol then there must be a function for it. We must ask ourselves what useful contribution does cholesterol make to human metabolism? What is it doing in atheromatous plaques? These questions are not usually asked and the general wisdom is only that it is dangerous; as a result therapeutic evangelism attempts to reduce blood cholesterol in all people by as much as possible. The claim that most people are now said to be at risk from high cholesterol that requires treatment has led to the publication of a book entitled *Overdosed America: The Broken Promise of American Medicine* [4].

It has been noted that people who have a particularly low serum cholesterol concentration have a high risk of cancer. The interpretation is usually that the cancer pre-dated the low cholesterol and effectively caused it, and the low cholesterol is thus absolved from a harmful role. But this assumption is not valid; people with a low cholesterol level are at a certain disadvantage from malignant disease, and an improved understanding of the function of cholesterol might help clarify this.

I have already pointed out that there is a new but growing understanding that an inflammatory process is involved in the development of atherosclerosis. It is difficult to imagine how the deposition of cholesterol, a physiologically simple substance, in arteries would produce inflammation that is not observed in other parts of the body. Cholesterol appears to have a role within the inflammatory process without causing it. There have been suggestions that blood lipids play an important role in immunity and the inflammatory process, and this subject has been reviewed very well in the *Quarterly Journal of Medicine* by the Swedish researcher Dr Uffe Ravnskov [5].

*Staphylococcus aureus* is well known as a cause of infection in human beings, infections that can be extremely serious. The most pathogenic strains of this organism produce a series of toxins that cause tissue damage and mediate certain aspects of disease. There is evidence that cholesterol can suppress the inflammatory process induced by *Staphylococcus aureus*. *In vitro* laboratory experiments have shown that the alpha toxin is almost totally inactivated by serum containing cholesterol, and in particular by purified LDL cholesterol, the low-density lipoprotein that is said to be bad for us [6].

If cholesterol were an inflammatory marker in a similar way to CRP, then we might expect it to increase in response to acute infection. This model conforms to observations of coronary heart disease, with serum cholesterol and CRP showing a similar pattern. There is, however, some evidence that cholesterol is removed from the blood in response to an acute infection, with the logical suggestion that this might be because of consumption of cholesterol [7]. The processes of increased synthesis and increased consumption can of course co-exist, and a balance between the two would determine the overall increase or decrease of the blood cholesterol level in response to infection.

A meta-analysis of 19 studies looked at 68 406 deaths from respiratory and gastro-intestinal diseases, most of which were infectious. It was found that the risk of death was lowest in those people who had previously been identified as having high serum cholesterol, and there was generally an inverse relationship between death from these conditions and serum cholesterol [7]. High serum cholesterol appears to be protective, and this can be seen in Figure 43.1.

**Figure 43.1  Specific mortalities related to serum cholesterol [7].**

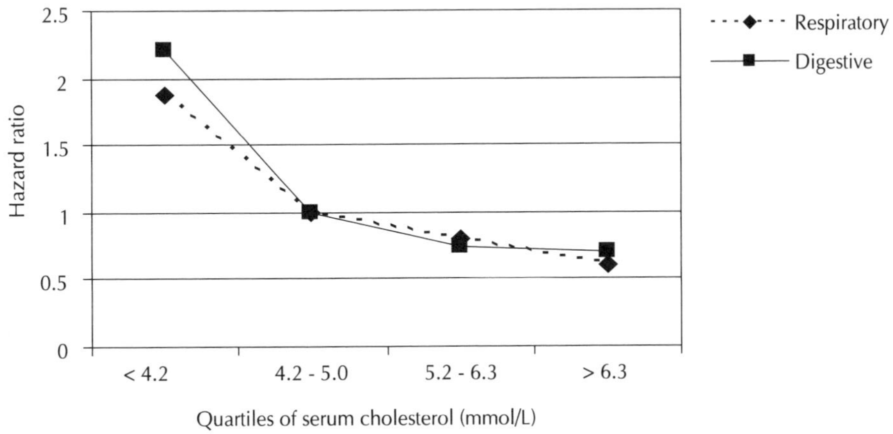

Quartiles of serum cholesterol (mmol/L)

*Adapted from Circulation with permission from Lippincott, Williams and Watkins.*

A further study was a 15-year follow-up of 120 000 individuals, recording the serum cholesterol at the beginning of the study and the health risk subsequently. Once again, there was a strong inverse association between the total cholesterol and the risk of hospital admission because of infectious disease [8]. In other words, a high cholesterol level appeared to be protective against acute infections, compatible with it having a role to play in a defensive inflammatory process. Figure 43.2 shows the relationship between serum cholesterol, expressed as quartiles, and the incidence of all infectious diseases in men and women.

**Figure 43.2 Relationship between serum cholesterol and infectious disease [8].**

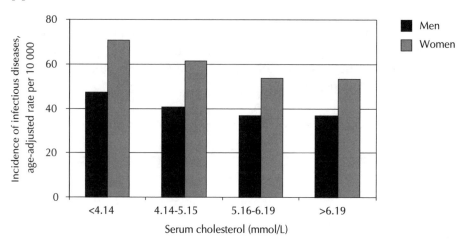

A similar study looking at 100 000 individuals over a period of 15 years showed that those with high serum cholesterol had the lowest hospital admission rate as a result of pneumonia and other respiratory tract infections (Figure 43.3) but this did not apply to the non-microbial respiratory conditions of chronic obstructive pulmonary disease and asthma [9].

**Figure 43.3 Relative risk of respiratory infection based on serum cholesterol [9].**

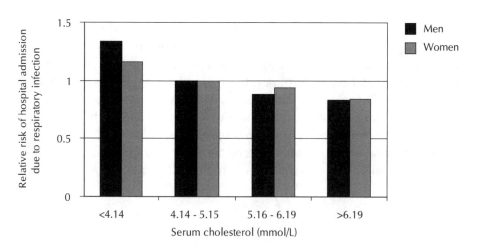

It has also been shown, from a study of 2446 unmarried men with a history of liver or sexually transmitted disease, that those with a low blood cholesterol level had the highest risk of subsequent HIV development, the viral infection that is the precursor of AIDS. The relative risk was 1.66 in the lowest quartile of serum cholesterol compared with the next highest quartile [10]. The follow-up time was 14 years and, to exclude the possibility of HIV causing low cholesterol, those who became HIV positive during the first 4 years of the study were not included in the analysis. This is another example of the protective effect of cholesterol.

A surgical study investigated patients who had to undergo emergency surgery because of infection within the abdomen. Post-operative mortality was almost three times higher in those with low blood cholesterol; the results are shown in Figure 43.4 [11]. A low albumin component of protein in the blood similarly predicted a higher mortality. In both cases, it would appear that metabolic consumptions of cholesterol and albumin are greater than synthesis.

**Figure 43.4  Post-operative mortality and serum cholesterol [11].**

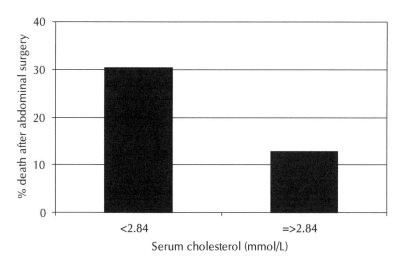

It could therefore be the case that the relationship between a high blood cholesterol level and subsequent clinical expression of coronary heart disease is because of the continuing subclinical latent inflammatory process in the arteries stimulating an elevated cholesterol level in the blood and, in exactly the same way, CRP and other inflammatory markers such as fibrinogen. The association between cholesterol and subsequent coronary heart disease must not be causative and indeed there is compelling evidence to suggest that it is a phenomenon secondary to the development of the disease.

It is possible that cholesterol is a component of the inflammatory process and has a defensive function; if the inflammatory process continues without completion, a build-up of cholesterol in the wall of the coronary artery can be expected. This would lead to occlusion of the arteries concerned, a process that has nothing to do with diet but that explains the association between cholesterol and coronary heart disease. In a similar way the inflammatory process of a condition called cranial arteritis can also lead to occlusion of the artery with, in this case, loss of vision or stroke. The inflammatory process in Crohn's disease (to be reviewed later) can lead to obstruction of the intestine. Inflammation of the tonsils in acute tonsillitis can obstruct the upper respiratory tract, and inflammation of the appendix can lead to acute obstructive appendicitis with rupture. There is thus a pattern in which a defensive inflammatory process creates bulk and can cause occlusion to part of the body. The atherosclerotic process with the coronary arteries conforms with this.

We have seen that there is a seasonal variation of serum cholesterol, and I have interpreted this as a diversion of the metabolism of 7-dehydrocholesterol in the skin from vitamin D into cholesterol synthesis, in the absence of sunlight of adequate energy content. Although this is plausible, there is a weakness in the model. The increase of cholesterol in the winter is greater than the diminution of vitamin D synthesis. Something else linked with winter, and probably vitamin D metabolism, appears to be driving cholesterol synthesis. We know that during the winter there is an increase in inflammatory markers such as CRP and fibrinogen in response to winter infections, and this in turn is a result of reduced vitamin D synthesis. If cholesterol is an inflammatory marker with a defensive role, then the winter increase in serum cholesterol would be part of the same process of response to infection.

It is appropriate at this point to revisit the statin trials and, in particular, the WOSCOPS study [12] described as the Scottish paradox in Chapter 28. We have seen that statins are undoubtedly helpful, not only in the natural history of coronary heart disease but also in the prevention of clinical manifestations of other atherosclerotic syndromes, cerebral infarction and peripheral arterial disease. As is quite clearly described in Chapter 28, statins have a benefit that is independent of their undoubted ability to reduce blood cholesterol levels. The mechanism behind their beneficial effect is not understood and, despite the evidence readily available, statin drug therapy is still often equated with 'cholesterol-lowering therapy'.

It has been noted that statins have an anti-inflammatory effect, the precise nature of which is at present unknown. I propose that the clinical effectiveness of statin therapy is mediated by this anti-inflammatory effect and that the cholesterol-lowering effect is unimportant and effectively an epiphenomenon. Like so many advances in medicine, such as the introduction of bromide for the treatment of epilepsy, the introduction of statins has been serendipitous. It is important in practical terms to dissociate statin therapy from its cholesterol-lowering action and simply talk about statin therapy *per se*.

# PART 8

# MICRO-ORGANISMS AND THE HEART

# 44

# COULD CORONARY HEART DISEASE BE CAUSED BY MICRO-ORGANISMS?

We saw in Chapter 5 that the fundamental causes of disease fall into very few categories. They include genetic factors, congenital birth defects, trauma, deficiency states, poisonings, psychological factors and micro-organisms. I propose that adequate exposure to the sun provides a high but not an absolute level of protection against coronary heart disease. The plausibility of this depends on our view of the major cause of this condition, something that is either generally mistaken or far from clear.

We have noted that coronary heart disease tends to run in families but that, in the vast majority of cases, it is a non-genetic form of family transmission. The epidemic nature indicates an environmental factor and not a genetic disorder. It is not congenital. It does not appear to be a deficiency state, although we have seen that insufficiency of vitamin D increases susceptibility. Suggestions of cholesterol poisoning do not seem to be sustainable and no other poisonings are obvious. The weakness of invoking a psychological cause has also been revealed.

By exclusion, we are forced to consider whether coronary heart disease might be caused by a micro-organism. This might sound extraordinary, but it is a suggestion that some people have been taking seriously for some years. We have already seen that syphilis and tuberculosis are chronic microbial diseases but their cause was not suspected for many years. They both show features of non-genetic family transmission and the pathology is inflammation.

We have established that coronary heart disease is inflammatory, this being the pathology or mechanism. There are a number of causes of inflammation, one example being a foreign body or irritant. Most inflammations, especially chronic diseases over a long period of time, are the result of infections, caused by viruses, bacteria, protozoons, yeasts or fungi. If coronary heart disease is inflammatory, then we must consider a causative micro-organism.

We can therefore envisage a possible model in which a micro-organism is the cause, inflammation is the mechanism and coronary heart disease is the disease:

micro-organism $\longrightarrow$ inflammation $\longrightarrow$ coronary heart disease

I have already described the traditional model of infection, with an acute onset followed by either death or gradual recovery, and we saw this in the example of hepatitis. We saw that the clustering of cases of cholera indicated a transmissible agent. This is an important part of the model, and clustering also applies to hepatitis, which was accepted as being a microbial disease several decades before the causative viruses were identified.

I have also indicated the difficulty in establishing a microbial model for chronic diseases such as tuberculosis and syphilis. In both of these the associated micro-organisms were ultimately identified, and it was not until this occurred that the models were generally accepted. Whereas hepatitis caused by A and B viruses is an acute disease with an abrupt onset followed by recovery (or occasionally death), the C virus causes a different type of disease, a chronic inflammatory process over many years, occasionally with a malignant end.

Peptic ulcer is a recent example of a chronic disease that has turned out to be caused by a micro-organism, which came as great surprise; it was never considered to be microbial until *Helicobacter pylori* was identified. It was quite remarkable how readily the microbial cause was then accepted, and if peptic ulcer can turn out to have a micro-organism as its cause, perhaps so can virtually any chronic disease.

Is it plausible that coronary heart disease can be caused by a micro-organism? To answer this question it is not essential to identify a micro-organism, it is the principle that needs to be clarified. First, is there a better model? The answer to this is 'no', but conventional wisdom is still firmly entrenched in the diet–cholesterol–heart theory. As stated by Earl Benditt and James McDougall, pathologists from the University of Washington, USA [1]:

*If we accept that aberrations in cholesterol metabolism provide the whole aetiological basis for coronary and other vascular occlusive disease, we need hunt no further. On the other hand, we think there is still a great deal to be explained and that viruses may well hold some, if not all, of the missing pieces of the puzzle.*

They also stated [1]:

*The rise and fall of coronary heart disease (CHD) in a number of Western countries in this century has been dramatic ... The shape of the CHD mortality curve reminds one of the rise and fall of epidemic diseases due to microbial agents.*

Coronary heart disease is an inflammatory process and inflammation usually has an infective cause. As with tuberculosis, syphilis and peptic ulcer, there is clustering in families that does not conform to a genetic pattern but indicates an environmental agent. There is an association with peptic ulcer and also an association with respiratory infections. The social and physical geography of coronary heart disease matches that of peptic ulcer and tuberculosis.

We have seen in respect of tuberculosis that there appears to be protection by exposure to the sun, implying immuno-enhancement and increased resistance against infection. The same appears to be the case with coronary heart disease, and as there is no clear cause we need to be open-minded and consider that it might be infection.

Shortly before 1977 it was noticed by astute clinical observation that [2]:

*a considerable proportion of the patients admitted to the coronary-care unit of the King Edward VII Hospital, Midhurst, Kent, gave an unsolicited history of an influenza-like illness before admission.*

This led to a structured research project, the result of which was the observation that 10 out of 38 patients admitted with an acute myocardial infarction had positive antibodies indicating recent infection with Coxsackie virus. It was already known that Coxsackie B virus could cause myocarditis, an infection of the heart muscle (well reviewed in an editorial in *The Lancet* in 1979) [3], but myocardial infarction is a different disease, although there can be some clinical confusion between the two in individual cases.

A similar and subsequent study was undertaken at the nearby Crawley Hospital, Sussex, UK. Serum samples were obtained from 93 survivors of myocardial infarction but only three showed a significant antibody rise to Coxsackie B virus [4]. This result did not support the findings from Midhurst, and so the role of the virus became very doubtful. However, 10% of the patients had experienced a 'flu-like illness immediately preceding the myocardial infarction, and so a microbial cause remained a possibility. The problem was identifying a causative micro-organism.

The Bayler College of Medicine, Houston, Texas, USA, has been a pioneering centre of vascular surgery, led by the charismatic surgeon Michael DeBakey (1908–2008). A study from his department looked at antibody levels against viruses in patients with atherosclerosis undergoing arterial surgery. High levels of antibodies to cytomegalovirus were found in 57% of surgical patients, compared with 26% in a control group [5].

Coronary heart disease is a particular problem in a transplanted heart, for reasons that are not clear but might be related to therapeutic suppression of immunity. We will review this in a later chapter. However, I would like to draw attention to a report of cytomegalovirus being detected in 62% of patients with coronary artery disease developing after heart transplantation, compared with its detection in only 25% of those without coronary heart disease [6].

The possibility of a viral cause for coronary heart disease was reviewed in an editorial in the American journal *Circulation*, with the observation [7]:

*Despite the fact that atherosclerotic vascular disease is the major cause of morbidity and mortality in developed countries, there are wide gaps in our understanding of its cause … the primary inciting events in the atherosclerotic process remain poorly defined.*

The authors go on to make the interesting comment [7]:

*Likewise it is interesting to speculate whether viral infection may have a role in the clinical problems of restenosis after angioplasty and the accelerated atherosclerosis seen in patients on immunosuppressive doses of corticosteroids, both of which remain largely unexplained.*

The accelerated atherosclerosis in patients on immunosuppressive therapy is a subject that I will deal with later. For now let us remember the likelihood that an immuno-enhancing effect of sunlight protects against coronary heart disease, and so we would expect immunosuppression to increase susceptibility and severity.

The same process was undertaken in Helsinki, Finland, this time looking at patients with cerebral infarction (stroke). The study was of 54 consecutive patients with stroke, all aged less than 50 years, compared with 54 community-based age and sex-matched controls [8]. Nineteen patients had evidence of a febrile illness during the previous month, compared with three controls. In 80% of cases the infection was respiratory and mainly bacterial. This study again indicates an infection preceding an atherosclerotic event.

Subsequent research has provided evidence that the bacteria *Chlamydia pneumoniae* and *Helicobacter pylori* have a strong association with coronary heart disease and are possible contenders for its cause. If one or both of these bacteria cause coronary heart disease, then antibiotic therapy might be expected to be helpful. Clinical trials have been conducted and these will be reviewed later. A group from Boston, USA, approached this in a different way and felt that incidental antibiotic therapy might also be helpful [9]. They studied 3315 patients aged 75 years or younger with a diagnosis of a first myocardial infarction, and 13 139 matched controls without myocardial infarction. The result was that those who had taken tetracycline or quinolone antibiotics on one or more occasion during the previous 3 years had a significantly reduced risk of developing a myocardial infarction. This benefit was not conferred by other antibiotics. The relative risks are shown in Figure 44.1.

**Figure 44.1 Antibiotic monotherapy and subsequent myocardial infarction (MI) [9].**

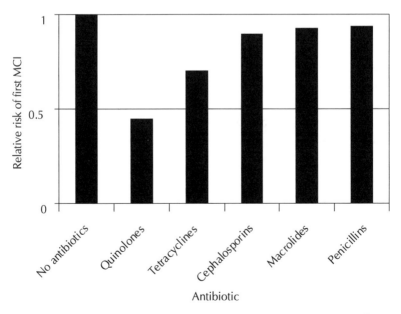

This supports a proposition that bacteria cause myocardial infarction. The quinolone antibiotics, which appear to have the greatest protective effect against myocardial infarction, include ciprofloxacin, ofloxacin, levofloxacin, moxifloxacin, norfloxacin and nalidixic acid. Of these, ciprofloxacin is at present the most widely used in the UK.

It might be expected, as with *Helicobacter pylori* and peptic ulcer, that the medical–scientific community would have embraced this interesting work and looked positively at the possible causative role of micro-organisms in coronary heart disease. The speed of development of antibiotic therapy in the treatment of peptic ulcer was quite remarkable, and also very effective. But that has not happened with coronary heart disease. The general attitude is summarised by an editorial entitled 'Antibiotics for prevention of myocardial infarction? Not yet!' [10].

There are three attitudes that can be taken towards a microbial cause of coronary heart disease. One is denial; another is to look for a specific micro-organism, along the lines described above; a third approach is what has been termed the 'dirty chicken' hypothesis [11]. This is the suggestion that a variety of micro-organisms can trigger myocardial infarction, with a lifetime of recurrent infections and thus an increasing burden of inflammation damaging the arteries. It has some attractions; it would certainly fit in with a protective role of immuno-enhancing factors such as sunshine. It does not, however, fit in with the epidemic nature of coronary heart disease in the 20th century, which suggests a specific micro-organism, as with tuberculosis or syphilis. The dirty chicken hypothesis is based on a non-specific burden of a range of microbial diseases.

We must remember that microbiology is still a developing science. *Chlamydia pneumoniae* and *Helicobacter pylori* have only been recognised in recent years. We do not know the microbiological discoveries that lie ahead and we must remain open-minded. For now, we need to find out more about *Chlamydia pneumoniae* and *Helicobacter pylori* and their relationships with coronary heart disease.

# 45
## *CHLAMYDIA PNEUMONIAE*

We have noted that myocardial infarction is preceded by a febrile respiratory infection more often than would be expected by chance. We are uncertain as to whether this might be just a precipitating event or whether it might be causing the underlying coronary heart disease.

Acute infections result in an inflammatory reaction, and as a consequence of this we find the appearance of non-specific inflammatory markers in the blood, such as erythrocyte sedimentation rate (ESR) and C-reactive protein (CRP). Another inflammatory marker is fibrinogen, the natural precursor of fibrin that creates a blood clot. Following an acute infection the coagulation of the blood increases. In theory this could precipitate a blood clot on the surface of an atheromatous plaque that is already causing critical stenosis of a coronary artery, and the result would be myocardial infarction, perhaps with sudden death. What we need to know is whether infection just precipitates a coronary event, a myocardial infarction, by inducing a blood clot or whether it might be involved in a more fundamental and long-term process of causation of coronary heart disease itself.

Coronary heart disease has been a very serious public health problem in Finland for many years and in particular in Karelia, the most northern part of Finland. This comes as no surprise to us, as we are dealing with an area that is far distant from the equator and effectively at sea level. We now know that insufficiency of sunshine leads to susceptibility to coronary heart disease, and we are still searching for the cause. A great deal of work has been undertaken in Finland and much of it has centred on a possible microbial factor.

A study from Helsinki published in 1988 looked at 40 male patients who survived acute myocardial infarction, 30 with chronic coronary heart disease, and 41 matched controls [1]. They were all tested for antibody evidence of infection with a newly discovered organism, *Chlamydia TWAR*, subsequently reclassified as *Chlamydia pneumoniae*. It had been initially identified as a respiratory pathogen and the study was stimulated by the link between respiratory disease and coronary heart disease, a link that we have seen in a previous chapter. The critical serological test turned out to be IgG antibodies in a titre greater than 1 in 128 plus IgA antibodies in a titre greater than 1 in 32; the results can be seen in Figure 45.1.

**Figure 45.1 Serological evidence of *Chlamydia TWAR* infection [1] ].**

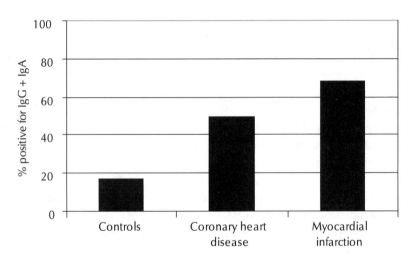

© *1988, adapted from* The Lancet *with permission from Elsevier.*

It can be seen that there is a very significant association between *Chlamydia pneumoniae* and coronary heart disease, both in its chronic dormant phase and, in particular, at the time of instability with acute myocardial infarction. This suggests that infection, like inflammation as we have seen, appears to be a fundamental part of the development of coronary heart disease and not just the precipitating event of a final coronary artery occlusion.

But only 50% of those with coronary heart disease had positive antibodies to *Chlamydia pneumoniae* (*TWAR*) at the titres mentioned above. A lower titre of IgG antibodies, greater than 32, was positive in 87% of patients with coronary heart disease but also in 61% of controls. Infection with this organism is therefore very common and, if it does have a causative role in coronary heart disease, progression from the initial respiratory infection does not always occur. This might depend on the resistance or, alternatively, the susceptibility of individuals to the infection.

A group from St George's Hospital Medical School, London, UK has been very active in trying to identify a microbiological cause of coronary heart disease; we have already seen some of their work and we will see more of it. This group investigated antibodies to *Chlamydia pneumoniae* in coronary heart disease, by studying 213 male survivors of myocardial infarction [2]. The presence or absence of antibodies is shown in Table 45.1, and we can see that most patients (72%) were antibody positive, indicating current or past infection with *Chlamydia pneumoniae*.

**Table 45.1** *Chlamydia pneumoniae* **antibodies and myocardial infarction (MI) [1]**

|  | MI |
| --- | --- |
| No antibodies detected, % | 27.7 |
| Antibodies detected, % | 72.3 |
| Weak positive, titres 1/8 to1/32, % | 34.7 |
| Strong positive, titres >1/64, % | 37.6 |

© *1988, adapted from* The Lancet *with permission from Elsevier.*

A question remains regarding the relevance of the positive antibodies. Respiratory infection with *Chlamydia pneumoniae* in the community is so common (but not routinely identified) that a causal association with coronary heart disease is by no means clear. The next stage was to see whether the presence of antibodies has any bearing on future coronary events. The way to determine this would be to compare the future outcome of a group of patients strongly positive for antibodies with a similar group to which antibiotic treatment would be given to eradicate the organism.

Eighty patients (37%) had strongly positive antibodies, more likely to represent active infection than intermediate positive antibodies. Sixty of these were recruited into the antibiotic phase of the study [2]. Twenty were given a placebo tablet as controls; 40 received one or two courses of azithromycin.

The antibody titre decreased in 17 of the 40 patients who received azithromycin, but in only two out of the 20 taking placebo. This clearly suggested that the high antibody titre represented an active rather than historical infection, and that the antibiotic treatment was effective in controlling or eradicating the infection. The cardiovascular outcome of the groups can be seen in Figure 45.2.

**Figure 45.2** *Chlamydia pneumoniae* **antibodies and risk of coronary heart disease [2].**

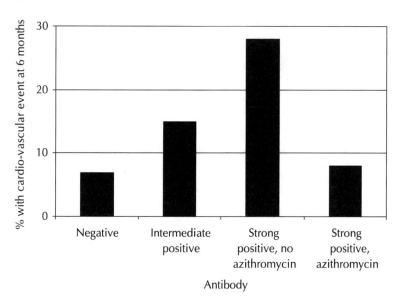

The titre of antibodies had a bearing on outcome; those with the highest titres (strong positive) had the greatest number of cardiovascular events, 28% after 6 months compared with 7% in those with negative titres and 14% in those with intermediate titres. The antibiotic therapy with azithromycin, given to those with high titres, had a dramatic effect on outcome, reducing the cardiovascular event rate more that three-fold, from 28% to 8%.

The conclusion that we can draw from this important study is that the hypothesis that *Chlamydia pneumoniae* causes coronary heart disease is strongly supported; but it cannot be the only cause, and this puts the proposal on a rather shaky foundation. We like to see one disease related to one organism, for example tuberculosis and *Mycobacterium tuberculosis*, syphilis and *Treponema pallidum* and AIDS and HIV. However, other mycobacteria can cause atypical tuberculosis, and hepatitis can be the result of a range of viruses; coronary heart disease might also have more than one microbial cause. It might be the case that coronary heart disease is really coronary heart diseases, but there is no attempt to subclassify at the present time. Sometimes the disease is patchy and localised, sometimes it is diffuse. Are these two patterns the same disease with the same cause, or are they perhaps two diseases with different causative micro-organisms? At this stage we must remain open-minded but, in the study described above, a course of azithromycin given after myocardial infarction had an extremely beneficial effect, irrespective of the micro-organism or the mechanism.

1997 saw a similar study, this time from Buenos Aires, Argentina; 102 patients who survived myocardial infarction (in this study ECG changes without q-waves) were randomly allocated to receive a course of the antibiotic roxithromycin and the outcome was compared with that of 100 controls [3]. There were fewer deaths and cardiac events in the treated group and the details can be seen in Figure 45.3.

**Figure 45.3 Effect of azithromycin on outcome after myocardial infarction (MI) [3].**

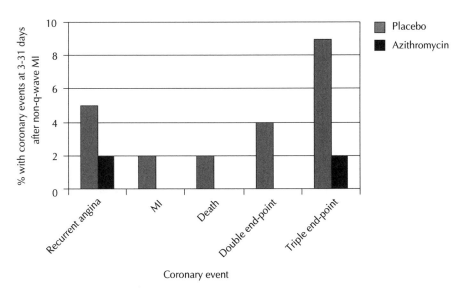

*© 1997, adapted from* The Lancet *with permission from Elsevier.*

389

Once again we can see a beneficial effect from antibiotic therapy, this time with roxithromycin. In this study there was no attempt to identify *Chlamydia pneumoniae* infection.

But other studies have shown conflicting results. A recent study of azithromycin therapy in patients admitted to hospital with acute coronary syndromes has taken place in Slovenia, Israel, Germany, Austria and the USA (Los Angeles) [4]; 716 patients were randomised to receive azithromycin for 4 days and the outcome at 6 months was compared with that of a control group of 723 who received a placebo tablet. The results are shown in Figure 45.4.

**Figure 45.4 Azithromycin after acute coronary syndrome [4].**

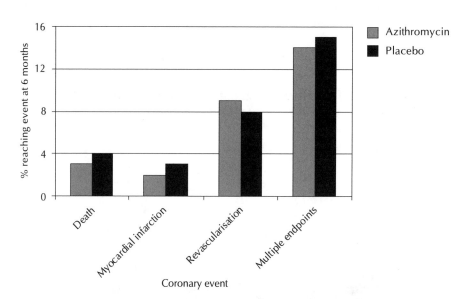

We can see that there were no significant differences between the two groups and that overall the outcome for all was good. Revascularisation means that the patients developed further cardiac events and, as a result, either coronary angioplasty or coronary artery bypass surgery was performed. This study did not identify the presence of antibodies to *Chlamydia pneumoniae*, which might be the key to effectiveness.

A study of roxithromycin undertaken in Germany looked at recurrence of coronary artery narrowing (restenosis) after insertion of coronary artery stents [5]. It investigated the use of the antibiotic in those with high titres of antibody against *Chlamydia pneumoniae*. Overall the rate of restenosis was 31% in the 506 patients who received roxithromycin for 28 days, not significantly different from 29% in the placebo group. However, as shown in Figure 45.5, there was a better response to treatment in those with higher antibody titres. The higher the titre, the greater the amount of antibody detected.

**Figure 45.5  Restenosis of coronary arteries with roxithromycin [5].**

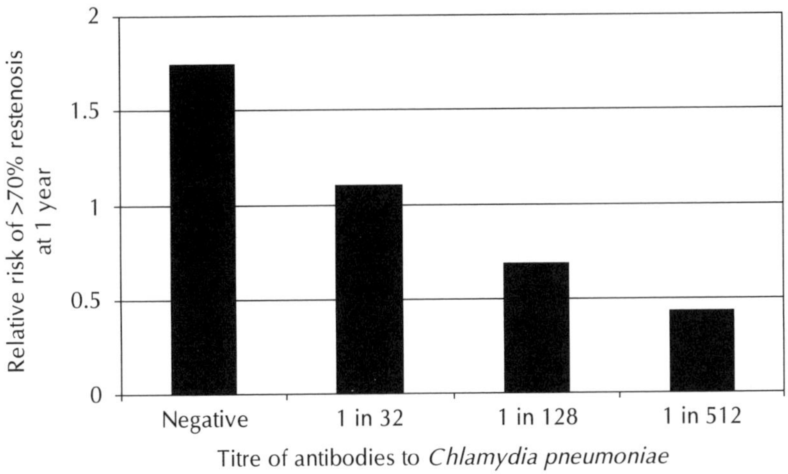

*© 2001, adapted from* The Lancet *with permission from Elsevier.*

It can be seen that the restenosis rate was much lower after treatment when titres were higher. Although *Chlamydia pneumoniae* might be actively causing disease in some patients, in others there appears to be a different cause.

The method of detection of *Chlamydia pneumoniae* in these studies has been by identification of antibodies. Although the organism is known to be most strongly associated with respiratory infections, especially acute tracheobronchitis, the whereabouts of the organism in the body at the time of the coronary heart disease studies is unknown. Is it influencing the atherosclerotic process from a distance, or is it acting locally? It is not possible to answer these questions in a clinical study.

A group from Johannesburg, South Africa, looked at atherosclerotic tissue obtained at autopsy, and in about half the cases they were able to identify *Chlamydia pneumoniae* by the technologically advanced methods of immunohistochemistry and polymerase chain reaction (PCR) [6]. Many similar studies have been undertaken since then, a total of 27 by 1998 [7]. These studies have been undertaken in a number of countries, and in only one study, in Brooklyn, New York, USA, was there a failure to detect *Chlamydia pneumoniae* in atheromatous tissue.

The association between *Chlamydia pneumoniae* and coronary heart disease appears to be greater when tissue specimens are examined than with antibody studies. The organism is a very small bacterium that has an intracellular existence; it cannot be cultured in the laboratory in the way that larger bacteria can be. Direct identification is therefore extremely difficult and remains generally a research subject rather than a routine clinical test. The studies that identify *Chlamydia pneumoniae* in atheromatous tissue must provide a great deal of support to the suggestion that the micro-organism is the cause of the disease. Or perhaps one cause of coronary heart disease. Other organisms have been implicated and one of these is *Helicobacter pylori*.

# 46
# *HELICOBACTER PYLORI*

In Chapter 9 we looked at peptic ulcer, recognising a social variation with a high prevalence among the poor. We also noted a decline in incidence similar to that seen with coronary heart disease and stroke.

It had long been thought that peptic ulcer might be caused by an impairment of blood supply to the stomach, but the work of Barry Marshall and Robin Warren in Perth, reviewed in Chapter 9, identified *Helicobacter pylori* as the cause in the great majority of cases, although not all [1]. Recent work in Glasgow, UK, has suggested that *Helicobacter pylori* is 'the commonest bacterial infection of mankind' and identified it as being present in 34% of the most deprived children compared with 16% of the most affluent in that city [2].

An editorial in the *British Medical Journal* in 1974 drew attention to the greater than average frequency of peptic ulcer in patients with coronary heart disease [3]. It also commented on gastric ulcer being found with higher than expected frequency in people with atherosclerotic disease who had X-ray evidence of calcification of the aorta. Although there are common links regarding socio-economic status and cigarette smoking, the association between coronary heart disease and peptic ulcer remained at that time unexplained.

The identification of *Helicobacter pylori* as the cause of peptic ulcer did not help this understanding because it moved the cause of peptic ulcer away from the old vascular hypothesis. The work described in Chapters 42 and 44 bring to attention the inflammatory characteristics of coronary heart disease and the possibility of a microbial cause. The association with peptic ulcer leads to the suggestion that *Helicobacter pylori* might be the cause of coronary heart disease.

*Helicobacter pylori* can be identified by microscopy of biopsies taken from the stomach at the time of gastroscopy and it can be cultured on a plate in the laboratory. This was the method used by Marshall and Warren. If the culture is positive, it always indicates active infection but not necessarily disease causation. *Helicobacter pylori* can also be detected by antibody tests of a patient's serum, serological testing. The antibodies, once produced, always remain in the serum, thereby conferring a level of immunity, but it means that a positive antibody test cannot distinguish between current infection and past infection that has cleared. This test is, however, very useful for community-based testing of untreated people.

The research group based at St George's Hospital Medical School in Tooting, south-west London, UK, was the first to investigate a proposed association between coronary heart disease and *Helicobacter pylori* [4]. The subjects of the study were 111 men aged between 45 and 65 years known to have coronary heart disease, together with 45 controls recruited from a community setting in a general practice; 59% of those with coronary heart disease were found to have positive antibodies to *Helicobacter pylori*, compared with 39% of the controls (Figure 46.1). This showed a definite but fairly weak association, and clearly further work needed to be undertaken.

**Figure 46.1** *Helicobacter pylori* **detection in coronary heart disease (CHD) [4].**

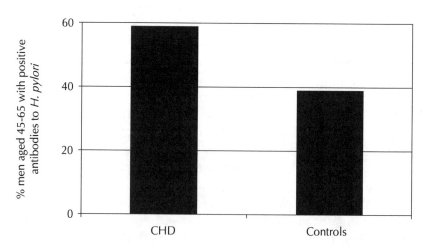

*Adapted with permission from the* British Medical Journal Publishing Group.

The British United Provident Association (BUPA) undertakes screening of people who consider themselves to be fit and healthy. As a result of data collection from such people, the centre has improved our understanding of normal ranges, for example regarding levels of ESR. Much of the screening is through blood testing, and for this purpose serum samples are stored; 21 520 men aged 35–64 years were examined between 1975 and 1982, of which 648 subsequently died from coronary heart disease. Serum from these men was tested for antibodies against *Helicobacter pylori*, as was serum from 1296 age-matched controls. The result was positive for 47.5% of the coronary deaths and 45.9% of controls; this difference was not significant (Figure 46.2). In this study *Helicobacter pylori* did not appear to be associated with coronary heart disease [5].

**Figure 46.2** *Helicobacter pylori* **detection and death from coronary heart disease [5].**

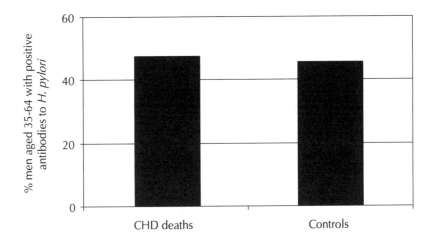

*Adapted with permission from the British Medical Journal Publishing Group.*

A similar study looked at 1122 survivors of myocardial infarction aged between 30 and 45 years and the same number of matched controls. All were tested for antibodies to *Helicobacter pylori*; 42% of the survivors tested positive and 24% of the controls, as shown in Figure 46.3 [6].

**Figure 46.3** *Helicobacter pylori* detection and myocardial infarction [6].

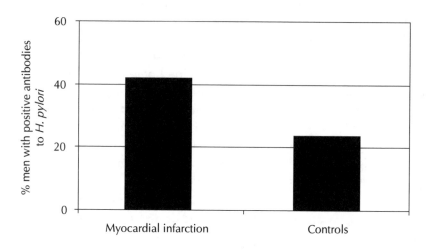

*Adapted with permission from the British Medical Journal Publishing Group.*

This study indicated a significant relationship between coronary artery disease and *Helicobacter pylori* but no conclusion was possible regarding whether this relationship was causal. This was similar to a large number of other studies reporting this association and referred to by John Danesh *et al.* [6]. The conclusion of the paper included the comment: 'randomised trials of anti-infective interventions may be needed to help determine causality'. One was to follow shortly.

In 2002 the group from St George's Hospital Medical School, London, UK, published a controlled trial of standard antimicrobial regimes to eradicate *Helicobacter pylori* and *Chlamydia pneumoniae*. The regimes were given to patients with established coronary heart disease [7]. The study was of 325 patients admitted to four hospitals because of acute coronary events, either unstable angina or myocardial infarction. Within 48 hours of admission the patients were randomised to one of three treatment regimes, each for one week: omeprazole, amoxicillin and metronidazole; omeprazole, azithromycin (for 3 days) and metronidazole; or placebo.

The patients receiving antibiotic therapy had a better outcome than those receiving placebo. Although the study endpoint was after 1 year of follow-up, the benefit from antibiotic therapy was apparent after the first week. The results at 1 year can be seen in Figure 46.4.

**Figure 46.4 Event-free survival after acute coronary event [7].**

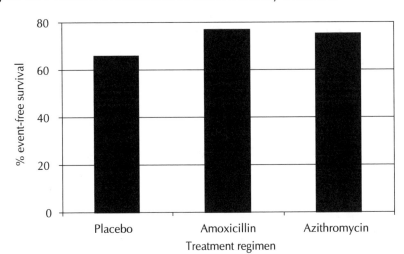

*Adapted from* Circulation *with permission from Lippincott, Williams and Watkins.*

There was a benefit from antibiotic therapy. The patients were then divided into groups according to whether they were positive or negative for antibodies to *Helicobacter pylori* and *Chlamydia pneumoniae*. The benefit of antibiotics was similar in each group.

The antibiotic regimes were given (with omeprazole to suppress acid secretion by the stomach) with the intention of eradicating *Helicobacter pylori* and *Chlamydia pneumoniae*, but the antibiotics are not specific to these organisms and will kill other bacteria. The study thus strongly supports a microbial cause of coronary heart disease, but it cannot conclude that the causative organism is *Helicobacter pylori*, neither can it rule it out.

Using a highly sensitive PCR method that detects specific DNA, researchers in Argentina were able to identify the presence of *Helicobacter pylori* in atherosclerotic plaques obtained at surgery. Testing was positive in 20 out of 38 cases, compared with none of seven normal controls obtained at autopsy [8]. This study strengthens the case for *Helicobacter pylori* being a cause of coronary heart disease. The strength of association is not as strong as with *Chlamydia pneumoniae*, but both remain possible causes of coronary heart disease. An association between *Helicobacter pylori* and the heart cannot be entirely discounted, even though it cannot be viewed as the sole cause of coronary heart disease.

A recent study from Italy has shown that men with the heart irregularity atrial fibrillation are more likely to have antibodies to *Helicobacter pylori* than controls [9]. The patients with atrial fibrillation were divided into those in whom it was persistent and those in whom it was paroxysmal. It was seen that, although the average serum cholesterol was the same in both groups and in controls, CRP was elevated in both atrial fibrillation groups, and more so in those in whom it was persistent, as shown in Figure 46.5.

**Figure 46.5  Cholesterol and CRP in atrial fibrillation (AF) [9].**

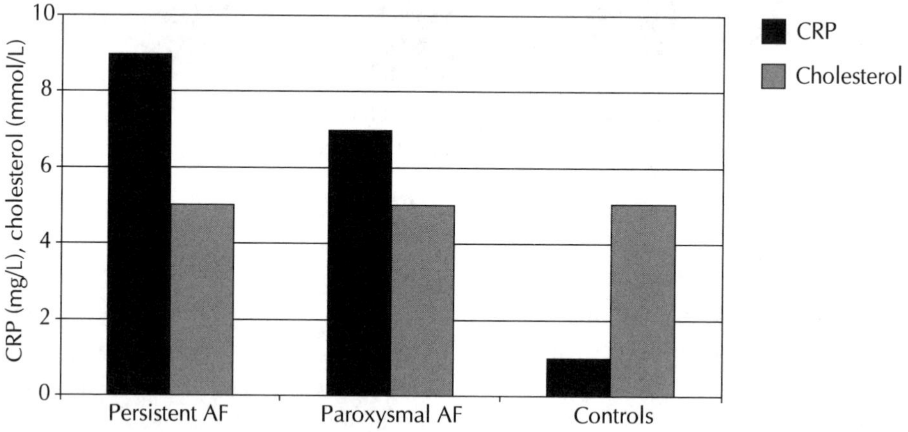

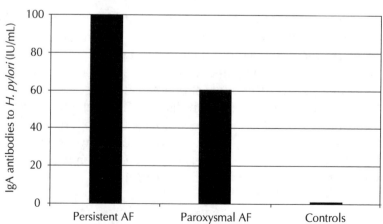

It thus appears that atrial fibrillation is associated with inflammatory features. We can see in Figure 46.6 that there is a high level of antibody to *Helicobacter pylori*, the positive serology being measured as IgG and expressed as international units per ml (IU/mL).

**Figure 46.6  *Helicobacter pylori* serology in atrial fibrillation (AF) [9].**

The high level of IgG antibody to *Helicobacter pylori* indicates a very strong association that can be reasonably interpreted as a causative role for this organism. What is happening with regard to heart pathology is impossible to judge at present, especially as biopsy material is not readily available for this fairly common condition. A repeat of this study is necessary for corroboration and it would, of course, be interesting to see the effect of *Helicobacter pylori* eradication therapy on atrial fibrillation, especially on recurrences of the paroxysmal variety. At present, however, we can see another relationship between infection and the heart.

The benefit of antibiotic therapy has been demonstrated in a number of studies and several antibiotics have been used. It is assumed that antibiotics have only anti-microbial effects, but it is theoretically possible that they have effects not against the bacteria but directly on the metabolism of the human body. It would need to be an anti-inflammatory effect but no such general property has been demonstrated during many years of antibiotic development. In the absence of such information it is reasonable to assume that response to antibiotic therapy indicates that a disease has a microbial cause. In respect of coronary heart disease, it looks as though the search for a causative organism must continue. There is another source of infection that has been investigated over the past few years and we will look at this in the next chapter.

# 47

# DENTAL HEALTH AND CORONARY HEART DISEASE

It has been noticed for several years that there is an association between coronary heart disease and poor dentition, both dental decay and periodontal disease. In an editorial of the *British Medical Journal of* 1985, Neil Jenkins, Emeritus Professor of Oral Physiology at the University of Newcastle upon Tyne, UK, informed us that 'In the past 10 to 15 years dental caries has declined by 35–50% among children in most industrialised countries' [1].

The decline thus started in the early 1970s, at exactly the same time we saw a decline in deaths from coronary heart disease, not explained by conventional wisdom. Jenkins is of the opinion that dietary hypotheses do not explain dental health improvement, nor is dental hygiene a satisfactory explanation. The only factor that he thought might provide the explanation was fluoride supplements, to either toothpaste or drinking water. He does not mention the possibility of clean air and increased vitamin D synthesis, enabling the body to develop strong teeth, as it does bones.

If we look at the distribution within the UK of adults with no natural teeth, we see a familiar pattern, shown in Table 47.1. It is assumed that having no teeth is the result of serious dental caries or periodontal disease.

**Table 47.1 Percentage of adults in the UK with no natural teeth [2]**

|  | % |
| --- | --- |
| Scotland | 28 |
| North | 26 |
| Yorkshire & Humberside | 24 |
| North-west | 23 |
| Wales | 23 |
| East Midlands | 20 |
| South-west | 20 |
| West Midlands | 18 |
| East Anglia | 18 |
| South-east | 15 |

*Crown © 2005, adapted with permission.*

Once again we find a health disadvantage for those who live in Scotland, where 28% of the adult population have no natural teeth, compared with the English average of 18%. Within England we find a gradient from south to north and another from east to west; those who live in the south-east are most likely to retain their natural teeth.

The geographical similarity between the prevalence of dental disease and mortality, especially from coronary heart disease, within the UK is thus obvious. We can then look at the association by using mortality data that we have already seen. Figure 47.1 shows a scattergraph and the association is very strong, with $R^2 = 0.7766$.

**Figure 47.1 Mortality and no natural teeth in the UK. SMR, standardised mortality ratio [2,3].**

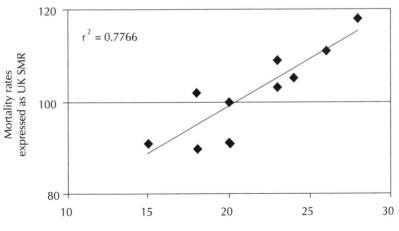

% of adult population with no natural teeth

*Crown © 2005, adapted with permission.*

We are as usual able to offer two possible explanations for this strong association. The first is that they share a common cause or common susceptibility. By now we are able to recognise that this might be caused by variation in sunshine exposure, with insufficiency of vitamin D in the northern parts of the UK.

The other possible explanation is that dental and periodontal disease cause coronary heart disease. This has been proposed and is a perfectly reasonable hypothesis now that we know that coronary heart disease has an inflammatory and probably a microbial basis. Precedence is relevant, as history reminds us that rheumatic heart disease has been the result of infection in the mouth and throat. We are searching for a causative micro-organism and its entry into the body, specifically into the arteries and the endothelial cells that line them. We have looked at *Chlamydia pneumoniae*, which enters the body via the respiratory tract. We have also looked at *Helicobacter pylori*, which enters through the stomach. Is it plausible that a causative organism could enter the body through the teeth and gums?

Even though it is easy to appreciate that periodontal disease is microbial, the cause of dental caries is not quite so easy to understand. Popular belief is that it is entirely chemical, the result of sugar in food. The general informed view is that it is microbial with chemical co-factors: 'Dental caries (tooth decay) is a chronic infectious disease in which the active agent or agents are members of the indigenous oral flora' [4].

It appears, therefore, that bacteria inhabiting the mouth in all of us can cause disease; when this happens it implies that body defence mechanisms have broken down and susceptibility has increased. James Shaw of the Department of Nutrition, Harvard School of Dental Medicine, Boston, USA, goes on to mention that the largest increase in the incidence of dental caries in England occurred after the middle of the 19th century, thus predating by half a century the epidemic of coronary heart disease [4]. This would coincide with a major move of the population to an industrial environment, with reduced vitamin D levels resulting from atmospheric pollution and long hours of indoor working.

The main organism that appears to be related to dental caries is *Streptococcus mutans*. Spirochaetes have also been found in periodontal disease and *Helicobacter pylori* has been found in dental plaque [5] but the relevance to coronary heart disease is by no means clear.

The first report of an association between dental health and coronary heart disease came from Finland [6]. A subsequent study of 9760 adults in the USA showed that, in those with periodontitis, the incidence of coronary heart disease was 25% higher than with those without [7].

A more recent study from Finland confirmed that dental disease is a major predictor of coronary heart disease [8] and the results of this study are shown in Figure 47.2.

**Figure 47.2 Dental and other characteristics [8].**

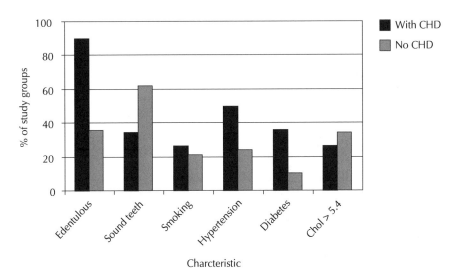

*Adapted from Circulation with permission from Lippincott, Williams and Watkins.*

This study shows that having no teeth was the most powerful risk indicator of coronary heart disease in those studied, far greater than other major risk factors; having sound teeth was clearly a great health advantage. Hypertension and diabetes were also strong indicators; smoking showed little increased risk. In this study high cholesterol appeared to give a slight advantage, with serum cholesterol greater than 5.4 mmol/L being more common in those without coronary heart disease.

As dental decay shows a historical perspective, social gradient and geographical variation similar to those seen in coronary heart disease, it would seem reasonable to accept that dental disease and coronary heart disease must have something in common. We must not lose sight of the fact that coronary heart disease could be the result of dental disease earlier in life, but there is no direct evidence to support this at the present time. An intervention study would be helpful, looking at the effects of treatment, specifically eradication of dental disease on the subsequent development of coronary heart disease.

Removal of all teeth obviously removes all dental decay, and brings periodontal disease to an end. If dental and periodontal disease were the cause of coronary heart disease, then total dental clearance would be expected to be followed by an improvement in coronary risk. However, this is not the case: we have seen in Figure 47.1 that having no teeth is most strongly related to coronary heart disease. A definitive study looked at 11 348 USA adults followed-up for 17 years [9]. The results can be seen in Figure 47.3.

**Figure 47.3  Coronary events and dental status [9].**

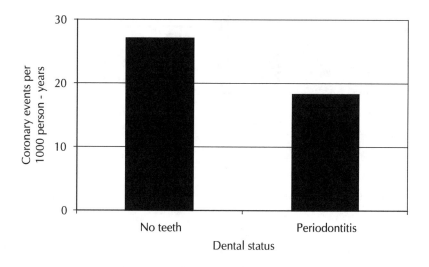

It is quite clear that that those who had dental clearance for dental and periodontal disease did not gain a cardiovascular advantage from that procedure. We have seen in preceding chapters that there appears to be an early advantage when infections thought to cause coronary heart disease are treated. This is not the case with dental disease.

We can conclude that dental disease does not cause coronary heart disease and the mouth is unlikely to be the route of entry into the body of micro-organisms that could cause it. Dental and periodontal diseases are associated with coronary heart disease but this appears to be an association by common susceptibility. We have seen that vitamin D appears to give protection against coronary heart disease and respiratory diseases including tuberculosis. It is distinctly possible that vitamin D is necessary for good dental health.

# 48

# INFECTIONS OF THE HEART

The proposal that coronary heart disease might be caused by a micro-organism is based on plausibility. Does it make sense? The answer to this must be based on existing experience and knowledge that infections of the heart do occur, which is indeed the case.

Infective endocarditis is a condition in which bacteria directly colonise heart valves, causing damage to the valves themselves and also widespread effects as a result of septicaemia and immune reactions. The condition is occasionally caused by a very high pathogenicity organism such as *Staphylococcus aureus*, in which the timescale of the illness is very short, with rapid destruction of valves and, if untreated, death within a few days. More commonly, the condition is subacute and can last for several weeks or months, often with very non-specific clinical features that delay the diagnosis. The offending bacteria can usually be isolated from the blood and are most often a low-pathogenicity *Streptococcus* from the mouth. Endocarditis can also be caused by *Coxiella burnetii*, which must be identified by antibody tests. This organism is very similar to *Mycoplasma pneumoniae* in that it is an obligatory intracellular organism and cannot be grown by normal culture methods. Another micro-organism that has been shown to be responsible for endocarditis is *Chlamydia psittaci*, which is acquired from parrots and other birds. Antibiotic therapy usually cures infective endocarditis but the surgical replacement of a damaged heart valve is sometimes necessary. Infective endocarditis is generally an opportunistic infection, occurring on heart valves that are congenitally abnormal or damaged, and it can occur on artificial heart valves.

Rheumatic fever is also a bacterial disease affecting the heart but the way in which the disease happens is puzzling. The starting point is an infection of the throat with a pathogenic *Streptococcus*. This is followed by a generalised illness characterised by joint inflammation (hence the term rheumatic) and damage to the heart, which is not immediately obvious because it develops gradually over a number of years after the initial event. The bacterial infection is restricted to the throat and the damage to the heart valves is thought to be mediated by an unidentified chemical toxin produced by the bacteria or perhaps through an immune-mediated mechanism.

I have already mentioned that syphilis in its late tertiary phase can cause damage to the heart, in particular to the aorta and the ring of the aortic valve from which the aorta arises. I mention it again here as a reminder that it is another form of infection of the heart, in this case a continuing low-grade active infection over a number of years.

It is also possible for viruses to cause an acute illness called viral myocarditis, an infection of the heart muscle, and the Coxsackie virus group is particularly well known as the cause of this disease. It is extremely difficult to diagnose viral myocarditis clinically and it could be far more common than is actually realised. The characteristic features are usually acute heart failure in a young person, sometimes with chest discomfort and usually with ECG changes. On an echocardiograph it can be seen that the heart muscle is not functioning well. A differential diagnosis from myocardial infarction can be difficult, especially in an older person who has risk indicators of coronary artery disease. We need dwell on this no further, but just observe that this is another form of heart disease arising from an infection.

Kawasaki disease is an intriguing condition that has emerged relatively recently. It was first recognised in 1961 by Tomisaku Kawasaki, working in the Red Cross Hospital, Tokyo, Japan, and it has been identified in the USA and the UK and other parts of Europe since the mid-1970s [1]. It is a disease that affects young children and it is characterised initially by a fever and a rash with desquamation of skin. This initial phase looks very much like a virus infection or toxic reaction to a bacterium, but following this the child might exhibit a characteristic cry and sudden death can occur. The treatment is with aspirin, a medication that is generally to be avoided in children but is essential if Kawasaki disease is suspected. The diagnosis is based on the clinical features, thus on the judgement of the doctor. There is no diagnostic test but non-specific inflammatory markers may be positive. It is likely that Kawasaki disease is both under-diagnosed and over-diagnosed at different times and an excellent up-to-date review appeared recently in *The Lancet* [2].

An illness of acute fever with rash and rapid spontaneous recovery has all the features of a viral infection, as seen quite commonly in children. However, in about 25% of children with Kawasaki disease there are early or late features of coronary artery disease, leading to myocardial infarction. This might be delayed until early adult life, presenting as coronary heart disease, the initial fever and rash having been forgotten or even not recognised [3]. In this respect it is like rheumatic fever, with the initial streptococcal sore throat that initiated the disease not being regarded as anything out of the ordinary at the time.

I mention Kawasaki disease because it is a disease of the coronary arteries. The pathology of the coronary arteries in this condition is undoubtedly inflammatory, but the precise details of the pathological mechanism of the disease are not known. There are many features that suggest a viral infection, which is generally thought to be the initial trigger event. We must not forget the lesson of viral hepatitis, that many decades can elapse between a disease being recognised as having a microbial pattern and the identification of the causative virus.

There are other micro-organisms and indeed worms that can cause heart disease but the point I wish to make is that it is well established that infections can cause heart disease, and thus the concept that coronary heart disease might be caused by one or more micro-organisms must be considered to be valid. I have emphasised the inter-relationship between the sun and microbial disease. To provide a model for the interaction between the sun and cardiac health it is important to develop the concept that coronary heart disease might be caused by a micro-organism.

Once again I must return to the example of viral hepatitis. The first step was to recognise that the disease had features suggesting a microbial cause. At a later stage not just one but several causative viruses were identified. It was universally accepted that viral hepatitis had a viral cause before the identification of the viruses. Why was this? What do we accept as proof? This will be the subject of the next chapter.

# 49

# KOCH'S POSTULATES AND THE CONCEPT OF PROOF

Robert Koch (1843–1910) was not just a great pathologist but he became a great medical philosopher. He worked for a short time with the great pathologist Rudolf Virchow (1821–1902) in Berlin, but his important work on anthrax was undertaken while he was a medical officer during the Franco-Prussian War. At the time when Koch was formulating his ideas, the cause of tuberculosis (consumption or phthisis) was not in doubt. It was common, it ran in families and it was thus constitutional. I hear similar attitudes today concerning coronary heart disease: it is common; it tends to run in families; it is more common in the poor and in those who smoke; it is caused by an interaction between inherited factors and an unhealthy lifestyle. This is generally accepted now in the way that assumptions about tuberculosis were accepted in the mid-19th century.

But Koch felt differently about tuberculosis, in a similar way as a minority of people today think about coronary heart disease; we have seen much of their work. Koch identified the micro-organism that became known as *Mycobacterium tuberculosis* but his next challenge was to prove to the world that this was the cause of the disease tuberculosis. He set himself criteria of proof and these ultimately became known as Koch's postulates, a major contribution to medical understanding. The postulates are as follows.

1. *The specific organism should be shown to be present in all cases of animals suffering from a specific disease but should not be found in healthy animals.*

2. The specific micro-organism should be isolated from the diseased animal and grown in pure culture on artificial laboratory media.
3. This freshly grown micro-organism, when inoculated into a healthy laboratory animal, should cause the same disease seen in the original animal.
4. The micro-organism should be re-isolated in pure culture from the experimental infection.

Koch set himself the task of fulfilling these postulates before he would be satisfied that the tubercle bacillus (*Mycobacterium tuberculosis*) was the cause of consumption.

The concept of proof was first defined by Euclid, a Greek philosopher and mathematician. I am old enough to have been taught Euclidian geometry at school, but it was more than 40 years later that I appreciated its universal importance. Euclid started with a proposition (theorem) and then applied criteria that, if met, would lead to proof. For example, the proposition that two triangles are identical would be accepted as proven if the following minimum criteria were met: that two sides of each triangle are of equal length and that the angles between these two sides are also equal.

Proof therefore demands a prior statement of the criteria that must be met for the proposition (theorem or hypothesis) to be accepted. The principle was summarised by Euclid as *quad erat demonstrandum*, usually abbreviated to QED, meaning 'that has been demonstrated', indicating that the predefined criteria have been met.

It is very important to understand that proof is not absolute. Something that is 'proven' at one time might subsequently become 'unproven', meaning that new evidence has emerged that is paradoxical and conflicts with the underlying hypothesis. It might be that a newly defined criterion cannot be met. As a result a new hypothesis needs to be developed and new criteria of proof applied to it.

Koch's postulates are extremely rigorous and Koch himself realised this. They have a very high level of specificity, which means that when the postulates are fulfilled, as with tuberculosis, the chance of producing a misleading result is extremely unlikely. The organism can then be confidently accepted as causing the disease. It can be 'ruled in'.

However, because of the high rigour, the postulates are not very sensitive. In other words if the postulates are not fulfilled, it does not necessarily mean that the disease concerned is not caused by a micro-organism. It cannot be 'ruled out' and thus the postulates cannot be used to disprove the proposed causative micro-organism.

An example of this is cholera. We have already seen how this was considered to be a water-borne disease. With the new science of microbiology, Robert Koch himself felt that a micro-organism was probably the transmissible agent, and he identified the bacterium *Vibrio cholera*. He felt that this was the cause of cholera but, because he could not culture the organism in the laboratory, his attempts to apply his postulates failed. However, despite this *Vibrio cholera* was not rejected as the cause of the disease: the proposal remained unproven but accepted.

Koch's postulates are well established in medical education but their limitations are not usually taught. Many doctors still regard the postulates as the only concept of proof but this shows a poor understanding of the meaning of proof. The application of Koch's postulates demands a certain level of investigative technology that we have not always achieved. Let us consider the postulates applied, for example, to *Chlamydia pneumoniae* as a possible cause of coronary heart disease.

1. *The specific organism should be shown to be present in all cases of animals suffering from a specific disease but should not be found in healthy animals.*

Evidence of infection with *Chlamydia pneumoniae* as judged by antibody tests is not present in all patients with coronary heart disease, and so this micro-organism cannot be judged to be the only cause of the disease (or diseases). Similarly with hepatitis A virus, it is one cause of viral hepatitis but it is not the only causative virus.

We now know that many micro-organisms can be found in the bodies of normal people but might not cause disease. This is the carrier state; it was not known to Koch, but its recognition makes his first postulate rather too constrained. It does not take into account nosocomial infections, diseases caused by low pathogenicity micro-organisms that are normal contaminants of the human body. When they cause disease it is because of a breakdown of a body's defence mechanisms.

2. *The specific micro-organism should be isolated from the diseased animal and grown in pure culture on artificial laboratory media.*

Culture on an artificial laboratory medium cannot be achieved with many micro-organisms identified within recent years, including *Chlamydia pneumoniae*. Diagnosis is frequently by antibody tests or specific DNA recognition using PCR. This postulate is too rigorous for present-day widespread application.

3. *This freshly grown micro-organism, when inoculated into a healthy laboratory animal, should cause the same disease seen in the original animal.*

410

It is now realised that most infections are restricted to a single animal species. Whereas guinea pig inoculation was an important part of the diagnosis of tuberculosis, the same process cannot be applied to most microbial diseases. It is also known that an infecting agent might cause a different disease in different species. It took a long time to realise that *Mycobacterium lepra*, a micro-organism causing leprosy, would grow in the armadillo but no other non-human host.

4. *The micro-organisms should be re-isolated in pure culture from the experimental infection.*

It follows from postulates 2 and 3 that there are also serious constraints regarding the application of postulate 4. We therefore have a situation in which Koch's postulates cannot always be used to prove the microbial cause of a disease, meaning that the postulates cannot be fulfilled to a level of scientific acceptance. The disease might still be accepted as being microbial, for example as with virus hepatitis, and the failure to fulfil Koch's postulates cannot be used to disprove the microbial cause of a disease. We must be very clear about this regarding the possibility of *Chlamydia pneumoniae* or other micro-organisms being the cause of coronary heart disease and it is important not to reject a microbial hypothesis prematurely.

Koch's postulates were ground-breaking at the time and have been of immense importance. With the advancement of medical science, their relevance has diminished and unfortunately they are not always understood. They can be seriously misused, leading to confusion and false claims. For example [1]:

*The epidemiology of the major risk factors – high serum cholesterol, cigarette smoking and raised blood pressure – shows characteristics which indicate that they are causes of coronary heart disease; in the case of cholesterol, even Koch's postulates are fulfilled.'*

We can see the absurdity of this statement, which was made in the *Journal of the Royal College of Physicians of London* by Professor Barry Lewis of St Thomas's Hospital, London, and Professor Geoffrey Rose of the London School of Hygiene and Tropical Medicine, UK, highly respected clinical scientists who should have known better.

Clinical science has missed opportunities for appreciating the potential of micro-organisms to cause disease by the failure to appreciate Koch's postulates in the way that Koch understood them. Koch realised that if the postulates were fulfilled then the proposal being developed would be 'ruled in' or effectively proven. Since Koch, there has been a tendency for the failure of Koch's postulates to be fulfilled as 'ruling out' a proposal. This is an incorrect interpretation of decision-making, as was appreciated by Koch regarding the microbial cause of cholera.

Inference or deduction can generally be represented by what is called a two-by-two contingency table. This is illustrated in Table 49.1.

**Table 49.1 Koch's postulates and microbial cause of disease**

|  | Koch's postulates fulfilled | Koch's postulates not fulfilled |
|---|---|---|
| Disease caused by micro-organism | 1 | 2 |
| Disease not caused by micro-organism | 3 | 4 |

The truth is that a disease is either caused by or not caused by a specific micro-organism. If Koch's postulates were universally applicable, then they would be fulfilled in all diseases caused by micro-organisms, that is they would all be in box 1. If, on the other hand, a disease was not caused by a micro-organism then Koch's postulates would not be fulfilled, and they would fall into box 4.

However, Koch's postulates are not universally applicable because of low sensitivity. This means that even if Koch's postulates are not fulfilled, a disease can still be caused by a micro-organism, and thus fall into box 2. This could be called a false negative, in that the testing is negative but the disease is in truth caused by a micro-organism. An example is again *Vibrio cholera,* in the experience of Robert Koch.

The high specificity of the postulates means that there are no false positives. If the postulates are fulfilled then this is accepted as proof and this would not happen in a disease not caused by the micro-organism. In other words, no results fall into box 3.

We have to live with the problem that many diseases fall into box 2, in that they are thought to be caused by a micro-organism but Koch's postulates have not been fulfilled. This was the case with viral hepatitis for many years and the postulates were only fulfilled with human transmission studies that would not be acceptable today. The suggestion that *Chlamydia pneumoniae* is the major cause of coronary heart disease would also currently be placed in box 2 because Koch's postulates have not been fulfilled but the suggestion is powerful. The proposal is not proven but also it is not generally accepted, mainly because the alternative diet–cholesterol theory is generally accepted.

Most, if not all, statisticians appear to be aware of the nature and limitations of Koch's postulates, but unfortunately few clinical scientists.

The eminent British statistician Sir Austin Bradford Hill felt that proof of causation could be made using different criteria than Koch's postulates, and he felt this to be necessary in cases of inanimate causes of disease, for example cigarette smoking as the cause of carcinoma of the lung. He identified the following criteria as being necessary for proof to be established, recognising, as mentioned earlier, that proof is pragmatic, not absolute, and might change with the passage of time [2].

1. *Strength of association*
2. *Consistency of association*
3. *Temporality*
4. *Biological gradient*
5. *Plausibility*
6. *Coherence*
7. *Experimentation*
8. *Analogy*

Koch's postulates identified absolutes: a bacterium did or did not grow. Hill's criteria (we should really call them 'Hill's postulates') are not absolute and all criteria can be regarded as judgemental.

The strength of association has been identified in a number of studies that we have reviewed. It is the relative risk that is important and this has been a common method of presentation of data. However, relative risk is obviously not absolute and it cannot be regarded as proof.

Consistency is important. We have many examples of conflicting results from a number of studies, especially regarding the relationship between serum cholesterol and coronary heart disease. We have seen that whereas most studies have shown a relationship between *Chlamydia pneumoniae* and coronary heart disease, one study failed to show this.

Temporality indicates that an association at one point in time does not indicate a cause–effect relationship; we must look at the association over a time-line. We have seen many studies that have identified a possible cause and then followed-up the subjects over a period of time to record the subsequent development of disease. This has been particularly important with coronary heart disease, recording the development of its clinical manifestations. We have noted the difficulty of temporal relationships in a disease that has a long latent period, for example syphilis.

A biological gradient was demonstrated in the studies of *Chlamydia pneumoniae*, which identified that the higher the titre of antibodies to the micro-organism, the greater the risk of coronary heart disease and the greater the benefit from antibiotic therapy.

All these add up to construct plausibility. Does it make sense? Is there a coherent pattern: does it all hang together? Are there parallels: do micro-organisms cause heart disease? Does the assembly of the pieces of the jig-saw puzzle create a picture that we can recognise as sensible?

Experimentation is limited by ethical considerations. It might be possible to transmit the disease to others, if not in experimental animals then in other human beings. This sort of experiment has been undertaken in the past, the subjects usually being unsuspecting prisoners, residents of institutions or minority groups. Such research would not be tolerated today.

The other type of experiment is to eliminate the disease or infection in a group and compare future illness with untreated controls. We have seen this with antibiotic therapy in people with coronary heart disease. If the treatment is not part of the usual management of the illness, and as long as safety is assured, the experiment can receive ethical approval. We have also seen the fate of people following dental clearance, looking at the incidence of heart disease. The dental clearance was not in itself an experiment but performed for clinical purposes and thus ethical, a form of natural experiment.

Finally there is analogy. I have used this very frequently, using the geographical, social and ethnic patterns of rickets and tuberculosis to indicate similarities with coronary heart disease and the importance of the sun and vitamin D. Analogies with tuberculosis and syphilis have emphasised the distinct possibility that coronary heart disease is caused by a micro-organism. Analogy with hepatitis indicates that a disease can be accepted as being microbial before the causative micro-organism has been identified. Analogy means recognising a pattern that can be transferred from one disease to another.

Hill's criteria of causation have been reviewed and refined by researchers at the National Institutes of Health (NIH), Bethesda, Maryland, USA [3], to look at the possibility of a micro-organism causing a disease, in this particular case Crohn's disease, which we will touch upon later. The principles are equally applicable to a possible microbial cause of coronary heart disease.

All the experiments, studies and criteria described in this book so far have helped us develop an understanding of the possible factors leading up to coronary heart disease, but have we reached a conclusion? What do we mean by conclusion? This leads us into another concept, that of the paradigm.

# 50
# SCIENCE WORKS BY PARADIGMS

Science means knowledge and the purpose of science is to develop an understanding of the world or indeed the universe about us, whether it is mathematical, physical, chemical or biological. Understanding can, however, only be a best guess.

An example of this is the physical force of gravity, explained to a level of scientific satisfaction at the time by Sir Isaac Newton (1642–1727). For 300 years his theories were accepted as explaining the nature of the universe but there were certain inconsistencies or paradoxes, by which I mean exceptions to expected behaviours, that cast doubt on the model that Newton had developed.

The accumulation of paradoxes meant that a new explanation was necessary, and a major step in this direction was taken by Albert Einstein (1879–1955) in his general and special theories of relativity. The next step was the clarification of quantum mechanics, in particular by Werner Heisenberg (1902–76), and these developments provided a better explanation of the nature of the universe. They were theories but, as they provided the best model, they became a paradigm, the accepted wisdom of the time, accepted and shared by the key workers.

Einstein himself felt that his conclusions were not adequate and he was searching for a unified field theory, to combine the forces of gravity and electromagnetism into a single model. This has not yet been achieved but, if it is, there will be a change of paradigm to something new and beyond the best model produced so far by the mathematicians and scientists of the 20th century.

An important paradigm concerned our understanding of combustion, the nature of which had baffled people for a long time. The major observation was that, when something burned, heat and light were given off, and the best explanation before the scientific enlightenment of the late 18th century was that everything contained something called phlogiston. When combustion took place it was believed that phlogiston was given off in the form of light and heat energy. This was accepted and moved from being a theory to being a paradigm, the difference being that of widespread academic acceptance.

But many theories or paradigms produce a number of anomalies or paradoxes that have to be explained away in rather elaborate ways, in a series of subordinate theories. A theory thus becomes ever more complex, and the English philosopher William of Ockham (1285–1349) warned about this tendency. His plea was to avoid convoluted theories and to keep thinking as simple as possible. This is encapsulated in what has become known as Ockham's Razor, *entia non sunt multiplicadem praetor necessitatem*: 'do not produce new concepts unless absolutely necessary'. The term razor represented William's desire to cut down elaborate and untenable theories.

Antoine-Laurent Lavoisier (1743–94) in France and Joseph Priestley (1733–1804) in England made the simple observation that, when a substance burns, it becomes heavier. If it was giving off phlogiston then it should become lighter. This paradox was explained away by the adherents of the phlogiston theory (in a process that in political circles today is called spin) by the argument that phlogiston must have a negative mass, but this obviously defies the laws of physics. Using Priestley's observations and more of his own, Lavoisier identified that combustion was the process of combination with oxygen. In the face of compelling evidence and too many paradoxes, the paradigm of combustion ultimately changed from that of phlogiston to that of oxidation. It is interesting to note that, to the end of his life, and despite evidence to the contrary, Priestley would not abandon the phlogiston theory; the change in paradigm was achieved by Lavoisier.

It must be recognised that every paradox strikes at the foundations of a theory and weakens it. The more convolutions of thought and complexities to accommodate a paradox, the greater the need to reconsider the paradigm. Thomas Kuhn (1922–96), the influential American scientific philosopher of the 20th century, points out in his book *The Structure of Scientific Revolutions* [1] that no theory can be perfect and explain everything, otherwise research would stop. An inconsistency might be accepted without abandoning a paradigm but a point is reached when the number of inconsistencies or paradoxes becomes too great for the paradigm to be sustainable.

This is the reality for the diet–cholesterol–heart paradigm of the causation of coronary heart disease: too many paradoxes have been identified by a considerable number of clinical scientists. We have seen many inconsistencies: the London banking and transport paradox that those consuming the highest proportion of fat have the fewest deaths from coronary heart disease; the Leningrad paradox that people subjected to starvation have a high incidence of coronary heart disease; the French paradox that people consuming a diet high in fat and cholesterol have a low incidence of coronary heart disease; the first Albanian paradox that the most socio-economically deprived population in Europe has a very low incidence of coronary heart disease; the second Albanian paradox that the population with the lowest wine consumption in Europe has a very low incidence of coronary heart disease; the Scottish (west of Scotland) paradox that the benefit of statin therapy is unrelated to initial serum cholesterol level or its reduction; the Northern Ireland paradox that a population with about the highest incidence of coronary heart disease in Europe has lifestyle characteristics that are very similar to the population of Toulouse; the elderly paradox that a high serum cholesterol is a positive advantage; and several others. Each paradox can generate a subordinate theory, but I believe that the weight of paradoxical evidence means that the paradigm must change: we must look for a new model.

A paradigm is a theory that is embedded within society and has become accepted wisdom. We now have government actions and directives that are based on the diet–cholesterol–heart paradigm, and we have a huge pharmaceutical and nutritional industrial complex that is carried in its wake. Why should the paradigm change even if there is a better explanation available? Why dislocate our research and industrial roller-coaster? What, therefore, must be necessary for us to change the direction in which there is so much institutional confidence? The situation is very different from the time of Lavoisier and Priestley, whose challenge was to alter the thinking of a very small scientific community. Today it is necessary to influence not only a huge international medical community but also national governments and multi-national industries.

People in general, including scientists and politicians, feel comfortable with a paradigm that is within their experience and understanding. The stress–psychology–heart hypothesis appealed to people who worked within psychology and behavioural sciences, including Sir Michael Marmot, who expressed his interpretation of coronary heart disease in his book *The Stress Syndrome* [2]. But this model does not find much support among people who work within an environment of pathology. The diet–cholesterol–heart theory is comfortable for people who have some sort of understanding of food, and this includes the general population; dietary manipulation therefore falls on receptive ears. Those whose work involves cholesterol metabolism also feel comfortable with this hypothesis, especially when it is supported by a large and profitable industry.

It might be suggested that, in the course of this book, I have been unfair in the way in which I have presented the two sides of the diet–cholesterol–heart story, that I have concentrated on papers and findings that have challenged the hypothesis and that I have given inadequate attention to those that have supported the hypothesis. To take such a view is to regard the strength of the hypothesis to be determined by a sort of vote, a majority of evidence. This is not the way that science should work, as was pointed out eloquently by the scientific philosopher Karl Popper (1902–94). He indicated that the purpose of scientific experiment is to disprove the hypothesis: the principle of falsification. In other words, we are trying to find inconsistencies that challenge a theory or paradigm. The important part of science is then to make certain that such challenges are themselves robust and not the subject of either error or fabrication.

An example, presented by London-based freelance journalist Michael Cross in the *New Scientist*, after Popper, is that a statement might be made that all swans are white. An individual might observe tens, hundreds or even thousands of white swans and this would tend to support the hypothesis. However, the observation of a single black swan would immediately invalidate this supposed truth [3]. Kuhn noted that scientists become wedded to a theory and that their efforts are generally to add to the weight of accumulated support, like continuing to count white swans [1]. He regards this as normal science and points out that it is comfortable for research establishments in which science and research have become institutionalised. He does not regard it as good science.

A paradigm is of great importance as a framework, as expressed by Mark Buchanan, physicist and author, in his remarkable book *Ubiquity* [4]:

*Without a paradigm, a scientist would drown in a bewildering sea of natural phenomena, unable to tell which facts are important and which are not.*

In other words, within science there must always be a paradigm, a conceptual framework. Even in a critical state a paradigm will not collapse until there is an alternative to take its place, and the overlap time might be several years or even decades. The stress–psychology–heart and the diet–

cholesterol–heart hypotheses are effectively paradigms in critical states; they will not collapse until an alternative becomes accepted by a critical mass of scientific opinion.

A relatively new method of dealing with controversies in clinical medicine is to have a consensus conference, to create an accepted and usually majority understanding within the scientific community. There has been much criticism of the consensus method in that it can be used as a way to silence critics or to create a majority view. If there is controversy, then it should only be met by further research.

The basis of the consensus conference has been criticised particularly regarding the careful selection of the participants [5], and another criticism concerns vested interests. A consensus conference has taken place regarding the diet–cholesterol–heart hypothesis that was openly organised and funded by a pharmaceutical company (Parke-Davis) [6]. This can hardly be expected to create independent thought and we must not forget the vast amount of money to be made by pharmaceutical companies in lowering the blood cholesterol levels of the majority of the fit and healthy British population. Similarly, the Diet and Health Symposium II, organised in 2003 by the Hyperlipidaemia Education And Research Trust (a self-perpetuating group with the clever acronym HEART), was funded by Alpro, manufacturers of soya-based alternatives to dairy products [7]. This is a good example of pseudo-science working closely with industrial interests. The whole concept of the consensus conference can be seen as a way of perpetuating the *status quo*, of continuing the paradigm and opposing the advancement of science.

If a paradigm is to be abandoned, there must be a new paradigm to put in its place. Using the criteria of Sir Austin Bradford Hill [8], is the theory that coronary heart disease is caused by a micro-organism strong enough? In practice it is the weakness of the old paradigm that is probably more important than the strength of the new paradigm, and this depends on the state of public knowledge and the comfort of the scientific community. To quote again from Mark Buchanan's book *Ubiquity* [4]:

*In every paradigm, scientists discover a logical structure that makes sense of a portion of the world and gives them an intellectual foundation to which they cling – until the discrepancies and inconsistencies grow so unsettling as to force them to break with tradition and alter some of their cherished ideas.*

In coronary heart disease and its treatment, tradition clings to the weak and unstable diet–cholesterol–heart paradigm, and is supported by the politicisation of health care, including government health policies that are based on the diet–cholesterol–heart hypothesis. Altering cherished ideas is much easier than altering institutionalised policies and directives.

Several teams have suggested that coronary heart disease is caused by a micro-organism but we have seen that so far no single micro-organism has been identified with consistency. I have mentioned the dirty chicken hypothesis, that a variety of infections provide a burden of inflammation that initiates the disease [9]. This theory has its attractions and fits with many of the observations that we have encountered, but there is one observation that does not fit, akin to the single black swan. We have noted an epidemic of coronary heart disease with an abrupt beginning; this immediately suggests a specific micro-organism. An epidemic of hepatitis would be caused by just one of the hepatitis viruses, not all of them simultaneously.

On the other hand, an epidemic could be caused by a new susceptibility rather than a new micro-organism. For example, was the emergence of AIDS because of a mutant virus or a lifestyle change? Perhaps it was a combination of the two, but the sudden emergence suggests that a mutant virus was the most important factor.

And so with coronary heart disease: if we accept that a microbial cause is most likely, then I believe that the search for a causative micro-organism must continue. If coronary heart disease is caused by a micro-organism, we can envisage a model that allows relative protection by sunlight that, via vitamin D, enhances immunity. This model also incorporates the paradoxes that we have encountered.

Having paused to consider the nature of proof and the concept of the paradigm in scientific thought, it is time to look at more evidence concerning the pivotal role of sunlight and vitamin D in a range of aspects of human health.

# PART 9

# ASPECTS OF IMMUNITY

# 51
# SOUTH ASIAN ETHNICITY AND CORONARY HEART DISEASE

In the last chapter we have seen the criteria proposed by Sir Austin Bradford Hill for assessing causation when the application of Koch's postulates is not appropriate, and the last of these criteria is analogy. Moving away from considering specific micro-organisms, I would like to use the process of analogy to look at health risks of the South Asian population of the UK.

South Asian immigrants into the UK have an increased risk of rickets and osteomalacia, the bone effects of vitamin D deficiency. We have also noted the increased risk of tuberculosis, with a maximum incidence at about 5–8 years after arrival in the UK(see Chapter 10) [1]. This and the partial protection by meat in the diet has led to speculation that susceptibility to tuberculosis is caused by vitamin D insufficiency, the result of inadequate exposure to sunlight and exhaustion of vitamin D reserves.

Michael Marmot and colleagues from the London School of Hygiene and Tropical Medicine, UK, reported that in England and Wales in 1970–72 the mortality from coronary heart disease was 20% higher in men and women who had been born in South Asia than in the general population [2]. They later reported that, in London, Asian men and women had a mortality rate from coronary heart disease 50% higher than the national average [3]. This clearly presents a major public health issue, but also an intellectual challenge to understand the reason for the excess mortality.

A study undertaken in Harrow, UK, compared 54 Asian men with 77 white men presenting with a first myocardial infarction [4]. The Asian men were found to have an average age of 50.2 years, which was significantly younger than the average age of 55.5 years for the white men. Cigarette smoking was very similar, the mean daily cigarette consumption being 16.5 for Asian men and 17.5 for white men. Diabetes was more common in the Asian men, 18% compared with 3% in the white men, and this is a theme that we will review in more detail in a later chapter. Death rates immediately following myocardial infarction were similar.

The study also looked at the severity of coronary heart disease in the two groups, as assessed by subsequent coronary angiography. Figure 51.1 shows that single-vessel disease was found twice as frequently in the white men as in the Asian men. The more severe three-vessel disease was more than twice as common in the Asian men.

**Figure 51.1 Ethnic differences in the severity of coronary heart disease [4].** MI, myocardial infarction.

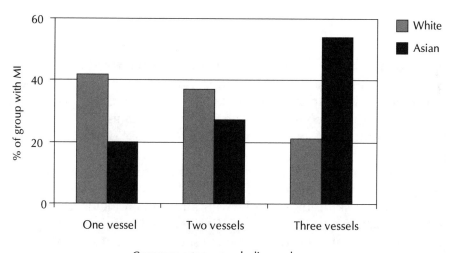

*Adapted with permission from the British Medical Journal Publishing Group.*

The authors then looked in detail at the population of Harrow in the 1981 census, to compare the age structure of the ethnic groups and to match this with the onset of coronary heart disease. It can be seen in Figure 51.2 that coronary heart disease was much more common in men of South Asian ethnicity and this was obvious at an early age, before 40 years.

**Figure 51.2 Ethnic differences in the age of onset of coronary heart disease [4].**
MI = myocardial infarction.

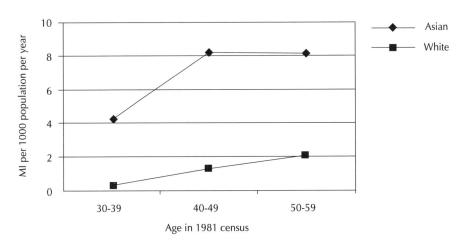

*Adapted with permission from the British Medical Journal Publishing Group.*

It is quite clear, therefore, that not only is coronary artery disease more common in men of South Asian ethnicity living in England, but it is also more severe and occurs earlier in life. There is both a serious problem and a puzzle.

To add to this, we have already noted the decline in the incidence of coronary heart disease since 1970. Between 1970–72 and 1979–83 in England and Wales the mortality from coronary heart disease fell by 5% in men and 1% in women. During this time the mortality rate in South Asians increased by 6% in men and by 13% in women [5].

Things seem to be getting worse from one generation to the next for South Asians in the UK. With a reference hazard ratio of 1.0 in whites born in England and Wales, we find a slightly lower hazard ratio in South Asians who were born in Asia but we see an increased overall mortality rate in their children born in the UK, as shown in Figure 51.3. The data represent men aged under 65 years at the 1991 census, with follow-up to 1997 [6].

**Figure 51.3  All causes of mortality of first and second generation ethnic groups within the UK [6].**

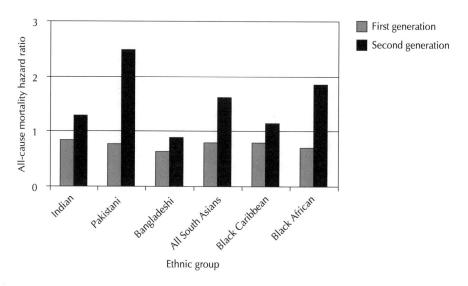

*Crown © 2002, adapted with permission.*

Despite upward socio-economic mobility, something is clearly going wrong regarding the health of people of South Asian ethnicity living in the UK. We can see that they share it with immigrants from Africa and the Caribbean. What might be the answer? Might it have a link with the development of tuberculosis?

The differences between the religious and dietary groups within the South Asian community that we saw with tuberculosis do not appear to feature with coronary heart disease. The risks of death from coronary heart disease among Hindus and Muslims living in South London are very similar, with a just a marginal increased risk for Hindus (relative risk of 1.08) [7]. Although there are cultural differences between the many ethnic groups that come from South Asia, all have an increased susceptibility to coronary heart disease. P. M. McKeigue and Michael Marmot made an interesting comment [3]:

*Any general explanation of the high rates of coronary heart disease in South Asians must invoke some factor that is common in the diverse communities that make up the Asian population in Britain.*

Such a factor cannot be dietary because of the great variations of diet within South Asian groups. Could it be that the common factor is skin pigmentation?

426

Raj Bhopal, Professor of Public Health at the University of Edinburgh, UK, wrote an editorial recently in the *British Medical Journal* with the title 'Epidemic of cardiovascular disease in South Asians' [8]. The increase is worrying because we have seen a major reduction of the epidemic in the population overall [8]. The epidemic of coronary heart disease started its decline in the UK just after 1970, and that of stroke 10 years earlier in about 1960. The UK government has projected an end to the epidemic by 2015 (Figure 18.4) [9] but now we see that an epidemic is currently developing in the South Asian population of the UK. In his editorial, Bhopal identified the greater susceptibility of South Asian people but, in a long list of possible causes, he did not mention, and perhaps had not even considered, vitamin D insufficiency.

I propose that the high incidence of coronary heart disease in the South Asian population of the UK is because of a high level of susceptibility, probably to one or more of the as yet unidentified micro-organisms that cause the disease. The susceptibility is thus analogous to the pattern of tuberculosis, with the risk increasing with time spent in the UK, vitamin D reserves gradually becoming exhausted. Insufficient synthesis of vitamin D is a result of the genetic and biological factor of skin pigmentation in a climate that has very low levels of sunshine. Evolution has selected fair-skinned people to live in the north-western margins of Europe, at latitudes further north than anywhere in China. The absence of skin pigmentation maximises vitamin D synthesis from the sun in an area where the sun is low in the sky, with consequent poor intensity at ground level. South Asian people are not only biologically but also culturally adapted to living much closer to the equator; they cover their bodies extensively with clothes, especially Muslim women. They have no need to expose their bodies to obtain a sun-tan. During pregnancy in Europe, South Asian women will inevitably pass an inadequate amount of vitamin D to their off-spring, hence the early age of development of coronary heart disease in the next generation and the observation that mortality from it worsens with successive generations in the UK.

In Chapter 6 we saw how genetic factors can have a major influence on susceptibility or resistance to infection. The inherited factor of skin pigmentation is of great advantage to a person living in or close to the tropics, but it creates susceptibility to disease in a person living in the north-west fringes of Europe.

In discussing the high incidence of coronary heart disease in South Asians, Professor Bhopal states that 'Prevention must start in childhood' [8], but he is starting too late. Prevention is close at hand if we can identify the susceptibility factor of South Asians living in the UK as vitamin D insufficiency. Prevention should start before conception, not in childhood.

There is of, course, a tendency to look at coronary heart disease alone, trying to find explanations for the ethnic features among traditional risk indicators derived from the traditional diet–cholesterol–heart hypothesis. None fits, and we must look at the big picture. If we do, we find that it is not only coronary heart disease that is more common among those of South Asian ethnicity, and the problem is shared by those from Africa and the Caribbean.

'Why is there so much end-stage renal failure of undetermined cause in UK Indo-Asians?' This is the title of a review from the renal unit of St Mary's Hospital London, UK, serving the populations of Brent and Harrow [10]. The incidence of end-stage renal (kidney) failure in South Asians was four times that of the white population of the same area. The incidence was three times higher among the Afro-Caribbean population, as shown in Figure 51.4.

**Figure 51.4  End-stage renal failure and ethnicity [10].**

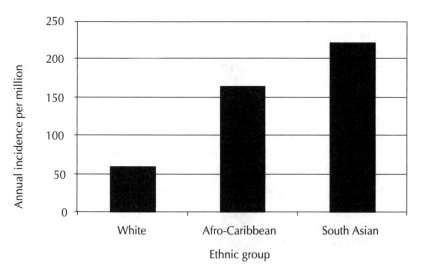

*Adapted from the QMJ with permission from Oxford University Press.*

428

The link between South Asians and Afro-Caribbeans can only be the genetic characteristic of skin pigmentation. It is not obviously dietary and is unlikely to be cultural. South Asians probably have a more indoor lifestyle and a greater tendency to cover their skin with clothes.

Among the South Asians there was a high incidence of end-stage renal failure as a result of diabetes, with a relative risk of 6.2 [10]. The relative risk was even higher, at 7.8, for kidney disease of undetermined cause, meaning presentation with advanced renal impairment and small kidneys, without diabetes or hypertension. The causes are shown in Figure 51.5.

**Figure 51.5  Cause of end-stage renal failure and ethnicity [10].**

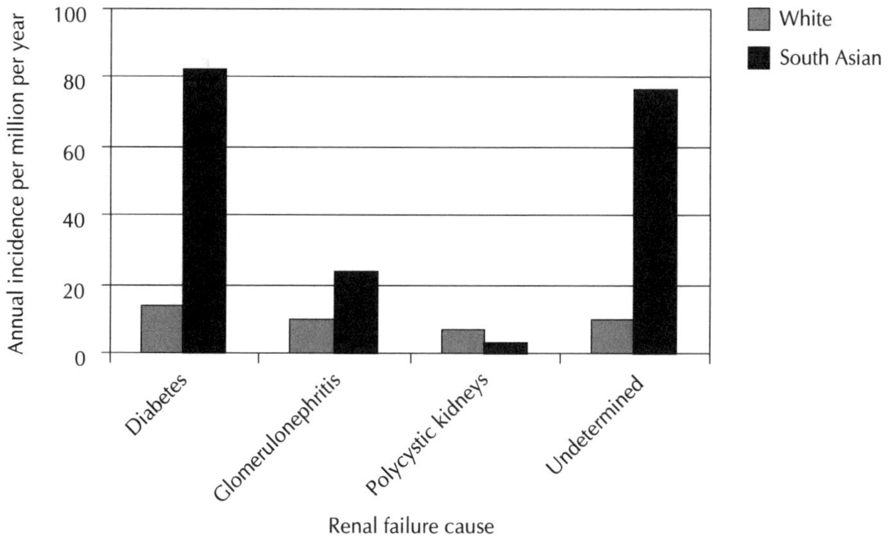

*Adapted from the* QMJ *with permission from Oxford University Press.*

South Asians whose origins are Bangladeshis appear to have the worst health profile, and there is a particularly large community in Tower Hamlets, London. Table 51.1 shows the relatives risks, recorded as standardised mortality ratios (SMR), with 100 as the national average [11].

**Table 51.1  Patterns of mortality among Bangladeshis in England and Wales [11]**

|                           | SMR |
|---------------------------|-----|
| Coronary heart disease    | 148 |
| Cerebrovascular disease   | 267 |
| Diabetes                  | 685 |
| Cirrhosis of the liver    | 254 |

We can see a particularly high mortality from diabetes, and this is a characteristic that we now expect to see in South Asian groups. We will look in more detail in later chapters at diabetes and renal failure, considering ethnic background and relationships with coronary heart disease. Before doing so, I would like to look at other aspects of immune suppression and susceptibility to coronary heart disease.

# 52
# THE SPLEEN AND
# CORONARY HEART DISEASE

The spleen is found in the upper abdomen, beneath, and protected by, the lower ribs on the left side. It is a very vascular organ and subject to injury, especially when enlarged, for example because of chronic malaria. Bleeding from a spleen injury can be fatal and surgical removal of a damaged and bleeding spleen (splenectomy) is an important emergency operation. Once the bleeding spleen has been removed and the injured patient is well and discharged from hospital, it used to be thought that everything was then fine.

The spleen was considered to have no obvious function in the human, and it was thought to be vestigial, that is rendered redundant by evolution. In the dog it appears to be a reservoir of blood that can be mobilised at times of blood loss, but in human beings it is not considered large enough to have such a function. The spleen is known to remove old red cells and platelets from the blood, and after splenectomy older red cells can be identified by microscopic examination of the blood. The platelet count increases following splenectomy. The spleen has been considered to be a bit of a nuisance and has sometimes been removed at surgery to facilitate surgical resection of the pancreas or stomach.

It was first reported in 1952 that there is a significant disadvantage to not having a spleen [1]. People that have undergone a splenectomy are particularly susceptible to infections caused by the respiratory pathogenic micro-organism *Pneumococcus*, also called *Streptococcus pneumoniae*. They are particularly prone to rapid death from meningitis caused by this organism. Although *Pneumococcus* is responsible for about half the microbial deaths following splenectomy, there is also an increased risk from several other organisms [2].

It is clear that the absence of a spleen increases susceptibility to infections. The spleen is a lymphatic organ and it is now realised that it is involved in the development of immune defence mechanisms. Following splenectomy, patients should be given regular immunisation against *Pneumococcus* and life-long daily penicillin [3].

Splenectomy for trauma was undertaken on a relatively large scale during the Second World War, with at the time no thought of long-term consequences and without long-term antibiotics. An investigation was undertaken of 740 USA war veterans whose spleens had been removed. After a 30-year follow-up, 108 had died and the analysis of those deaths came up with interesting results that have effectively been ignored and not become generally known [4]. The results are summarised in Figure 52.1, indicating the relative risks of death in those who have undergone splenectomy compared with the same number of age-matched controls with a relative risk of 1.

**Figure 52.1  Relative risk of death after splenectomy [4].**

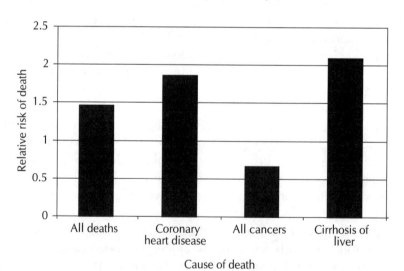

© *1977, adapted from* The Lancet *with permission from Elsevier.*

The overall risk of death is the most important outcome, and if it were 1.0 we might just be looking at a change in the cause of death, as a result of splenectomy. It can be seen, however, that the risk of all causes of death is about 50% higher than the average population, indicating that, far from being vestigial, the spleen is an organ of considerable importance. If something causes the overall risk of death to be increased by 50%, it is serious and cannot be ignored.

Out of 108 deaths from all causes in these 740 men, 41 were the result of coronary heart disease. The comparable number of coronary heart disease deaths among controls was 23, showing a greatly increased (almost double) death rate from coronary heart disease following splenectomy. This had not previously been known. There was also an increased risk of death from pneumonia (6 versus 0 deaths), as we would now expect, but this cannot be displayed as a relative risk; with zero deaths in the control group, the relative risk in the splenectomy group would be infinity. There were more deaths from cirrhosis of the liver, 12 versus 6. There were fewer deaths from cancer, 14 versus 22, for reasons that are not clear.

The increased risk of death from coronary heart disease following splenectomy can be explained in two ways. The first is an increased clotting tendency as a result of a rise in the platelet count of the blood, but we have seen that coronary heart disease is inflammatory and not caused by excess blood clotting. If we look at deaths from blood clotting effects (thrombo-embolism) among this group of Second World War veterans, we find only one death among those who had a splenectomy [4]. The blood clotting explanation is thus not acceptable.

The second explanation is suppression of immunity, leading to an increased risk from infective processes; it conforms with the observation of an increased risk of death from pneumonia. It makes a great deal of sense coupled with our knowledge that the risk of coronary heart disease is increased with immunosuppression (to be expanded later) and that it is likely to be caused by a micro-organism.

This important study appears to have had no impact on medical thinking. However, it was followed 20 years later by a similar study [5]. This time the reason for splenectomy was elective removal for treatment of hereditary spherocytosis. In this condition, the red blood cells are malformed and fragile, and are removed prematurely from the blood stream by the spleen. This leads to low-grade anaemia, and treatment can be removal of the spleen to improve the survival of the red blood cells.

A study from Wisconsin, USA, looked at the outcome of 144 patients who had hereditary spherocytosis treated by splenectomy and who had reached an age of 40 years [5]. They were compared with 88 patients with the same condition who had not had the spleen removed. The comparison was based on the number of atherosclerotic events occurring in the total number of years after the age of 40 in each group. The event rate was 5.9 times higher in the splenectomy group than in the control group (Figure 52.2).

**Figure 52.2 Atherosclerotic events after splenectomy [5].**

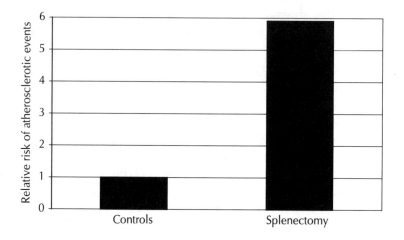

A practical message is that splenectomy is to be avoided if at all possible, but the relationship with subsequent coronary heart and other atherosclerotic disease is not widely known. Another important message concerns the nature of the relationship, with support of the hypothesis that immunosuppression (as with sunlight and vitamin D insufficiency) increases susceptibility to infection and thus to coronary heart disease.

# 53
# SEX AND CORONARY HEART DISEASE

In Figure 18.3 we saw that mortality rates from coronary heart disease in the USA had declined by more than 50% between 1970 and 1990 [1]. We have also seen that the incidence of death from coronary heart disease in women is only about one-third of that in men [1]. Figure 18.4 showed the same sex difference in the UK [2]. This is the general pattern: being male is a powerful risk indicator of coronary heart disease.

The very active Bristol University Epidemiology Unit has made the extraordinary comment [3] 'The 20th century epidemic of coronary heart disease affected only men in most industrialised countries'. Perhaps there was a script error and the word 'only' should have been 'mainly'. The data presented in the paper demonstrate that the epidemic occurred in both sexes but the incidence was much greater in men, in accordance with other studies. The authors concluded that this was the result of lifestyle differences, in particular a higher fat intake and cigarette consumption in men. But did these factors explain the epidemic? Almost certainly not.

We need to investigate the general observation that coronary heart disease at a given age is more common in men than in women, and we return to the concept of illness being a product of disease and behaviour. Is the sex difference of coronary heart disease a result of misbehaviour by men? Conventional wisdom, as expressed by the Bristol group, would support this view, that coronary heart disease is caused by lifestyle characteristics. But we have found this approach lacking in conviction and we are drawn to the view that it is caused by a micro-organism. We must also remember that disease is a product of its cause and susceptibility; perhaps men have a greater susceptibility to infection.

The behaviour of men compared with women does have an influence on mortality. War, the result of humans being unable to settle their differences without resorting to violence, results in a large number of male deaths. Historically this has been balanced by deaths in women arising from the risk of childbirth. Young men have a much higher risk of death from industrial and agricultural accidents and, in more recent times, from road traffic accidents. Although driving a car too fast would appear to be a behavioural phenomenon, we might ask whether such behaviour is genetically determined and therefore could indirectly be thought of as a disease. However, for now we will regard it as behavioural. Even though behavioural factors influence survival, is this the case for the sex difference in risk of coronary heart disease?

It is clear that a female advantage regarding illness, disease and death (excluding childbirth) is not confined to behavioural trends, coronary heart disease or the human species. An overview of 38 published studies indicated that infestation by parasites is much higher in males of about 50 mammalian species [4] and the cause is not believed to be behavioural. The observation is true for studies in the wild and in controlled experimental studies. A particularly important observation is the absence of sex difference in juveniles, that is before sexual maturation, implying that sexual maturation and the appearance of sex hormones at adolescence is a critical factor.

The authors of this study felt that the sex differences are mediated by immune advantages of the female, and this was the hypothesis being tested by the design of the study. We are considering in this book that competent immunity is protective against coronary heart disease; perhaps the higher incidence of the disease in men is a result of a lower level of immune competence compared with women.

The suggestion is that a female's protection against coronary heart disease is mediated by female sex hormones (oestrogen) rather than by genetic influences. This would predict that the post-menopausal female (exclusively human) could lose the advantage gained during reproductive life. The prediction would continue that in later human life the incidence of microbial disease, and coronary heart disease, will be the same for men and women. This is indeed the case.

Anil Ananthaswamy, a science writer based in San Francisco, USA, stated in the *New Scientist* [5]:

*The key to women's longevity may lie with their stronger immune systems. Traditionally, men's shorter lives have been put down to the greater risks they take, but researchers have come up with a tantalising new theory after finding that women produce more new immune cells than men.*

436

This was a review of research undertaken at the Imperial College School of Medicine, London, UK, which studied T cells produced by the thymus gland, important components of the immune system that help to provide immune competence. The observation was that T-cell production was higher in women than in men and that in both sexes the production rate declined with age [6].

The influence of sex and sex hormones on immunity is far from fully understood [7]:

> *The influence of sex hormones on hetero- and auto-immune reactivity cannot be denied. In general terms androgens and progestogens seem to dampen immune responses while oestrogens show the opposite tendency. The mechanisms behind this influence are still unknown.*

The risk of coronary heart disease increases after the menopause in women and this is most obviously explained by the loss of oestrogen and its immune-enhancing effect. Could this post-menopausal disadvantage be reversed by hormone replacement therapy (HRT)? Data from observational studies indicate that this might be the case. In a large meta-analysis the relative risk of coronary heart disease for women taking oestrogen-only HRT was 0.7 and for those taking combined HRT 0.66, as shown in Figure 53.1 [8].

**Figure 53.1  HRT and risk of coronary heart disease (CHD) [8].**

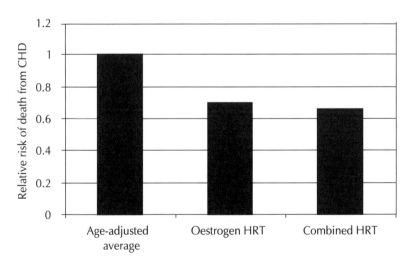

In another study the relative risk of women with coronary risk factors taking HRT was 0.57 compared with those not on HRT [9]. We have seen previously that observation studies can be influenced by behavioural characteristics that are not part of the main investigation. For example, are women taking HRT a special group with features that might influence the risk of coronary heart disease, perhaps not smoking? These biases can be minimised in prospective randomised controlled clinical trials. Such a trial was undertaken in Alberta, Canada, the subjects being 1017 women aged 50–69 years who had survived a first myocardial infarction [10]. Oestrogen-only HRT was given to half the women but it produced no advantage over the control group, as judged by the frequency of clinical endpoints.

An alternative approach is to investigate the effect of oestrogen on coronary heart disease itself, rather than its clinical expressions. Three-hundred and nine women with coronary artery disease, demonstrated by coronary angiography, were randomised to receive either oestrogen/progesterone HRT or placebo. At follow-up angiography after about 3 years there was no significant difference between the two groups. Clinical events were also similar [11].

The sex difference of incidence of coronary heart disease, although real, cannot be explained with confidence. There are features that support the hypothesis that coronary heart disease is caused by a micro-organism and that women have an enhanced immune system that gives them some protection. It is unclear whether this is mediated by oestrogen. Immune competence might well be important in protection against coronary heart disease and we need to explore this further.

# 54

# IMMUNE SUPPRESSION AND CORONARY HEART DISEASE

The main thesis presented in this book is that lack of sunlight and consequent insufficiency of vitamin D results in impaired immunocompetence. Several diseases result, in particular tuberculosis and coronary heart disease. Are there any precedents for this assertion?

We have seen that men might have a mildly but significantly lower level of immunocompetence compared with women. Immunodeficiency is currently most well-known through the acquired immune deficiency syndrome (AIDS), arising from infection with human immunodeficiency virus (HIV). AIDS sufferers develop a series of life-threatening infections that are opportunistic, meaning that the infecting micro-organisms would be unlikely to cause significant disease in normal healthy people whose body defence mechanisms are intact. The micro-organisms cause infection when the opportunity arises, that is when the body defence mechanisms are impaired because of a malfunction of immune mechanisms. One of the most important infections complicating AIDS is tuberculosis, which has therefore made an important international resurgence. Tuberculosis is an infection that can lie dormant for many years. We have seen that insufficiency of vitamin D can cause its activation.

A major problem after heart transplantation is severe coronary heart disease [1]. It appears that the transplantation process itself initiates the coronary heart disease, or some process linked to the transplant, rather than the original disease that necessitated the transplant. The same thing happens after kidney transplantation; it is the transplantation process that is important, not the organ.

A body naturally rejects transplanted tissue via its immune mechanisms. To enable a transplanted organ to survive, recipients are given powerful immunosuppressant therapy with medications such as prednisolone (corticosteroid), azathioprine, ciclosporin (previously cyclosporin), tacrolimus, sirolimus and mycophenolate. We know that opportunistic infections can occur as a result of suppressing immunity and it is distinctly possible that such infections bring about severe accelerated coronary heart disease.

Cancer can be treated with surgery and radiotherapy. A third modality of treatment used with increasing frequency is chemotherapy and the medications concerned are very powerful. They are designed to kill cancer cells but they inevitably kill other rapidly dividing cells, especially those of the bone marrow, including cells that are responsible for immunity. The outcome of testicular cancer has been transformed with the introduction of radiotherapy and chemotherapy to supplement surgery, with present-day survival rates of more than 90% (greater in those with socio-economic advantage) [2]. Nine-hundred and ninety-two men were treated at the Royal Marsden Hospital, London, UK, and follow-up assessment was undertaken after 10 years. It was noted that the men who had received treatment with radiotherapy and chemotherapy had developed a higher risk of heart disease than those who received surgery alone [3]. The results are shown in Figure 54.1.

**Figure 54.1  Heart disease after treatment for testicular cancer [3].**

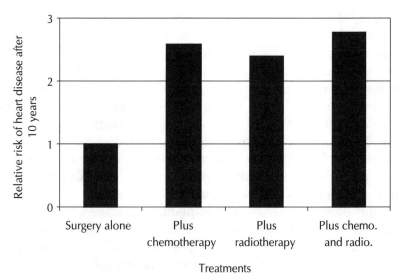

We can see that those treated with chemotherapy and radiotherapy had a risk of heart disease about two-and-a-half times higher than those who had only surgery. The authors indicated that this was not because of any change in conventional risk factors. I suggest that it might be the result of damage to and suppression of the immune system.

We saw in Chapter 43 that statin drugs have anti-inflammatory effects unrelated to the cholesterol-lowering effects. Statins have been given in order to minimise coronary heart disease following heart transplantation, and there is a major benefit that was not foreseen: a dramatic reduction of rejection episodes in recipients taking pravastatin therapy [4]. Figure 54.2 shows the results from a randomised clinical trial undertaken in Los Angeles, USA.

**Figure 54.2 Benefit of pravastatin after heart transplantation [4].**

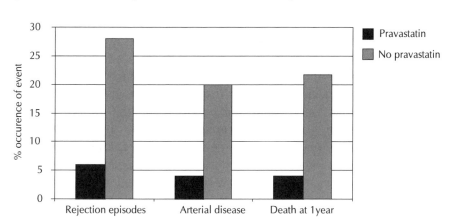

We can see a dramatic reduction of untoward events in those taking pravastatin, organ rejection episodes falling from 28% to 6%, arterial disease from 20% to 4% and death at 1 year from 22% to 4%. Statins thus appear to be not just anti-inflammatory but also immune-modulating. It is clear that statin drugs have many more properties than the known one of HMG-CoA reductase inhibition (Figure 27.1), responsible for the cholesterol-lowering property, which does not appear to of clinical importance. We have seen that cholesterol might be an advantage in the inflammatory process, and it would follow that inhibition of cholesterol synthesis might be a disadvantage. At present we can only assume that statins give a benefit that outweighs any possible disadvantage from inhibition of cholesterol synthesis. However, it is important to note recent information concerning ezetimibe, a different class of cholesterol-lowering medication. Ezetimibe certainly lowers blood total and LDL cholesterol levels but it appears to worsen atherosclerotic plaque development in the carotid artery. This indicates a very special therapeutic property of statins unrelated to effects on cholesterol [5].

As immunosuppression appears to increase susceptibility to coronary heart disease, it might be expected that patients with AIDS would have an increased risk of developing coronary heart disease. When AIDS is untreated, death from other microbial complications occurs at an early stage; when it is treated with effective anti-retroviral drugs an increased risk of developing coronary heart disease has been demonstrated. A programme in Denmark enrolled 23 468 people positive for HIV and reported its findings in 2003. Those who had received a combination anti-retroviral treatment had a 26% increased risk of myocardial infarction each year of treatment for the 4–6 years of follow-up [6].

The authors could not explain this finding, but they pointed out that the absolute risk of myocardial infarction was low and that in practice the treatment was of far greater benefit than danger. The point that I would like to make is that this is another example of immunosuppression increasing the risk of coronary heart disease, thus supportive of a microbial cause. There is then the issue of whether the risk is a result of the immunodeficiency of AIDS, moderated by treatment to diminish complications of other infections, or is caused by a direct effect of the antiviral therapy. This cannot be answered by the data, but the study is continuing.

In the Prologue to this book we saw that Abdul developed end-stage renal (kidney) failure and subsequently developed coronary heart disease at an early age. This is a well-recognised association and a cause for concern. Abdul's kidney transplant failed because of disease in his new kidney, leading to his unfortunate death (he did not receive statin therapy at that time). Immune mechanisms are closely associated, and our next step is to explore the important relationship between kidney failure and coronary heart disease.

# 55

# CHRONIC RENAL FAILURE, VITAMIN D AND CORONARY HEART DISEASE

In Chapter 2 I mentioned Bright's disease, which we now call acute glomerulonephritis, historically an important condition and today a significant cause of death from kidney failure. Following the initial illness, the kidney damage can be fatal over a short or long period of time, but at the time of Richard Bright (1789–1858), a physician at Guy's Hospital, London, UK, the mechanisms were not understood. We now know that the damage is immune-mediated, but the concepts of infection and immunity were unknown until recent years, and it was not possible to measure routinely the function of the kidneys until the mid-20th century.

I was very fortunate to receive my medical education at Manchester University, UK, where in the latter half of the 20th century important advances were made in the understanding of kidney disease. This was initially under the influence of Robert (later Sir Robert and then Lord) Platt. He was a man of remarkable wisdom; I remember in particular his comment that 'From the patient's viewpoint, a major operation is an operation performed on "me". A minor operation is an operation performed on someone else'.

His point was to identify with patients, who are sensitive and often frightened people, whose concerns must be respected by their doctors. Platt became the first president of the Royal College of Physicians of London, UK, to come from outside London, and he was responsible for transforming the college into a national and indeed international medical educational facility. While Professor of Medicine at Manchester, he initiated the study of kidney disease that was developed by his colleague and successor Sir Douglas Black, who also became president of the Royal College of Physicians of London. We have already encountered him as the co-author with Peter Townsend of what became known as the Black Report, concerned with the social dimensions of health and illness in the UK (see Chapter 38) [1]. Douglas Black, like Robert Platt, was a man of great intellect and humility, a great scientist as well as a kind doctor.

Manchester became an important centre for research into kidney disease and it became obvious that bone complications of chronic renal failure occurred much more frequently in patients in Manchester than in similar units in Australia and the USA. The third successive professor of medicine during my time in Manchester was S. W. (Bill) Stanbury, who developed the line of research into metabolic bone disease to an international reputation. It was a lecture given by Stanbury in about 1980 that first alerted me to the wide range of activity and potential importance of vitamin D.

The subject of the bone disease that occurs with chronic renal failure is rather complicated and we must remember Abdul, whose medical history we encountered in the Prologue to this book. He developed end-stage chronic renal failure requiring dialysis and then kidney transplantation. At the same time he had biochemical features of osteomalacia and was given treatment with vitamin D. He also developed tuberculosis.

When vitamin D is deficient, the calcium level in the blood tends to fall. The body compensates for this by increasing the secretion of parathyroid hormone (PTH), produced by the four parathyroid glands that are embedded in the thyroid gland in the neck, a process called hyperparathyroidism. The serum concentration of PTH increases above its normal range; PTH mobilises calcium from the bones, thus restoring the serum calcium levels back into the normal range, but usually at the lower end of the range (2.2–2.6 mmol/L). The mobilisation of calcium from the bone is mediated by activation of bone cells called osteoclasts (literally 'bone destroyers'); the cells that put calcium into bone are called osteoblasts, 'bone creators'. In hyperparathyroidism, both production and destruction of bone are increased. The resultant increased turnover of bone can be estimated by an increase within the blood of the enzyme alkaline phosphatase.

The vitamin D content of blood is not measured in normal clinical practice, mainly because the importance and frequency of vitamin D insufficiency is vastly underestimated. Its measurement as calcidiol and calcitriol is new and is mainly a research activity, but it can be made available to clinical services. In the diagnosis of rickets and osteomalacia, deficiency of vitamin D is assumed by the finding of low or low-normal serum calcium, together with an elevated alkaline phosphatase (not essential) and an elevated level of PTH. This was the initial finding in Abdul, who had a PTH level of 522 pg/L, the upper limit of the normal range being 70.

The elevation of PTH in this circumstance is a measure of what is called secondary hyperparathyroidism, which means an increased activity of the parathyroid glands secondary to a reduced calcium concentration in the blood, itself the result of deficiency in vitamin D. Primary hyperparathyroidism occurs when the parathyroid glands become overactive without an obvious stimulus, and the serum calcium level then becomes higher than normal.

Abdul developed vitamin D deficiency with osteomalacia and secondary hyper-parathyroidism. The overactivity of the parathyroid glands subsequently became excessive and, as a result, the serum calcium level rose to greater than the normal range. This is called tertiary hyperparathyroidism. It is the combination of osteomalacia and tertiary hyperparathyroidism that gives rise to the specific condition of renal osteodystrophy, bone disease associated with chronic renal failure. When tertiary hyperparathyroidism occurs it is no longer possible to use the serum PTH level as a measure of vitamin D deficiency. Abdul's vitamin D supplements were stopped without it being known whether or not he was still deficient in vitamin D. The over-riding imperative at this stage was to control the elevated serum calcium level.

It is this phenomenon that Platt, Black and Stanbury encountered in Manchester much more frequently than researchers working in other countries. The special feature of the population of Manchester compared with those of cities in Australia and the USA was a fundamental insufficiency of vitamin D as a result of high latitude, long winters and almost constant cloudy weather.

Abdul provides an example of the association between osteomalacia and chronic renal failure, but what is the nature of this association? We noted in Chapter 16 that vitamin D goes though two phases of enhanced activity. The first takes place in the liver, with the transformation of calciferol and cholecalciferol into calcidiol (Figure 55.1). The second phase is the further transformation into calcitriol, the most active form of vitamin D, and this process takes place in the kidneys.

**Figure 55.1 Activity of vitamin D.**

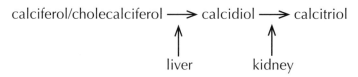

If this process is impaired by kidney failure, then osteomalacia as a result of a failure to produce calcitriol can be expected. This is the usual view, but it does not take into account the Manchester experience, that vitamin D deficiency is a local population phenomenon that perhaps pre-dates the renal failure. The above model indicates that, in osteomalacia of chronic renal failure, the expected finding would be a very low blood level of calcitriol but an elevated level of calcidiol. This is important: if calcidiol is not being converted into calcitriol, then the blood level of calcidiol will increase unless an alternative metabolic pathway is available.

These predictions are not realised in clinical practice; the blood levels of calcitriol and calcidiol are both usually subnormal in end-stage kidney failure. This indicates that vitamin D from the diet or sun exposure is deficient and low levels of calcidiol and calcitriol are the result. This is independent of the presence of kidney disease. We need to consider whether vitamin D deficiency could be a precursor, perhaps part of the cause of chronic renal failure, rather than a consequence.

We must look at chronic renal failure in a different way and we need to return to Bright's disease. Acute glomerulonephritis starts with an infection, historically mainly a streptococcal infection of the throat, in this way similar to rheumatic fever. We now know that it might be initiated by a variety of micro-organisms.

The normal immunological response to infection is rapid, and it should completely overwhelm and clear an invading bacterial or viral infection. The persistence of antibodies gives long-term immunity against a second attack. An alternative outcome is that the infection is overwhelming and the patient dies. This can be the result of either a highly pathogenic micro-organism or serious deficiency of immune mechanisms.

There is a third possible outcome. It might happen that the immune reaction is not completely successful, in that it controls the infection but does not eliminate it completely. The result is a continuing immune process that sets up a continuing inflammatory reaction, and this is often referred to as immune-mediated or sometimes auto-immune disease.

Persistent bacterial proteins, called antigens, combine with the corresponding and stimulated antibody together with a protein called complement in the blood, to produce immune complexes. They circulate in the blood and can become trapped in the capillaries within the kidney filtration units, the glomeruli. This causes an inflammatory reaction, with leakage of protein and red blood cells into the urine. The process can result in progressive destruction of the glomeruli over a period of time that can be days, weeks, months or years. Death from kidney failure is the result, but rescue therapy can be undertaken with treatment to suppress the inflammatory process and, if this fails, dialysis or kidney transplantation.

The incidence of glomerulonephritis or Bright's disease has declined significantly in this country, as has its counterpart, rheumatic fever. The reasons for this cannot be proven but they appear to be because of the improved living conditions of the population. It is my view that improved nutrition and clean air made a particular contribution; we know that both adequate food supply and vitamin D synthesis are necessary for immune competence.

Chronic renal failure has not disappeared. A major cause in the UK at the present time is diabetes, particularly as people with diabetes live for much longer than was previously the case.

We noted in Chapter 51 that South Asian and Afro-Caribbean residents of the UK have an increased susceptibility to end-stage kidney disease, and I refer you back to Figure 51.4. We also saw in Figure 51.5 that the major causes of the excess of kidney disease are diabetes, glomerulonephritis and 'undetermined', meaning that the disease was so advanced that its detailed pathology could not be identified.

We will see shortly that diabetes is particularly common in the South Asian population of the UK, and diabetes is a major cause of kidney failure. However, the problem of end-stage renal failure in the South Asian population cannot be explained on the basis of diabetes alone. We remember that Abdul developed diabetes, but 10 years after the kidney failure was recognised. In Leicester and west London in the 1980s, it was noted that the non-diabetic South Asian population had a risk of developing end-stage renal failure three times that of the background population. In the 1990s it was reported that in London there was a 3.5 times increased risk for the South Asian and 3.2 times increased risk for the Afro-Caribbean groups compared with the background population of developing end-stage renal failure [2].

Another study put the relative increased risk of death from chronic renal failure in the UK at 3 times for the overall South Asian population but 5 times for Bangladeshi men and Pakistani women and 4.5 times in Afro-Caribbeans [3]. The full spectrum of mortality from renal disease in the UK by country of birth can be seen in Figure 55.2.

**Figure 55.2 Mortality from renal disease for the population aged 20–69 years, by country of birth [3].**

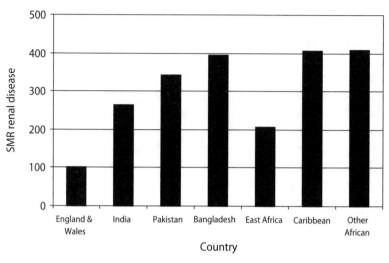

*Crown © 1996, adapted with permission.*

Feehally commented in 2003 [2] that 'The interaction of genotype and environment in the pathogenesis of this susceptibility to renal disease is not yet understood'. I would like to suggest that if we take the genotype (genetic factor) of skin pigmentation and the environmental factor of sunlight insufficiency as a starting point, then understanding might not be far away.

It has also been noted that there is a marked excess of tuberculosis among South Asians with renal failure, also exhibited by Abdul, and this can be interpreted in three ways. First, chronic renal failure predisposes tuberculosis; second, tuberculosis initiates chronic renal failure; third, there is a common factor, something that predisposes to tuberculosis also predisposes to chronic renal failure.

We come back to our knowledge that susceptibility to tuberculosis is increased by vitamin D deficiency and so we must consider that susceptibility to chronic renal failure is also increased by vitamin D deficiency. This conforms with the decline in the incidence of acute glomerulonephritis (Bright's disease) and our observation that South Asian people living in this country have a variety of illnesses resulting from low sunlight exposure and subsequent insufficient synthesis of vitamin D.

We return to analogy and plausibility, part of the process of proof identified by Sir Austin Bradford Hill. Is there a possible mechanism that might link vitamin D insufficiency with end-stage glomerulonephritis and kidney failure? The key must lie in the immune process. We need to understand what determines whether it is successfully completed, with an end to the disease, or it continues, with an immune-mediated inflammatory reaction and organ destruction that might lead to death. Inflammatory cells, and in particular macrophages, release a number of chemical signals called cytokines. One of these is transforming-growth factor-beta (TGF-β), which leads to completion of the disease process and healing, with restoration of normal body structure and function (Figure 55.3). An alternative cytokine is tumour necrosis factor-alpha (TNF-α), which promotes a continuing destructive process as part of continuing disease, often called auto-immune [4]. Medications that inhibit TNF-α are under evaluation and use in a number of chronic inflammatory diseases at present.

**Figure 55.3**

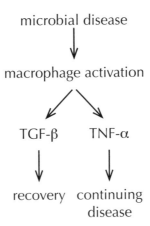

The key to the outcome of an inflammatory disease process that might have been initiated by an infection is whether TGF-β or TNF-α production is dominant. Perhaps vitamin D has an active role in this part of the inflammatory process, leading to TGF-β production and healing, rather than TNF-α production and continuing disease.

In the clinical condition of end-stage chronic renal failure, such as experienced by Abdul, rescue dialysis or kidney transplantation stabilises the patient's condition and death from renal failure itself is prevented or delayed. The disease might develop in a transplanted kidney, as with Abdul, but the major cause of death is the various manifestations of coronary heart disease. The excess mortality in those on maintenance dialysis is shown in Figure 55.4, using data from the USA [5].

**Figure 55.4 Cardiovascular mortality in dialysis patients [5].**

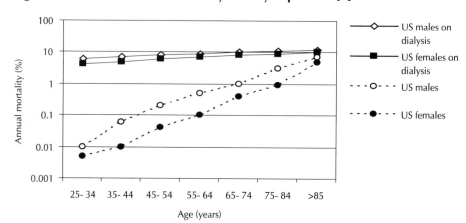

It can be seen from a longitudinal study by the Kaiser Permanante Health Maintenance Organisation (HM) of northern California, USA, that severe kidney failure is associated with premature death, especially from cardiovascular events [6]. An international group concluded that 'Even mild renal (kidney) disease should be considered a major risk factor for cardiovascular complications after a myocardial infarction' [7].

It therefore appears that, for reasons unknown, the development of coronary heart disease is markedly accelerated with chronic renal failure, similar to what we have seen for South Asians living in the UK. Could vitamin D deficiency be the common accelerating factor?

In their review of premature cardiovascular disease in chronic renal failure, Colin Baigent et al. from Birmingham [5] noted that death rates were five times higher if there was co-existing diabetes. We have a powerful association between coronary heart disease, chronic renal failure, type 2 diabetes, vitamin D deficiency or insufficiency, ethnicity and geography. Is vitamin D the common link? The association with diabetes means that we must investigate this complex disease further.

# PART 10

## DIABETES, ENVIRONMENTAL FACTORS AND CLIMATE

# 56
# DIABETES AND VITAMIN D

Diabetes mellitus is a condition defined by an elevated glucose concentration in the blood, but it is a very complex syndrome and blood glucose is only part of it. It would be better if it was defined in a different way, perhaps based on causation, but there is no clear understanding of this. In fact diabetes probably has several forms with a variety of causes.

There are two fundamental patterns to diabetes. The first is a primary impairment of insulin production by the beta cells of the islets of Langerhans within the pancreas, generally called type 1 diabetes. The second, type 2 diabetes, is caused by resistance to insulin within the body. Although insulin is produced in type 2 diabetes and although blood levels of insulin are normal or even greater than normal, the metabolic effects of insulin are inhibited by factors that have not been fully defined.

In type 1 diabetes, a crisis might be reached in which carbohydrate metabolism fails completely and metabolic pathways are switched into the breakdown of fat in order to provide energy. The metabolic result of this is the production of keto-acids and, if this exceeds excretion, the patient goes into a diabetic (keto-acidotic) coma. This will be fatal if the patient is not given insulin by injection. Insulin therapy is essential in type 1 diabetes, and so it is also called insulin-dependent diabetes mellitus (IDDM).

Type 1 diabetes is the major type among young people and so it is sometimes called juvenile-onset diabetes. It has thus been considered an inherited metabolic disorder but, in recent years, it has become quite clear that environmental factors are also important. It is a disease in which there is likely to be an interaction between genetic factors giving susceptibility and one or more environmental factors precipitating the disease.

The incidence of juvenile-onset type 1 diabetes increased world-wide in the latter half of the 20th century, especially in those below the age of 5 years. We have already discussed that such a rapid increase cannot be caused by a genetic factor but indicates one or more environmental factors.

The genetic risk of childhood diabetes is contained in what are called the tissue HLA haplotypes. A UK study showed that these genetic factors are little different in patients with diabetes born within the past 15 years compared with those who developed diabetes in childhood 50 years earlier. Although certain HLA haplotypes create susceptibility, it is the view of the authors that the increased incidence of childhood diabetes must be to the result of a major environmental factor rather than a change in the genetic factors [1].

There is a very significant international variation in the incidence of diabetes. For example, a child in Finland is almost 40 times more likely to develop type 1 diabetes than a child in Japan and almost 100 times more likely than a child in the Zunyi region of China [2]. We have already seen that a high incidence in one country compared with another might be the result of an environmental factor but could be genetic if that genetic variation creates some form of local advantage for the individuals concerned. We saw, as an example, in Chapter 6 that genetically determined haemoglobin variations create resistance to malaria. There would seem to be no genetic advantage to allowing the emergence of diabetes, and the rising incidence in recent years would therefore indicate environmental factors.

In Europe there has been a 3–4% annual rate of increase of type 1 diabetes, with larger increases in central and north-western European countries. The largest rate of increase is seen in children aged 0–4 years, and Figure 56.1 shows the annual increase of incidence of childhood diabetes for a number of countries [2,3].

**Figure 56.1  Relative increase in incidence of type 1 diabetes in children aged < 14 years [3].**

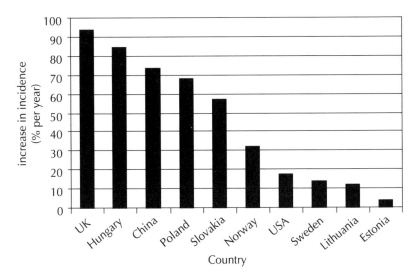

The rapid increase with clustering suggests that the cause might be a micro-organism, but this is by no means certain. Type 1 diabetes is thought to be caused by immune-mediated damage to the islets of Langerhans, clusters of cells within the pancreas in which insulin is produced. The immune reaction implies a trigger factor, and this could be activation by infection, as in certain other diseases.

There is an international geographical variation of childhood type 1 diabetes and we can see details in Table 56.1. The incidence of insulin-dependent diabetes in children is lowest in Japan and highest in Finland.

This pattern is something that we have seen with coronary heart disease, which has been noted by others. Professor David Matthews and his colleagues from the diabetes research laboratories in Oxford, UK [4], took things a stage further by plotting a scattergraph of the incidence of childhood diabetes against latitude [4]. The result is displayed in Figure 56.2.

**Table 56.1  Incidence of type 1 diabetes, age <14 years, per 100 000/year [4]**

| | |
|---|---|
| Finland | 30.3 |
| Sweden | 24.9 |
| Scotland | 21.6 |
| Norway | 20.8 |
| UK, Oxford | 18.5 |
| Australia, west | 14.9 |
| New Zealand, South Island | 12.7 |
| New Zealand, North Island | 10.1 |
| Estonia | 10.2 |
| Italy, Turin | 8.4 |
| France | 8.0 |
| USA, Colorado | 7.8 |
| Austria | 7.8 |
| Slovakia | 7.5 |
| Hungary | 6.9 |
| Germany, east | 6.7 |
| Poland | 5.9 |
| Algeria | 4.7 |
| Japan | 1.7 |
| China, Shanghai | 0.7 |
| Peru | 0.5 |

*Adapted with permission from the British Medical Journal Publishing Group.*

**Figure 56.2  Incidence of type 1 diabetes and latitude [4].**

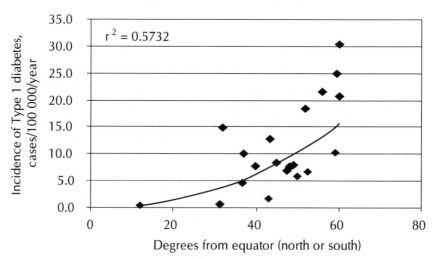

*Adapted with permission from the British Medical Journal Publishing Group.*

We see a scattergraph that is very similar to that of latitude and coronary heart disease (shown in Figure 33.1). There is a significant association, with $R^2 = 0.5732$; latitude therefore appears to have an influence on the development of diabetes in children. This could obviously be mediated by sunlight and vitamin D, as suggested by Matthews et al. [4].

Although sunlight variations might influence geographical variation, the increase of diabetes in children in Europe [5], shown in Figure 56.3, suggests that there is a different environmental factor. This might be a micro-organism but no consistent microbial association has been identified and only congenital rubella syndrome is definitely associated with type 1 diabetes.

**Figure 56.3 Trends in childhood diabetes in Europe [5].**

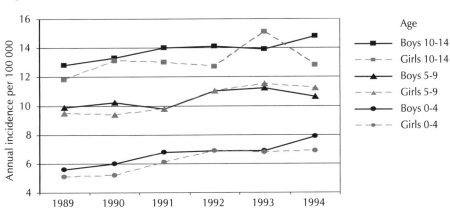

© 2000, adapted from The Lancet with permission from Elsevier.

A study from Bradford indicated a more or less constant background risk of childhood diabetes in the years 1978–90, with a rate of 10.5 per 100 000 [6]. However, during this time the incidence of diabetes in children of Asian ethnicity increased from a low level of 3.1 per 100 000 to 11.7 per 100 000, a more than three-fold rise. This indicates an environmental factor to which the Asian immigrants have become exposed. As with coronary heart disease, the incidence of diabetes in South Asian immigrants is increasing with successive generations. Those born in the UK appear to have a higher risk of diabetes than those born in South Asia.

The incidence of diabetes in children of South Asian parents has thus risen substantially above that of the background population, which conforms with the general observation of an increased risk in this ethnic group. This has been clearly identified in a UK study conducted in 1993–94, the results of which can be seen in Figure 56.4 [7].

**Figure 56.4  Relative prevalence of diabetes by ethnic group [7].**

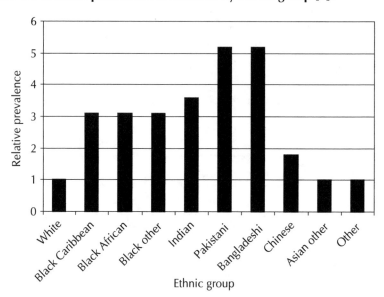

We can see the highest incidence is in those from Pakistan and Bangladesh, but diabetes is equally common among Africans and Caribbeans as among Indians. Clearly a dark skin is linked with a major risk of diabetes, best explained as a genetic factor of skin pigmentation interacting with environmental factors found in the UK.

We have seen in an earlier chapter that there is a social variation of diabetes, as reported from Liverpool, and diabetes is more common in areas with socio-economic deprivation (Figure 38.14). Putting the ethnic and social differences together with the latitude effect, as shown in Figure 56.2, we can see that insufficient sunlight and vitamin D is probably important in susceptibility to diabetes.

Although the health of ethnic minority groups has been studied in considerable detail in the UK, there are no good detailed epidemiological studies in their countries of origin. There are studies, but they are not entirely representative of the population. In the UK we have a regular census and virtually every person in the country can be identified; as a result population samples can be taken for a variety of research studies, health related or other. Think of achieving this in India, with its population of one billion; even though a head count has been undertaken recently, this does not allow the ready identification of every person.

A nationwide survey of diabetes in India was undertaken and reported in 2003 [8]. It was a study of 5516 people with diabetes, but was not really a representative sample of the diabetic population of India, which is estimated to be 32 million. Nevertheless, whereas in the UK diabetes is more common in the socio-economically deprived, in India it appears to be more common in the socio-economically privileged. However, it is also more common in urban than in rural locations. This can be seen in Table 56.2, which shows the background characteristics of the study group.

**Table 56.2  Diabetes in India [8]**

| | | |
|---|---|---|
| Educational status | Illiterate | 8.1% |
| | School | 64.6% |
| | College | 27.3% |
| Employment status | Not working | 7.2% |
| | Working | 54.3% |
| | Retired | 13.8% |
| | Housewife | 24.7% |
| Monthly household income (roubles) | <5000 | 29.3% |
| | 5000–10 000 | 33.2% |
| | >10 000 | 36.9% |
| Location | Rural | 23.6% |
| | Urban | 76.4% |

We have seen this pattern previously. In Chapter 15, we saw the work of Hutchinson and Shah, who investigated the epidemiology of rickets in the Nasik district of Bombay and published their work in 1922 [9]. They found that rickets was rare among poorer children, who spent a lot of time outdoors, and much more common among the wealthy children, who spent most of their time indoors. The same pattern was observed with tuberculosis. Exposure to the sun provided adequate vitamin D synthesis and was protective against rickets and tuberculosis, and it would appear that exposure to the sun also provides protection against diabetes. The prevalence of diabetes among South Asians living in England is greater than in those living in India. There are many ethnic Asian people living in the UK who frequently visit India and Pakistan; many tell me that when in South Asia they do not require insulin or tablet treatment for the diabetes and it remains stable without medication. When they return to the UK, the diabetes becomes uncontrolled and they require treatment once again.

In a study in 2000 it was noted that the children of women who took cod liver oil during pregnancy appeared to have a lower incidence of type 1 diabetes [10]. To investigate whether the beneficial effect of cod liver oil was the result of vitamin D supplement, a further study was undertaken in Finland. It involved 10 821 children born in 1966, of whom 81 developed diabetes; it was recorded whether the children had taken vitamin D supplements during the first year of life [11]. The results of the study are shown in Figure 56.5.

**Figure 56.5 Vitamin D supplements in infancy and subsequent diabetes [11].**

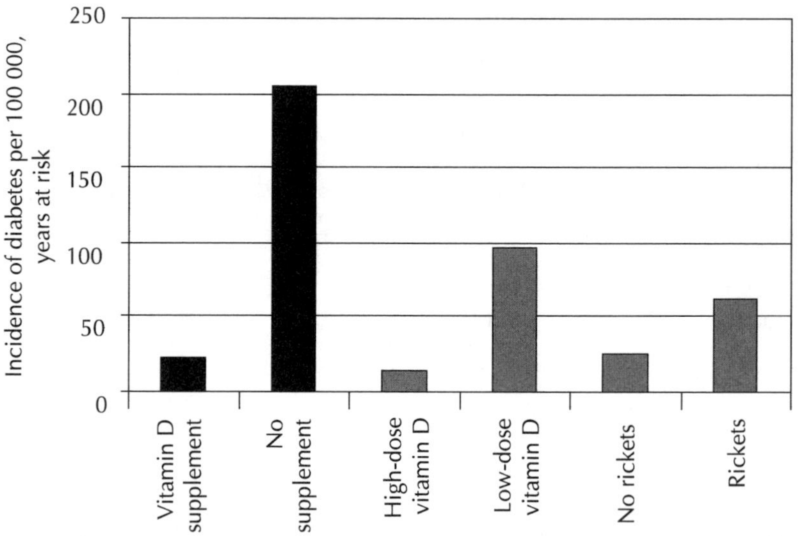

© 2001, adapted from The Lancet with permission from Elsevier.

The occurrence of diabetes at follow-up in 1997–98 was almost 10 times higher in those who had not taken vitamin D supplements regularly compared with those who had. There was also a dose effect; a higher dose of vitamin D was more effective at protecting against diabetes than a low dose. Some children were suspected as having rickets, a result of vitamin D deficiency, and they had a higher incidence of subsequent diabetes compared with those without rickets. This benefit of cod liver oil supplement during infancy was confirmed in a further large study undertaken by the Norwegian Childhood Diabetes Study Group [12].

Vitamin D appears to have an important role in protecting against diabetes. In this chapter, we have concentrated on childhood type 1 diabetes. In the study from India, of the 5516 people with diabetes, only 5.1% had type 1 and 94.9% had type 2 [8]. In the next chapter we will look at type 2 diabetes in more detail.

# 57
# THE METABOLIC SYNDROME
# AND INSULIN RESISTANCE

We are now going to look at evidence indicating that type 2 diabetes is not an isolated condition but just one component of a larger syndrome, called at the present time the metabolic (or dys-metabolic) syndrome. Its title changes with understanding. The concept is quite new but the fundamental feature is that the body tissues are somehow resistant to the action of insulin; the amount of insulin in the blood must therefore increase above normal levels to overcome this resistance. Diabetes occurs when, despite this, the body fails to produce enough insulin to overcome the resistance, allowing the blood glucose level to rise. It can be seen, therefore, that the rise in blood glucose is not the fundamental or perhaps the most important part of type 2 diabetes or the metabolic syndrome. The subject is very complex but I will try to illustrate the development of thinking and the influence of vitamin D regarding type 2 diabetes.

We have seen in the study from India that type 2 diabetes is much more common than type 1 [1]. The general perception is that type 1 diabetes is more severe or serious, based on its often dramatic and symptomatic onset, with excessive thirst (polydipsia), excessive urine production (polyuria), a tendency to go into a rapidly developing and potentially fatal coma and onset at an early age. Type 2 diabetes is insidious in its onset and usually without symptoms, often found incidentally by urine or blood testing.

There is no such thing as mild diabetes if we consider the long term. Diabetes has a number of so-called complications, by which is meant associated diseases that develop over a variable period of time. Table 57.1 shows the associations present at the time of diagnosis of diabetes in the study from India [1]. It can be seen that the burden of illness is much greater in those with type 2 diabetes, which is 94.9% of all those with diabetes.

**Table 57.1  Diabetes in India [1]**

|  | Type 1 (%) | Type 2 (%) |
|---|---|---|
|  | 5.1 | 94.9 |
| Hypertension | 8.5 | 28.5 |
| Heart disease | 3.9 | 11.9 |
| Eye problems | 16.3 | 27.0 |
| Kidney disease | 2.1 | 2.8 |
| Neurological disorders | 0.0 | 0.5 |
| Skin problems | 7.4 | 7.7 |

It has been noted for a long time that people with diabetes have an increased risk of coronary heart disease, and when myocardial infarction occurs it carries a higher mortality rate. In the Whitehall Study the risk of coronary heart disease was followed-up for 18 043 men aged 40–64 years for more than 7 years [2]. At the outset of the study the men were tested for diabetes with a standard glucose tolerance test, in which they were given 50 grams of glucose in water by mouth and the blood glucose concentration measured 2 hours later, by which time it should have returned to normal. The actual blood glucose recordings were sorted so that various groups could be identified. The 95% of the study group with the lowest 2-hour blood glucose (that is below the 95th centile) had similar coronary event rates at 7 years. The 5% with the highest blood glucose levels at 2 hours had about twice the mortality from coronary heart disease.

The reason for this is not really known. An editorial by Jukka Salonen, Professor of Epidemiology at the University of Kuopio, Finland, was entitled 'Non-insulin dependent diabetes and ischaemic heart disease: related, but how?' [3].

The diseases associated with diabetes have been called complications, and atherosclerotic disease is loosely grouped with these. The term complication implies that the diabetes comes first and the others follow as a consequence. This does not quite fit the evidence, as type 2 diabetes is often diagnosed after a person is admitted to hospital because of myocardial infarction. The time sequence is therefore not clear and perhaps the term association is more neutral and thus preferable to the term complication.

A study published recently compared the outcome of myocardial infarction in people with long-standing diabetes and those in whom it had just been diagnosed [4]. The outcome was equally bad in the two groups compared with those without diabetes, as shown in Figure 57.1.

**Figure 57.1 Mortality after myocardial infarction [4].**

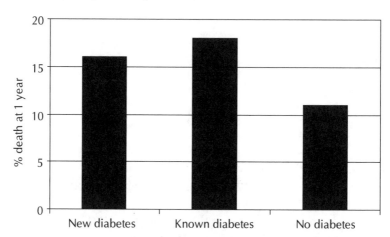

*Adapted from* Circulation *with permission from Lippincott, Williams and Watkins.*

If the poor survival of people with diabetes following myocardial infarction was the result of diabetes, it might be expected that the longer the diabetes had been present, the worse the outcome would be. This is the usual model with a complication, but this study shows it not to be the case.

The time relationships indicate that diabetes, as defined by elevated blood glucose, is associated with coronary heart disease and atherosclerotic disease by a common cause or susceptibility rather than by a cause–effect relationship. This has led researchers to look at a more fundamental cause and definition of diabetes, but without full success so far. The alternative models are shown in Figure 57.2.

**Figure 57.2  Models of type 2 diabetes and coronary heart disease.**

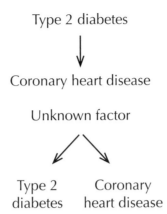

The discovery of insulin was a major step in the treatment of diabetes. Insulin is now produced industrially using bio-engineering technology but, until about 20 years ago, it was extracted from the pancreas of cows and pigs. At one time this had to be undertaken in hospitals and an excellent account of the early days of insulin treatment in Edinburgh has been provided by my former colleague Dr Rae Lyon [5]. The biological production of insulin means that its measurement is traditionally in units of biological activity rather than mass units.

The measurement of insulin in the blood by specific immuno-assay methods has allowed further research into the understanding of diabetes. It had been assumed that diabetes is the result of a failure of insulin secretion by the pancreas, but it became clear that this is not always the case. Patients with type 2 diabetes have higher levels of serum insulin 2 hours after a glucose drink compared with non-diabetic subjects [6].

It has also been discovered that obese subjects without diabetes have a high insulin response to a glucose load [7]. A study from Glasgow, Scotland, indicated higher insulin levels after a glucose load in patients with duodenal ulcer [8], another disease that we have encountered.

The same has been shown for patients with peripheral atherosclerotic disease [9]. In this study, 51 patients without diabetes were compared with 47 controls, obesity being the same in the two groups. The insulin response to a glucose load was greater in those with peripheral atherosclerotic disease [10]. This study was undertaken at Queens University Medical School, Belfast, Northern Ireland, and was part of a great deal of work carried out mainly by Robert Stout and John Vallence-Owen. They recognised that the serum insulin levels were higher in the disease group but that the blood glucose levels were also higher. If the insulin was functioning normally, the glucose levels should have been lower. It follows that the insulin was not functioning and therefore the patients, or rather their tissues, were resistant to insulin. Another important message from this study was that, in the group studied, obesity did not determine blood insulin levels.

It follows that, even if there is insulin resistance, insulin production should increase to keep the blood glucose level normal. If the blood glucose level rises above the normal level, that is if an individual develops diabetes, it means that insulin production has failed to be adequate. Diabetes always results from insulin insufficiency, either absolute (type 1) or relative (type 2).

A high blood insulin level, called hyperinsulinism or hyperinsulinaemia, is therefore associated with type 2 diabetes, obesity, coronary heart disease, peripheral atherosclerosis and duodenal ulcer. Further studies have associated it with classic coronary risk factors, including hypertension and hypercholesterolaemia [11]. It has also been noted that hyperinsulinism is an independent risk factor for coronary heart disease; it need not be associated with the classic risk factors and is not mediated by cholesterol or other lipid abnormalities [12].

We also find an association between cigarette smoking and insulin resistance, the details of which are shown in Figure 57.3. It can be seen that there is a greater insulin response to a 75-g oral glucose load in people who smoke [13].

**Figure 57.3  Insulin response to an oral glucose load [13].**

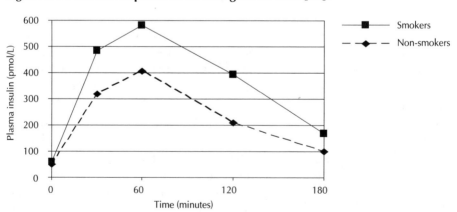

We can only speculate whether this is of fundamental importance. A research project that I undertook many years ago indicated that cigarette smoking induced the stomach to empty more rapidly [14]. This would lead to a more rapid absorption of glucose into the blood stream, and this would induce a greater insulin response. In other words, there are suspicions that cigarette smoking has a causative effect on increased blood insulin levels. I suspect that this would be only a tiny component of hyperinsulinism and would probably have no effect on insulin resistance.

We are often told that coffee is somehow bad for us, probably on the basis that it is a dietary characteristic of industrialised societies. It is also enjoyable, perhaps indicating that it must be undesirable as judged by self-appointed custodians of public health and morality. A study of 17 111 men and women aged between 30 and 60 years, living in the Netherlands, indicated that popular wisdom might not be correct [15]. During almost 10 years of follow-up, the relative risk of developing type 2 diabetes was substantially lower in those who drank plenty of coffee, as shown in Figure 57.4.

**Figure 57.4  Coffee consumption and the development of type 2 diabetes [15].**

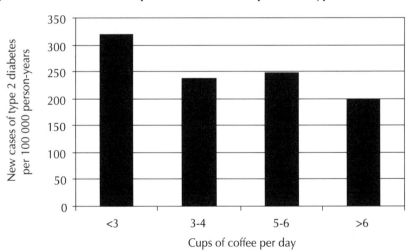

© 2002, adapted from The Lancet with permission from Elsevier.

Coronary heart disease, hypertension, obesity and hypercholesterolaemia are associated with insulin resistance and type 2 diabetes more frequently than can be expected by chance. This led Gerald Reaven, of the Department of Medicine at Stanford University, Palo Alto, California, USA, to develop the concept of a syndrome [16,17].

Insulin resistance is another way of looking at insulin sensitivity and it can be measured in a number of ways, reviewed clearly by Reaven in his 1983 paper in the *American Journal of Medicine* [16]. One way is to give subjects an injection of insulin, the dose adjusted to body weight, and observe the resulting reduction in blood glucose; the greater the sensitivity to insulin, the greater the fall in blood glucose. The disadvantage is that a rapid reduction in blood glucose to subnormal levels (hypoglycaemia) can be unpleasant and dangerous.

An alternative method had been used by Sir Harold Himsworth (1905–93) and his colleague R. B. Kerr at University College Hospital Medical School, London, UK in 1939 [18]. This was the first study to divide the diabetic population into two groups, according to whether they were insulin sensitive or insulin resistant (insensitive). They gave the subjects 50 grams of glucose as a standard glucose tolerance test but gave insulin by injection at the same time. In those sensitive to insulin, the blood glucose rose only minimally, but the blood glucose increased much more in those who were insulin resistant [18]. A calculation has been developed using the blood glucose and insulin levels to determine a value for insulin resistance. Insulin resistance = fasting insulin (miu/L) × fasting glucose (mmol/L)/22.5. This is called HOMA (the Homeostasis Model Assessment), developed by Professor David Matthews and colleagues at Oxford University, UK [19].

Reaven used the term 'syndrome X', the use of the word syndrome as usual indicating a lack of understanding of causation and the mechanism behind the association of the constituent disease processes. However, he was aware that association is a clue to cause and this is the important aspect of the syndrome. The term syndrome X became superseded by the term insulin-resistance syndrome, in the recognition that insulin resistance is perhaps the factor that links the diseases together. Because insulin resistance is not really understood, the term metabolic syndrome is coming into use at the present time, and also the term dysmetabolic syndrome, to emphasise that the metabolism is abnormal.

But the mechanism behind the metabolic syndrome remains a mystery and we are again tying to look for cause–effect relationships. Type 2 diabetes is often diagnosed at the time of admission of a patient with myocardial infarction, but it is often the case that on previous admissions diabetes was definitely not present. The relationship between the two appears to be a common cause or a common susceptibility, as suggested above.

In peaceful industrialised nations, we are in an era of plentiful food supply leading to overconsumption, with people eating for pleasure rather than out of necessity. Gluttony is felt to be a major problem at the present time and, as a result, obesity. It is suggested in the press that we are sitting on 'an illness time-bomb' and that our obese underactive children are going to be victims of a future epidemic of coronary heart disease. We have already seen the Leningrad paradox, that a population suffering from starvation has a particularly high incidence of coronary heart disease. We have also seen that the epidemic of coronary heart disease is well past its peak and is perhaps close to its end in the UK. The link between gluttony, obesity and coronary heart disease is far from clear.

Obesity is part of the metabolic syndrome and it closely associated with type 2 diabetes. The relationship needs to be explained; it is generally thought that it is cause–effect, but there is much more to it than the simple model shown in Figure 57.5.

**Figure 57.5  Development of type 2 diabetes.**

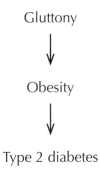

We will see that there are several other factors involved in the development of type 2 diabetes. Obesity is a condition of too much fat stored within the body, and the storage occurs in fat cells called adipocytes. There must be a difference between carrying fat within the body and carrying it in a shopping bag, even though both would make walking hard work. Somehow the body must know its weight and whether or not it is obese; the total mass of fat cells must exert an effect on the metabolism of the body. It has been identified that there is a hormone called leptin that is secreted by fat cells. It has an effect on the brain, and its function is to reduce appetite and thereby food intake [20].

If leptin is the link between fat cell mass and body metabolism, then we might expect it to have a role in the development of the illnesses associated with obesity, for example type 2 diabetes. The link is not clear, but if obesity is causing insulin resistance and type 2 diabetes, then the aim of treatment must be to reduce fat cell mass. This can be achieved in two ways.

The first is to eat less. If the effect on diabetes is beneficial, all is well and good for the patient, but from the scientific viewpoint of understanding things are not clear. Is it the reduced food intake that is directly important or is it the reduced fat cell mass?

The other way to reduce fat cell mass is by surgery, and this is being undertaken increasingly as liposuction. This can have a major effect on obesity and has been the subject of a recent study into metabolic consequences in 15 obese women [21]. The conclusion of the authors was:

*Abdominal liposuction does not significantly improve obesity-associated metabolic abnormalities. Decreasing adipose tissue mass alone will not achieve the metabolic benefits of weight loss.*

So the role of obesity as the cause of insulin resistance and type 2 diabetes must be in some doubt and we cannot yet form a definite conclusion.

Fat cells produce another polypeptide hormone, adiponectin, which appears to have beneficial effects, protecting against diabetes and atherosclerosis. The production of adiponectin is reduced when there is obesity and also when there is insulin resistance, but this is not really understood. When given to experimental animals, adiponectin increases insulin sensitivity [22]. Research into this hormone is in its very early stages and, although it is apparently beneficial, no other conclusions can yet be reached.

There is something about obesity that appears to be more fundamental to ill-health than the development of diabetes. We find insulin resistance among children who are obese and we also find that this relates to C-reactive protein (CRP), the inflammatory marker that we encountered in relation to coronary heart disease [23]. Figure 57.6 shows particularly high levels of CRP in severely obese children and adolescents with high levels of insulin resistance. This suggests that the pathogenesis of diabetes, whatever its cause, and like coronary heart disease, is inflammatory.

**Figure 57.6  CRP levels, obesity and insulin resistance in children [23].**

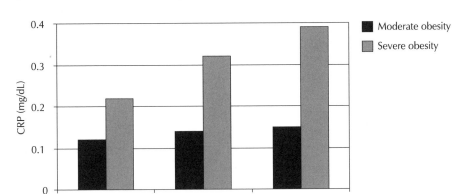

Obesity is not straightforward. Although food intake is of great importance, there are others factors, probably inheritance and one or more environmental factors.

*Obesity by itself seems not to be dangerous. Some disease-generating factor, in addition to the basic condition of central obesity, is required for associated diseases to become manifest [24].*

Certain people are particularly prone to obesity at times of plentiful food supply, examples being the Pima Indians in the USA and some aboriginal groups in Australia. We discussed this in Chapter 6 in relation to the thrifty gene, which provides a survival advantage in times of food shortage but a disadvantage in times of plentiful food [24]. Obesity is the result of more than gluttony, and so is the metabolic syndrome.

Abdul, whom we met in the Prologue, had some features of the metabolic syndrome, with coronary heart disease, cerebrovascular disease and type 2 diabetes, but he was not obese; on the contrary, he was underweight. This suggests again that obesity itself is not essential for the disease state from which Abdul and so many others suffer, and so the simple model given above cannot be correct. We have seen that coronary heart disease, diabetes and chronic renal failure are more common in the UK in those of South Asian ethnicity. The same is true of the metabolic syndrome, with obesity being characteristic but not always present [25].

There is a strong possibility that the high susceptibility of South Asians in the UK to coronary heart disease and diabetes is a result of vitamin D insufficiency. This is the result of the interaction between the genetic factor of skin pigmentation and the environmental factors of cultural sunshine avoidance and residence distant from the equator in north-west Europe. We must therefore ask whether insulin resistance might also be a manifestation of vitamin D insufficiency.

The suggestion has been made that vitamin D insufficiency is the fundamental feature of the metabolic syndrome, leading to its various clinical manifestations. This was based on an observation from a study in the Netherlands, once again involving Daan Kromhout of the National Institute of Public Health, whose work in that country has been exceptionally productive [26].

The subjects of this study were 142 elderly male citizens of Zutphen in the Netherlands, aged between 70 and 88 years, all with type 2 diabetes. Of these men, 39% had low blood vitamin D levels, and this was found to be related to a lack of outdoor activity rather than inadequate diet. It was also noted that, the lower the vitamin D level, the greater the intolerance to glucose. This means that after a glucose load the blood glucose was higher, as shown in Figure 57.7.

**Figure 57.7 Blood glucose response to an oral glucose load based on vitamin D status [26].**

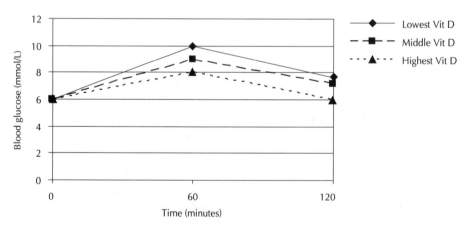

This was not because of insulin deficiency but because of insulin resistance. Figure 57.8 shows higher levels of plasma insulin in those with the lowest blood levels of vitamin D.

**Figure 57.8 Plasma insulin response to an oral glucose load based on vitamin D state [26].**

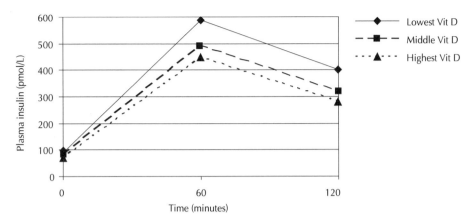

Those with the lowest levels of vitamin D had the greatest increase in insulin, indicating that they were the most resistant to insulin. This was independent of weight, age, physical activity, diet and season.

This study indicates that vitamin D is active in blood glucose control and is perhaps a co-factor in the activity of insulin. With insufficiency of vitamin D, there appears to be a resistance to activity of insulin. Vitamin D would appear to have a potential role in the prevention of diabetes and the metabolic syndrome.

One of the authors, Barbara J. Boucher from St Bartholomew's and the Royal London Medical & Dental School, UK, went on to develop the idea. She reminded us that there are vitamin D receptors (VDRs) in the insulin-producing beta cells of the islets of Langerhans within the pancreas and that insulin production depends on vitamin D [27].

A reminder about vitamin D receptors: they are complex proteins found within cells and they are basically genetically determined enzymes that are transcribed from RNA. However, at this stage the VDR molecule is in an inactive form; to become active it must combine with vitamin D as calcitriol, like a key (calcitriol) to undo a lock (VDR). The activated VDR can then enable the functioning of the targets cells, osteoblasts (in bone), immune cells, in particular macrophages, and the insulin-producing beta cells of the islets of Langerhans within the pancreas. If the VDR has certain mutations, then calcitriol will not be able to activate it, with resultant target-organ failure.

The role of vitamin D in the mechanism of insulin resistance is supported by a study of British men of South Asian ethnicity. Those with low levels of vitamin D demonstrated a particularly high serum insulin concentration after a glucose load, indicating an association between vitamin D insufficiency and insulin resistance. Boucher *et al.* [28] went on to investigate 65 east London Asians with diabetes and found that 44 of them were deficient in vitamin D, as judged by a blood level of calcidiol less than 11 ng/mL. The high prevalence of both diabetes and osteomalacia in British Asians has led to the comment 'Whether their vitamin D deficiency contributes to the pathogenesis of their diabetes is an area ripe for investigation' [29]. Almost 20 years later the opportunity for research remains ripe but undeveloped.

A further study of British South Asians living in London looked at the age at which the susceptibility to the metabolic syndrome first appears [30]. The comparison was between 1287 white children and 73 South Asian children. The South Asian children were found to be slightly slimmer, indicated by a lower ponderal index, a relationship between height and weight. They had higher plasma insulin levels when fasting and also after an oral glucose load, indicating insulin resistance. The relationship between plasma insulin and adiposity was stronger in the South Asian children, and this is the basis of the metabolic syndrome. It can be seen in Figure 57.9 that insulin levels increase with obesity but are always higher in the South Asians.

**Figure 57.9 Insulin response to glucose related to ponderal index [30].**

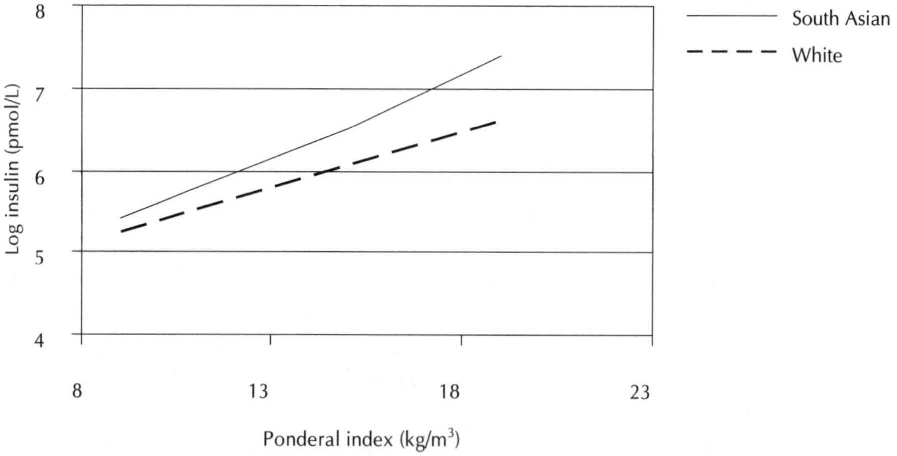

*Adapted with permission from the* British Medical Journal Publishing Group.

The roots of the metabolic syndrome in South Asians are thus present in childhood. We know of a familial tendency and the likelihood of an inherited factor, and perhaps we should look at circumstances before birth. These will be considered in the next chapter.

# 58
# THE MATERNAL FACTOR AND NON-GENETIC INHERITANCE

During the latter half of the 20th century it became clear that coronary heart disease tends to run in families. This was thought to be because of an inherited factor, presumably genetic, as this is the accepted way in which a disease characteristic can be passed from one generation to the next. However, we have seen with the experience of tuberculosis and syphilis that familial 'constitutional' diseases may not after all be inherited by genetic mechanisms. In general it is safer to use the term familial unless genetic abnormalities have been clearly identified. Occasionally the term 'polygenic' is used in an attempt to disguise ignorance, what might be called genetic spin.

It is as well to reflect on the mechanisms of inheritance, looking beyond the genetic inheritance first defined by the Austrian monk Gregor Mendel (1822–84). One of the most important factors that we inherit from our parents is money, and we have seen that this can have a major influence on health in childhood and adult life. We also inherit a place of residence; whether a child is to born to a family in Toulouse or Belfast has a major influence on life expectancy. Being born into a rural area provides an advantage over being born into an inner city environment. Being born into a family that has communal meals sitting around a table also provides a major health advantage. Similarly, being born into a family that attends church regularly will give a health advantage.

We have also seen that we inherit exposure to micro-organisms. A child born into a family in which tuberculosis is present has a relatively high risk of developing tuberculosis. The same applies to syphilis, hepatitis B and HIV/AIDS.

We have noted that insufficiency of vitamin D can increase susceptibility to disease. This can be because of inherited traditions of covering the whole body with clothing and sun avoidance as well as locations of birth and residence away from the equator.

These inherited factors occur after birth and they are generally called environmental factors. Genetic factors are determined at the moment of conception but there are other factors that occur between conception and birth. The environment of the uterus must not be forgotten and will form a major theme of this chapter.

The link between childhood environment and adult cardiovascular disease was first established by Anders Forsdahl, working at the University of Tromsø, Norway, in the 1970s [1]. Subsequent work in the UK has confirmed this finding [2] but, although the link is consistent, no-one understands the mechanism. There are non-genetic factors acting before birth, the main one being low birth weight. I have already mentioned the outstanding epidemiological work of Professor David Barker at the Medical Research Council Clinical Epidemiology Unit based at Southampton University, UK. He and his colleagues have searched birth records up and down the country and have related recorded birth weight and weight at 1 year to subsequent health [2].

Chronic obstructive lung disease and coronary heart disease are both related to weight at 1 year: the lower the weight, the greater the incidence of adult disease, as shown in Figure 58.1. These data are based on child health records of 5654 men born in Hertfordshire between 1911 and 1932 [2].

**Figure 58.1 Adult deaths from obstructive lung disease (COPD) and coronary heart disease (CHD) in relation to weight at 1 year [2].**

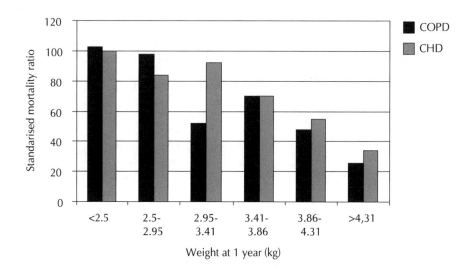

Weight at 1 year (kg)

It is quite clear from this work that low weight at 1 year, a reflection of gestational and early childhood factors, has been followed by a high risk of early death from coronary heart disease and chronic obstructive pulmonary disease in adult life. Barker points out that the same finding applies to birth weight, but a lower than average weight at 1 year gives a stronger prediction of adult ill-health.

Between December 1944 and April 1945 there was a famine in the Netherlands. The subsequent outcome of adults who were *in utero* at that time has been studied; it demonstrates that they have an increased risk of coronary heart disease, further evidence of foetal undernutrition being of great importance [3].

In further papers, Barker and colleagues have shown that the development of type 2 diabetes in adults (men aged 59–70 years) is strongly related to birth weight [4,5]. This is shown in Figure 58.2.

**Figure 58.2  Adult diabetes and birth weight [5].**

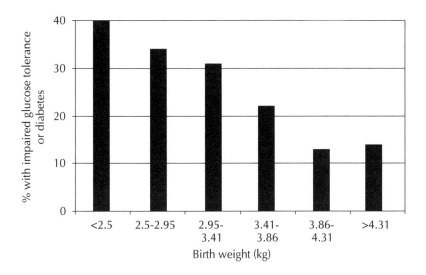

We can see a clear trend of high prevalence of adult diabetes or glucose intolerance affecting 40% of those with the lowest birth weights, compared with little more than 10% of those with high birth weights. The study also demonstrates a five-fold risk of the metabolic syndrome in those with a low birth weight compared with those with a high birth weight, as shown in Figure 58.3.

**Figure 58.3  Adult metabolic syndrome in relation to birth weight [5].**

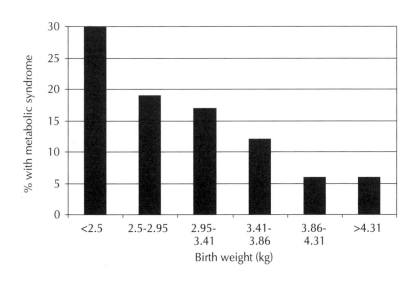

More recent research from New Zealand has confirmed a relationship between low birth weight and the metabolic syndrome in a study of 72 children aged between 4 and 10 years [6]. Those who were born prematurely were shown to have reduced insulin sensitivity, that is increased insulin resistance, compared with those born at term. We know that this is fundamental to the metabolic syndrome.

A study of 129 920 deliveries in Scotland looked at the subsequent health of mothers in relation to characteristics of their pregnancies [7]. It was found that pre-eclampsia, pre-term delivery and low birth weight were associated with a two-fold risk of symptomatic or fatal coronary heart disease during the following 20 years. These complications of pregnancy would also have an adverse effect on growth of the foetus and its weight at birth.

Recent research from Sweden has shown similar findings [8]. In a follow-up of 14 193 men and women born in Uppsala between 1915 and 1929, their birth weights and gestation dates were recorded. Subsequent deaths from coronary heart disease and cerebrovascular disease were also determined from records and were adjusted for age. Figure 58.4 confirms the increased mortality rates of those of low birth weight and a relative reduction of death rate in those with the highest birth weight.

**Figure 58.4  Risk of death from coronary heart disease (CHD) and cerebrovascular disease (CVD) on based on birth weight [8].**

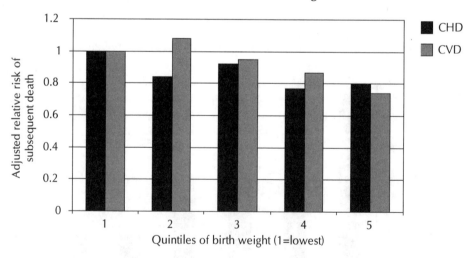

The gestation age at birth is shown in Figure 58.5. We can see a very strong association with death from cerebrovascular disease, with high death rates in those born early and a 40% relative reduction in those with the longest gestation ages. In this study there was no association with coronary heart disease [8].

**Figure 58.5  Risk of death from coronary heart disease (CHD) and cerebrovascular disease (CVD) based on length of gestation [8].**

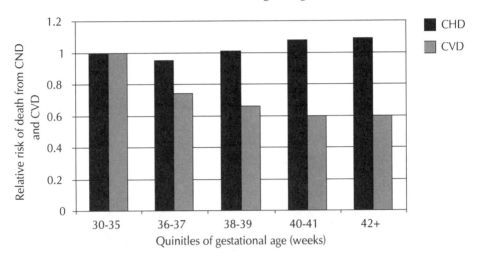

We have seen the detrimental effects of socio-economic deprivation on health, and in particular a high risk of premature death from coronary heart disease. Barker *et al.* [9] have demonstrated that a low birth weight acts together with poor living conditions in adult life to reduce life expectancy still further. A study of 3900 people born in England in 1946 has shown that those with low birth weight had on average poor educational achievement [10]. Maturation of the brain during gestation is of great importance and impairment of this might be expected to have a long-term effect on education and thus on subsequent socio-economic achievement.

Barker has clearly identified that inheritance of something from the mother is extremely important in adult life. He calls this 'the maternal factor' [2]; he has not identified its nature but I propose that it is vitamin D.

We have an association between low birth weight, childhood factors, socio-economic deprivation and serious health problems, particularly in South Asian groups. These conditions are now causing concern in the newly industrialising Asian cities. Might vitamin D insufficiency resulting from inadequate sunlight exposure be involved?

A study of pregnant Asian women in south London, UK, showed all of them to have low blood levels of vitamin D, measured as calcidiol, which is the best indicator of sunshine and dietary adequacy [11]. They had no obvious features of osteomalacia; 59 were given vitamin D supplement at a standard dose of ergocalciferol 1000 international units (IU)/day, and 67 acted as controls. Mothers in the treatment group gained weight faster in the last trimester (3 months) of pregnancy than those in the control group and, at birth, mothers and babies had normal blood levels of vitamin D (calcidiol). In contrast, mothers and infants in the control group had low levels of vitamin D in the blood, creating metabolic bone problems in some. Almost twice as many babies in the control group were small for their gestational age and the average birth weight was less, as shown in Figure 58.6.

**Figure 58.6 Effect of vitamin D supplement on birth weight [11].**

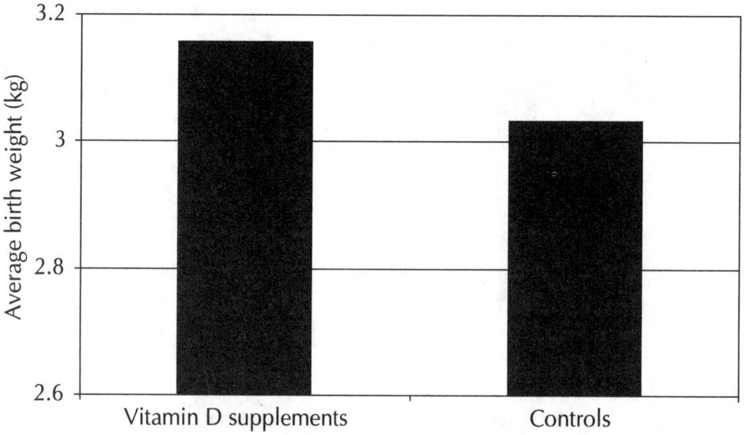

*Adapted with permission from the British Medical Journal Publishing Group.*

A recent editorial in the *British Medical Journal* expressed concern at the prospect of increasing the overall nutritional intake of pregnant women, especially South Asians, in an attempt to increase birth weight, as it might have a detrimental effect on the weight and health of the mothers [12]. It also expressed the view that small thin babies might actually have a moderate excess of fat and therefore tend to become obese adults. I propose that they tend to become obese adults as part of the metabolic syndrome to which they are prone because of vitamin D insufficiency during gestation.

However, in the search for the maternal factor, concern about birth weight and what to do about it, the simple and important study from St George's Hospital Medical School in south London, UK, illustrated in Figure 58.6 [11], seems to have been overlooked or prematurely forgotten. Rather than providing more food, the selective correction of vitamin D insufficiency by vitamin D supplement is effective.

In north-western Europe sun exposure is compromised and dietary sources of vitamin D become important. Consumption of fish has been shown to be protective against coronary heart disease and is also capable of healing rickets. A study from Denmark showed that low consumption of fish is a strong risk factor for pre-term delivery and low birth weight [13]. These factors in turn lead to a higher risk of subsequent development of the metabolic syndrome.

We have noted the relationship between low birth weight and average poor educational achievement. The New Scientist informed us in 2002 that 'Vitamin D's role in building healthy brains had been largely ignored, until researchers began to spot some curious epidemiological trends' [14].

This report was based on research undertaken in Australia by Professor John McGrath and his team at the Queensland Centre for Mental Health Research [15]. Later, experimental studies in rats indicated that deprivation of vitamin D during pregnancy resulted in abnormal structure and function of the brains of the offspring [16]. The report also commented on the increased likelihood of schizophrenia in Europe and North America in those born in the spring [15]. This time of birth is suboptimal as it means that the mother would have been pregnant during the winter and would thus have been unable to transfer adequate amounts of vitamin D to the developing foetus. We will see more evidence to support this view.

We have seen in Chapter 56 (Figure 56.5) that vitamin D supplements in the first year of life substantially reduce the risk of developing type 1 diabetes in childhood and early adult life [17]. Vitamin D also seems to have a role in the prevention of type 2 diabetes and other features of the metabolic syndrome; we must therefore acknowledge that vitamin D insufficiency is intimately associated with and precedes insulin resistance. It is very likely that vitamin D is the elusive maternal factor.

It is important to remember that during gestation the developing foetus receives a great deal of vitamin D from its mother, whose vitamin D requirements increase four-fold during pregnancy. It is thus an advantage to be pregnant during the summer months, giving birth during the late autumn or early winter. The baby born in the spring is at a disadvantage and breast milk contains virtually no vitamin D. Evolution expects that a baby's vitamin D reserves obtained from its mother before birth will last for several weeks, until it is old enough to lie in the sun and synthesise its own vitamin D. It is an advantage for the baby to be born in the early winter so that it will be 6 months old in the early summer, when it can lie outdoors, ideally in light shade.

Earlier cultures and traditions seem to have realised this. Easter is a festival that we associate with Christianity but it is much older and the name is derived from Eostre, the pagan goddess of fertility (the word oestrogen has the same origin). The implication is that the early spring is the optimal time for conception, with pregnancy during the summer months. The Maypole is another expression of spring fertility rites.

The metabolic relationship between vitamin D and insulin resistance needs to be clarified. We know that the insulin-producing beta cells of the islets of Langerhans in the pancreas have vitamin D receptors, and that vitamin D in its metabolically most active form of calcitriol appears to be a co-factor in the release of insulin. It must be remembered that insulin resistance on its own need not lead to an elevated blood glucose concentration, that is diabetes. The response of the body to insulin resistance, which would lead to a tendency to elevated blood glucose, would be to increase insulin production by the beta cells of the islets of Langerhans. It is only when this fails that diabetes develops. In other words, in both type 1 and type 2 diabetes there is an effective failure of appropriate insulin production [18]. Vitamin D is necessary for both insulin production and normal insulin activity; it is thus an important factor in protection against diabetes.

The maternal factor as the trans-placental passage of vitamin D would also explain the observation that we noted in Chapter 7, that season of birth predicts the development of childhood diabetes [19]. This shown in Figure 58.7.

**Figure 58.7  Month of birth and risk of childhood diabetes [19].**

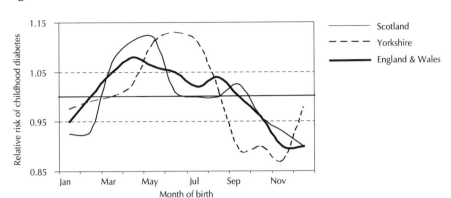

*Adapted with permission from the British Medical Journal Publishing Group.*

We can see that the risk of diabetes is highest with births in spring and early summer, the gestation having been during the winter with minimal transfer of vitamin D from the mother. The inclusion of data from Scotland and Yorkshire reflects the places of work of the various authors of the study [19]. The pattern is the same for these locations, without any significant differences. The relative risk in this study was calculated from observed incidence divided by the expected incidence (the annual average), greater than one indicating increased risk and less than one indicating reduced risk.

In early 2005, another study appeared that demonstrated the importance of the maternal factor, the link between the season of pregnancy and adult health. The age of normal menopause is later when a woman is born in the winter rather than in the summer, as shown in Figure 58.8 [20].

**Figure 58.8 Month of birth and age of menopause [20].**

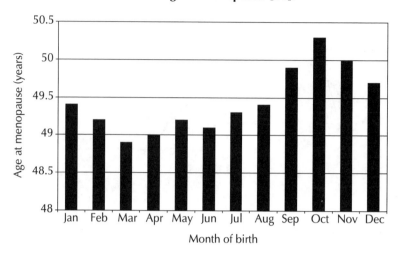

Although menstruation after completion of a family can be regarded as a nuisance, there are significant health advantages to the pre-menopausal woman and a later menopause is generally regarded as a good thing. Once again we see the advantage of pregnancy during the summer, probably mediated by improved vitamin D transfer from mother to foetus.

# 59
# HEPATITIS C VIRUS, DIABETES AND THE METABOLIC SYNDROME

We have seen that the metabolic syndrome is systemic. It affects multiple organs and systems within the body, including fat cells, coronary arteries, kidneys, cholesterol metabolism and insulin metabolism. Another organ can be added to the list, and it might turn out to be fundamental: the liver.

Blood returning from the intestine must pass through the liver on its way to the general circulation. Whilst the blood flows through the complex and specialised channels within the lobules of the liver, basic nutrients are removed by the liver cells (hepatocytes) and converted into complex chemical compounds for storage or use elsewhere in the body. For example, sugars are converted into the storage polymer glycogen, and amino acids are converted into proteins, including blood-clotting agents.

Poisons taken in by mouth, such as alcohol, are removed from the blood by the liver. Over a period of years a large amount of alcohol can damage the liver. An early feature of this is a build-up of fat within the liver, called in lay terms a fatty liver and in technical terms steatohepatitis. Cirrhosis is a later feature in which the structure of the liver is impaired and blood circulation through it is disrupted.

The current large number of blood tests performed 'routinely' on people who visit the doctor is probably apparent to everyone. Such tests, which may be undertaken on the fit and healthy, usually include a biochemical screen, part of which is a liver profile. A detailed description of this is not necessary at this stage; suffice it to say that minor unexpected abnormalities may be detected. If associated with a high alcohol intake, the corrective action is clear, but in the absence of alcohol excess referral to a liver specialist is the likely action. Although a number of disorders of the liver might be responsible for the biochemical abnormalities, a fatty liver is quite common. When not induced by alcohol excess, it is now termed non-alcoholic steatohepatitis (NASH), and the diagnosis is established with certainty by liver biopsy, a procedure not without danger. The presence of inflammatory cells as well as fat excess has led to it being classified as an inflammatory disease, hence – hepatitis [1].

NASH is often or indeed usually associated with obesity. It has also become clear that it can be associated with type 2 diabetes and hypercholesterolaemia; in other words it is now accepted as being part of the metabolic syndrome. It is not surprising, therefore, that, in the absence of diabetes, patients with NASH are found to be resistant to insulin, with elevated blood glucose levels after an oral glucose load. It is recognised that in the metabolic syndrome and NASH, liver cells lose their responsiveness to insulin and therefore their ability to remove glucose from the blood is impaired. It is thought that this is mediated by tumour necrosis factor-alpha (TNF-$\alpha$) acting on the liver cells [1]; TNF-$\alpha$ seems to be a key player in many disease processes. Its relationships with vitamin D and insulin resistance are crucial but as yet far from clear.

The insulin resistance factor that we have seen in the development of type 2 diabetes appears to be the result of chronic low-grade inflammation, important mediators of this being TNF-$\alpha$ and CRP. Suppression of these can be expected to increase insulin sensitivity and thus minimise diabetes. We have seen that vitamin D provides this action, especially in the developing foetus, with long-term importance. We have seen that pravastatin, used to reduce serum cholesterol, also suppresses CRP and TNF-$\alpha$. Certain tablets used in the treatment of diabetes act by increasing sensitivity to insulin, and these include metformin and the glitazone group. They reduce CRP levels by about 30%, similar to the effect of pravastatin, and it is likely that they help diabetes, at least in part, by suppressing the inflammatory process that is part of its causation [2].

In some people with NASH, the condition progresses from being a curiosity of which the patient is unaware, to cirrhosis of the liver, a life-threatening condition. In a smaller proportion, it progresses to liver cell cancer. It is likely that the progress of the condition is determined by the level of inflammatory activity, and once again we see the importance of TNF-$\alpha$ in the metabolic syndrome. It is a difficult subject that is not yet fully understood, but the present level of understanding is described well by Professor Anna Mae Diehl and her colleagues from the Liver Center at Duke University, North Carolina, USA [1].

The relationships between metabolic syndrome, TNF-α and the liver have been studied a stage further in a recent review from Jerusalem [3]. In an earlier chapter we looked at viral hepatitis, identifying A and B viruses in particular, and both viruses can cause acute hepatitis. Hepatitis B virus (HBV) can also cause long-term chronic liver disease and liver cancer, which is perhaps the most common cancer in the world. HBV is usually transmitted by blood or blood products and, in many countries, from mother to baby during the process of birth, when the bloods might mix. In the late 1960s there were outbreaks of viral hepatitis in renal dialysis units in the UK, and since then blood use has been strictly controlled. Blood for donation is checked by testing potential donors for the presence of HBV and using blood from only those who test negative.

However, it has been noted that, despite these precautions, some patients recovering from open heart surgery, in which large amounts of blood are used, still develop hepatitis. This observation led to the identification of the hepatitis C virus, HCV [4]. Its only known method of transmission is through blood and blood products but some people can be found to be positive for HCV without a history of blood transfusion or intravenous drug use.

Millions of people world-wide are infected with HCV and about 1 in 5 of these will develop cirrhosis of the liver, which might be fatal. A smaller proportion will develop primary liver cell cancer (hepatoma or hepatocellular carcinoma), and this is an example of the close association between inflammation and cancer, which we will see shortly. It also indicates the potential of viruses to cause cancer. Interesting work undertaken recently has identified *Helicobacter* species DNA in the liver of patients with HCV-associated liver cancer, suggesting that a greater burden of infection or inflammation may be responsible in the perplexing transformation of inflammation into cancer [5].

It has also been recognised recently that there is an association between HCV infection and type 2 diabetes. People with type 2 diabetes are more likely than expected to be HCV positive [6], and people who are HCV positive are more likely to develop diabetes subsequently than would be expected [7].

About 20% of patients with cirrhosis of the liver have diabetes, and the proportion is even higher if they are HCV positive. It has been observed that, whether or not they have cirrhosis, people who are HCV positive are about four times more likely to have diabetes compared with the general population [8]. This is not the case, however, with people who are HBV positive, indicating that the association with HCV is highly specific to this particular virus and is not just the result of liver disease [3]. We therefore see not just an association between inflammation and cancer but also the likely causative role of a specific virus in diabetes as well as in cancer.

The development of diabetes in HCV-infected people appears to be mediated by TNF-α, and the chain of events leads through insulin resistance to the metabolic syndrome. Studies in the USA have demonstrated that black ethnicity increases susceptibility to this development [3].

The model appears to be:

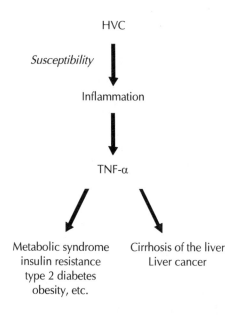

This conforms to the model that we have encountered earlier, with a micro-organism causing disease in susceptible people and TNF-α being involved in the process. The model shown here is based on the new findings that we have seen but research is far from complete. Black ethnicity increases susceptibility, and this could be the result of skin pigmentation and vitamin D insufficiency. We have seen that vitamin D is protective against type 2 diabetes and the metabolic syndrome; it might also be protective against the progression of NASH and HCV liver disease to cirrhosis and liver cell cancer. We can only speculate at present; the effect of vitamin D supplements in people with HCV infection is a research project that would be both simple and safe. It has yet to be undertaken.

# 60
# ATMOSPHERIC POLLUTION AND THE EMERGENCE OF CORONARY HEART DISEASE IN NEWLY INDUSTRIALISING COUNTRIES

In the recent past, coronary heart disease was unknown in countries such as India. We have seen that in South Asians it is a disease of migration to Europe, such that there is a greater susceptibility in the UK resulting in a mortality rate almost 50% higher than in the indigenous population. We have seen that the risk increases in subsequent generations, in the children born in the UK. I have explained this on the basis of vitamin D insufficiency, especially during gestation, increasing susceptibility to coronary heart disease by reducing immunity against a causative micro-organism, the identity of which remains uncertain.

Insufficiency of vitamin D comes about because of an interplay between genetic, behavioural and environmental factors. Inherited skin pigmentation reduces photo-synthesis of vitamin D; clothing and indoor living reduce the opportunities for exposure to the sun; the climate of north-western Europe, and particularly north-west Britain, provides much less sunlight energy at ground level than in South Asia.

Although Afro-Caribbeans experience a greater risk of the metabolic syndrome than the indigenous population of the UK, the risk to South Asians is even greater. This has been a puzzle but I suspect that the explanation is that Afro-Caribbeans are much more an outdoor people, in the UK and elsewhere, and in the UK they do not usually have the religious and cultural traditions of extensively covering their bodies with clothes. Although I have not seen this researched, I would anticipate that during pregnancy Afro-Caribbean women will pass on to their offspring more vitamin D than South Asian women do.

We have also seen that vitamin D deficiency expressed as osteomalacia is disturbingly common in South Asians living in the UK. This is sometimes precipitated by pregnancy [1], during which large amounts of vitamin D are passed across the placenta to the developing foetus. It can also appear as neonatal rickets in the South Asian ethnic groups [2], and this still occurs, perhaps the result of the veil or burkha being worn increasingly by Muslim women under the influence of current fundamentalist pressures. Osteomalacia resulting from vitamin D deficiency has been seen in India predominantly in the wealthy [3] but it has always been a feature of the poor in the UK, as reviewed in Chapter 15.

The World Health Report published in *The Lancet* in May 2001 was prepared by a team from the Global Programme on Evidence for Public Policy, part of WHO in Geneva, Switzerland [5]. The team assembled a ranked table of 191 countries based on healthy, or disability-free, life expectancy (DALE). Details of the data can be found in the very interesting original paper; some of the results are shown here in Table 60.1.

High neonatal death rates have a very important effect on the average age of survival from birth, and are likely to occur in hot countries with primitive industrial development. We saw in the early chapters of this book that water and sewage engineering had a profoundly beneficial effect on the health of the population of the UK. The same advances have occurred in other European countries and North America but they have not yet happened in many countries of the world. In the UK, Europe, USA, Japan and Australia, we owe our excellent health and life expectancy at the present time to a number of factors, perhaps the most important being peace and good government.

Not only do we have an ample supply of clean water, but there is an adequate, if not more than adequate, supply of food based on the efficiencies gained through the mechanisation of agriculture. In addition, we have advanced rail, road and air transport systems that enable food to be distributed with minimal delay and under hygienic conditions.

**Table 60.1 Disability-free life expectancy from birth in 1999 [5]**

|  | Rank | Years |
|---|---|---|
| Japan | 1 | 74.5 |
| Australia | 2 | 73.2 |
| France | 3 | 73.1 |
| Sweden | 4 | 73.0 |
| Spain | 5 | 72.8 |
| Italy | 6 | 72.7 |
| Greece | 7 | 72.5 |
| Switzerland | 8 | 72.5 |
| the Netherlands | 13 | 72.0 |
| UK | 14 | 71.7 |
| Finland | 20 | 70.5 |
| USA | 24 | 70.0 |
| Ireland | 27 | 69.6 |
| Denmark | 28 | 69.4 |
| Poland | 45 | 66.2 |
| Hungary | 62 | 64.1 |
| China | 81 | 62.3 |
| Russia | 91 | 61.3 |
| Albania | 102 | 60.0 |
| Bahamas | 109 | 59.1 |
| Pakistan | 124 | 55.9 |
| India | 134 | 53.2 |
| Bangladesh | 140 | 49.9 |
| South Africa | 160 | 39.8 |
| Sierra Leone | 191 | 25.9 |

© 2000, adapted from The Lancet with permission from Elsevier.

Clean water and adequate food were the main factors bringing about the health improvements in Europe during the 20th century. But Europe is a cold place in the winter: a supply of fuel for heating is essential, and also for cooking food and boiling water to minimise intestinal infections. Coal became the main energy source in the late 18th and early 19th centuries, initially being consumed at the place of need, in the home or at the workplace. This source of energy was essential for industrial development and the health of the public. Unfortunately the price to be paid was atmospheric pollution, and I have already indicated that this has been a major factor in the development of vitamin D insufficiency.

The second phase of the industrial revolution occurred in the latter half of the 20th century. It involved the centralisation of energy production in a network of major power stations, generating electricity mainly from coal, oil and gas and also water power (more correctly from gravity). Electricity is distributed to domestic and industrial users through a sophisticated power grid and a network of overhead and underground cables. The major effects are to improve the efficiency of coal combustion and reduce atmospheric pollution very substantially. There is the issue of invisible carbon dioxide emission but, although this might contribute to global warming, it is not a pollutant that interferes directly with the health of individuals.

Clean air following clean water and adequate food has made an enormous difference to the health of the population of well-industrialised countries. As it enables an increase in the incidental exposure of the population to the sun, I suggest that it has been the major factor in the decline of coronary heart disease. We can see from Figure 60.1 that the longest healthy life expectancy is in Japan. It might be asked why this is: the answer surely lies in peace, advanced industrialisation, clean air, clean water, obsessional cleanliness, abundant sea-food and a location of the main population centres much closer to the equator than those of Europe and North America. In addition there are no religious directives or cultural traditions to remain indoors.

It would not have been possible for the second industrial revolution to have occurred simultaneously with the first. The initial phase of industrial production allowed the technological development and manufacturing facilities necessary to develop wide-spread energy distribution. We now find the same two processes occurring in the newly industrialising regions of the world, mainly in Asia, especially China, and, to a lesser extent, India.

Many African countries do not know peace, have bad governments, little industrialisation and the additional burden of an epidemic of AIDS. But in Asian countries we see a worrying emergence of so-called western diseases, diabetes and coronary heart disease causing most concern, at the same time as industrial development. Even in urban Africa, coronary heart disease is appearing.

Countries industrialising at the present time do not produce comprehensive mortality and disease statistics, although they are being developed. It was just the same in the UK, and we have seen that such data collection was enabled by the process of industrialisation. In keeping with its virtual absence in the UK before about 1920, coronary heart disease was seen only rarely in Asian countries until the last years of the 20th century. It is now becoming common but data collection is not yet adequately sophisticated to allow accurate geographical presentation. We have seen some dramatic headlines: 'Global epidemic of cardiovascular disease predicted' (*New Scientist*); 'Global epidemic of cardiovascular disease predicted' (*The Lancet*); 'Cardiovascular disease in developing countries. An epidemic that can be prevented' (*British Medical Journal*).

It has been observed by those working with coronary heart disease in India that it is the higher social classes who are most at risk; this appears to the case currently with diabetes and historically with rickets. High-quality population surveys are not yet available or possible and so we must accept with certain reservations the opinions of those on the ground. Examples are Drs Singh, Verma and Niaz from the heart research centre in Moradabad [6] (Dr Verma was by chance a training grade doctor working with me in Blackburn in the late 1970s; Dr Singh's data on dietary treatment were eaten by termites, described in Chapter 21).

Observers inevitably look at lifestyle as the explanation: a sedentary lifestyle, more food, more dietary fat and less fruit and vegetables. Singh and colleagues noted no difference in fruit and vegetable intake between social classes but more fat eaten by the higher social classes, as shown in Figure 60.1.

**Figure 60.1 Dietary characteristics in India by social class [6].**

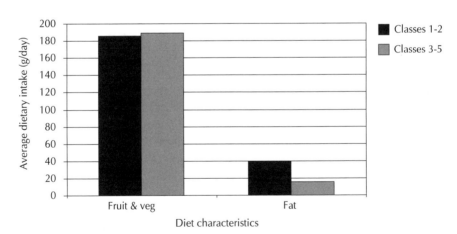

© 1999, adapted from The Lancet with permission from Elsevier.

We have seen from experience in Europe and the French paradox that a high-fat diet does not appear to equate to a high coronary risk, and explanations for an epidemic of coronary heart disease must be found elsewhere.

Industrialisation appears to be a feature that is associated with emergence of coronary heart disease, but the second phase of industrialisation, leading to an even greater food supply, is associated with its decline. I propose that the atmospheric pollution inevitably associated with early industrialisation is the important factor, but an enabling or susceptibility factor. I have suggested that coronary heart disease is caused by a micro-organism and that immunosuppression resulting from vitamin D insufficiency allows it to emerge. It is therefore necessary that the causative micro-organism is present in the population at risk; widespread air transport will make this inevitable.

There is evidence linking atmospheric pollution with coronary heart disease. There are three basic forms of air pollutant: suspended particulates, sulphur dioxide and nitrogen oxides. I will ignore carbon dioxide, of environmental rather than personal health concern, and carbon monoxide, high levels of which can kill individuals but only by local poisoning and not via geographical atmospheric pollution. Sulphur dioxide ($SO_2$) and the oxides of nitrogen (nitrous oxide $N_2O$, nitric oxide NO and nitrogen dioxide $NO_2$) are invisible but are irritants to the eyes and lungs. Suspended particulates create a fog and impair sunlight penetration to ground level. In practice the various pollutants are present simultaneously.

The process of industrialisation in eastern Europe has been slower than in the west, mainly because of failures to move from the dirty first phase into the cleaner second phase. The Czech Republic has a long industrial history and, because of the failure to change, it had in 1987 the second highest annual emission of sulphur dioxide in Europe [7]. A study was undertaken to assess a possible relationship between atmospheric pollution and neonatal mortality from respiratory disease, by looking at both factors in 46 of the 85 districts of the Czech Republic for which data were available [7]. The districts were arranged in quintiles (five groups), according to levels of atmospheric pollution. The three major pollutants were measured individually, particulates (TC-10), nitrogen oxides ($NO_x$) and sulphur dioxide ($SO_2$). The results are shown in Figure 60.2.

**Figure 60.2  Neonatal mortality and atmospheric pollution [7].**

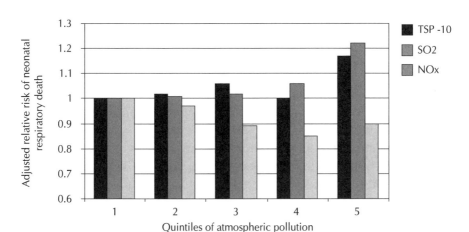

Neonatal mortality from respiratory disease increased with increasing amounts of sulphur dioxide and particles in the atmosphere, but oxides of nitrogen did not seem to have a detrimental effect. High levels of sulphur dioxide and particulate pollution were associated with a high level of neonatal death.

The mechanism of this is not clear. Perhaps sulphur dioxide has a direct toxic effect on the lungs of the neonate. Perhaps particulate pollution, which reduces sunlight penetration, has an adverse effect by reducing vitamin D synthesis by the mother and thereby vitamin D insufficiency in the neonate, leading to susceptibility to respiratory infection. However, these data from a former Eastern Bloc country do provide some insights into why it and neighbouring countries have higher than expected mortality rates.

A study from the USA, published in 1993, looked at mortality rates and atmospheric pollution in the following cities: Watertown (Massachusetts), Harriman (Tennessee), St Louis (Missouri), Steubenville (Ohio), Portage (Wisconsin) and Topeka (Kansas) [8]. There was an association between mortality and atmospheric pollution, most strongly with fine particulate pollution.

Long-term studies such as these seem to be relevant for a chronic condition such as coronary heart disease. A study from the active group at St George's Hospital Medical School in south London, UK, looked at daily atmospheric pollution and found that, as it increased, so did admissions to hospital on the following day presenting with acute myocardial infarction.

There was also an association between black smoke (particulates) and angina [9].

A multicentre study involving centres in Germany, Italy and Greece looked at short-term effects of sulphur dioxide and particulate pollution on mortality in 12 European cities [10]. It was found that an increase in atmospheric pollution was associated with an increase in daily mortality. The effects of both sulphur dioxide and black smoke (particulates) were greater in the summer than in the winter, suggesting that interference with sunlight was important.

The intervening mechanism involves an increase in inflammatory processes, as suggested by the observation from the University of Ulm, Germany, that plasma viscosity increases during times of increased air pollution. High viscosity is caused by increased amounts of circulating inflammatory proteins, for example CRP [11].

Further evidence for particulate air pollution being especially important in increasing susceptibility to fatal illness came from a study of 20 USA cities conducted by a team at the Johns Hopkins University, Baltimore [12]. Only particulate pollutants were significantly associated with mortality, indicating the importance of impeding the penetration of sunlight to ground level.

A further USA study, from Harvard, studied the relationship between air pollution and 772 episodes of myocardial infarction [13]. The conclusion was:

*The risk of MI [myocardial infarction] increased in association with elevated concentrations of fine particles in the previous 2-hour period. In addition, a delayed response associated with 24-hour average exposure 1 day before the onset of symptoms was observed.*

The decline of respiratory deaths following European smoke control legislation is well accepted, but the decline of deaths from coronary heart disease is generally considered to be a coincidence and not a consequence. It is very likely that smoke control legislation in the UK (the Clean Air Act 1956) led to a reduction of deaths from coronary heart disease, but such a possibility is unlikely to be considered seriously as long as it is felt that coronary heart disease is dietary in origin.

A group from Dublin, Ireland, investigated the effect of the smoke control legislation that was introduced in Ireland on 1 September 1990 [14]. Compared with the 6 years before the ban on the sale of coal, the following 6 years saw a 70% reduction in black smoke concentrations in Dublin. There was a corresponding reduction in all deaths (trauma excluded) by 5.7%. There was a reduction of age-related deaths from respiratory disease by 15.5% and from cardiovascular disease by 10.3%.

The reduction of respiratory and cardiovascular deaths occurred immediately after the ban on coal sales. It might be expected that there would be fewer respiratory deaths, as we are all aware of the detrimental effect of atmospheric pollution on our lungs, mediated by the toxic chemical effect of sulphur dioxide. The reduction of deaths from coronary heart disease, occurring in all seasons of the year in Dublin, cannot be explained on the basis of the traditional understanding, which is in reality, as we have seen, a misunderstanding. However, it fits into the models that we have defined, with coronary heart disease being a consequence of respiratory infection. Of more importance, susceptibility to both respiratory disease and coronary heart disease will be reduced by less atmospheric smoke, allowing better sunlight penetration and enhanced vitamin D synthesis.

The European and North American experience is that the first phase of industrialisation created reductions in infant mortality, but the appearance of atmospheric pollution and the emergence of coronary heart disease. The second phase saw clean air, more food, the decline of coronary heart disease and a much improved life expectancy. The newly industrialising countries, mainly in Asia, are experiencing improved infant mortality rates with a rapidly increasing population as a result, but also the appearance of atmospheric pollution and the emergence of coronary heart disease.

My holiday visits to Asia have been interesting and informative. Delhi is a bustling over-populated city but one thing struck me more than anything else. The sky was pale blue and the sun a pale object that I was able to look at in a way that I remember from my childhood in Manchester and Salford, before the smoke control legislation of 1956. Although industry is a major pollutant, domestic smoke production is of greater importance. Electricity distribution in Delhi is not as advanced as in western Europe and North America, and most cooking is performed over inefficient paraffin stoves with incomplete combustion.

Xian is the home of the terracotta warriors and is also one of the major industrial cities of China. It is surrounded by beautiful high mountains, but they have been visible from the city only very occasionally in recent years. The atmospheric pollution is much greater in Xian than in Delhi and in Manchester in the 1950s. The sky is a pale grey colour and, the sun is a vague pale object; visibility in the city centre is about 500 metres.

'Toxic smog shrouds Beijing', stated a headline in *The Guardian* on 11 October 2004 [15]. The article continued:

*According to the World Bank, 16 of the planet's 20 most polluted cities are in China ... For weeks on end this summer, yellowish-white clouds blocked the sun ... This is a common story in China's cities, where factories and homes rely on low-grade coal for about 80% of their energy needs and environmental protection has long taken second place to economic growth ... The health costs however are becoming apparent. Respiratory diseases are the leading cause of death in China.*

The atmospheric pollution appears to be in the usual major forms, sulphur dioxide being the acidic irritant, nitrogen oxides giving the yellow colour and particulates restricting sunlight penetration to ground level.

We can see that a large population in Asia is inevitably facing the same consequences of industrialisation as the population of western Europe in the 19th century. Not only is the sun obscured but the workers are moving from outdoor farm work in clean air to indoor factories, no doubt with long hours of work, few days off and little opportunity for holidays in a cleaner environment. Things are worse in Asia for two reasons. Western Europe, especially the UK and the other major industrial areas, have a strong south-westerly prevailing wind that brings a high rainfall off the Atlantic Ocean. The advantage of such intermittent cleaning of the atmosphere of pollution is not enjoyed in China, the industrial parts of which have still air and little rain. The second factor is that Asian people have pigmented skins that lead to less synthesis of vitamin D than the pale skins of the northern Europeans.

It is not only Asian countries that are experiencing atmospheric pollution as a consequence of economic development. We have seen the Albanian paradox, that people experiencing social deprivation do not necessarily have a high incidence of coronary heart disease. In the example of the Albanian population, the relative protection they receive is probably related to the high exposure to sunshine, but things are likely to change. Tiriana, the capital of Albania, can now be regarded as 'Europe's pollution capital' [16]:

*When Albania's communist dictatorship collapsed in the late 1980s there were only 2000 cars in the country ... In the past 15 years the city has paid the price of freedom. Choked with some 300,000 cars, lorries and buses which burn fuel banned in the EU, Tirana is now seen as the most polluted capital in Europe ... On an average morning, the volume of PM10s (particulate matter) is more than 10 times the World Health Organization limit.*

It has been calculated that, in the year 2000 in Tiriana, 35 000 tonnes of pollutants were emitted by traffic into the atmosphere, and this will undoubtedly reduce the exposure of the population to sunshine. The incidence of respiratory disease is already increasing. It is likely that the incidence of coronary heart disease will increase in the very near future.

The process of industrialisation will increase the amount of food available, as happened in western Europe and North America. However, I do not believe that this is the cause of the emergence of coronary heart disease in newly industrialising countries. I believe that the key factor is atmospheric pollution and the movement of people from outdoor to indoor work. If this is accepted, then there is a significant public health opportunity to correct vitamin D insufficiency and help maintain health. If public health initiatives are directed to dietary controls, then the efforts will be wasted.

It is likely that early industrialisation will inevitably result in atmospheric pollution and that this phase cannot be by-passed. However, the move to distributed natural gas and electricity is likely to occur much earlier than was the experience in Europe and North America.

# 61

# THE CLIMATE OF THE BRITISH ISLES

The health of the population of the UK is not good compared with that of most other countries in western Europe, despite the fact that the UK has the fourth largest economy in the world and one of the lowest infant mortality rates. According to WHO criteria, the health service of the UK is only the 18th best, as judged by criteria that are by no means universally applauded [1]. According to these criteria, France has the best health service, despite the fact that it is hugely overspent. That of the USA comes in at number 28, despite the fact that the USA has the world's largest economy.

We have already seen the distribution of disease within the UK. In the south east of England, the health of the population is comparable with that of northern France, whereas the health of the population in the north-west of England, Northern Ireland and Scotland is significantly worse. We have already looked at victim blaming and found, from data obtained mainly from the MONICA project [2] (see Chapter 35), that this high mortality rate cannot be explained by behavioural aspects such as cigarette smoking, diet, etc. I suggest that insufficient exposure of the population to the sun is responsible for the poor health profile. If there is something special about health in the north-western parts of the UK, and if sunshine deficiency might be an important factor, then we must try and explain this and look at the climate of the UK and how it might disadvantage the population.

It has long been recognised that the climate of the British Isles is unpleasant, especially that of Ireland, Scotland and the north-west of

England. A posting to Hadrian's Wall was thought to have been unpopular among the occupying Roman troops, and we must remember that the Roman name for Ireland was Hibernia, which means winter.

The British Isles lie well north of the equator, between 50 and 54 degrees latitude. The Shetland Islands are at the same latitude as Hudson Bay, Alaska and Siberia. The north-west of England, Northern Ireland and Scotland lie further north of the equator than any part of China. The similar latitude in the southern hemisphere skirts Antarctica and passes through Graham Land. It is well to the south of New Zealand and Australia or any other habitable part of the southern hemisphere; these features can be seen on the world map (Figure 61.1).

**Figure 61.1 Map of the world.**

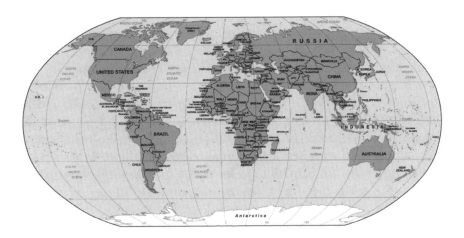

There are three major influences that determine the weather of western Europe and the British Isles in particular. The northerly location brings cold air from the Arctic, and this is noticeable even at modest heights. The Cairngorm plateau in Scotland has an altitude of about 1400 metres above sea level, modest by the standards of most countries, but it can be one of the coldest and most dangerous places in Europe. In the English Lake District in the spring, the weather can be pleasant in the valleys, close to sea level, but Arctic on the mountain-tops. at only 1000 metres.

The only thing that enables life and agriculture to flourish in the British Isles and Scandinavia is the Gulf Stream, and its extension the North Atlantic Drift, which carry warm water from the mid-Atlantic Ocean. The source of this warm water is a combination of the warming effects of the tropical sun and geothermal energy in the form of superheated water emerging from deep ocean vents. The intense energy created by the warm water building up in the central Atlantic Ocean and Caribbean Sea gives rise to the hurricanes and storms that cause devastation in Florida and the eastern seaboard of the USA. The same warm water feeds the Gulf Stream that crosses the Atlantic to the coast of north-west Europe.

There is an interaction between the cold Arctic air, which inevitably covers north-west Europe, and the warm air carried just above the warm water of the Gulf Stream. The warm air supports farming and life in Scotland and Scandinavia but only in coastal regions, and fishing continues all the year round. Because the warm air is present only close to sea level, human habitation in the winter in Scotland is generally not possible at more than about 50 metres above sea level.

Warm water creates evaporation and the air above the water is therefore very moist. When the Gulf Stream arrives in the North Atlantic, the warm moist air rises to meet the cold air from the Arctic. Rising air is already at relatively low pressure, with a tendency for the water to precipitate out as cloud and rain. The further the air rises, the lower become both the pressure and temperature, and therefore the greater the precipitation. The reason for the poor levels of sunshine in the north-western parts of the British Isles is the presence of cloud cover for much of the time, and this in turn is because of the unique location with Arctic air and warm sea. The mixing of the Gulf Stream and the Arctic air is similar to boiling a kettle in a cold kitchen in the winter: a great deal of condensation results.

The British Isles are to mainland Europe a group of off-shore islands that force the warm moist air up to an altitude that causes precipitation, taking a great deal of the water out of the air. But there is a third climatic factor at play, leading to continental Europe having a drier and sunnier climate than that of the British Isles. High-pressure areas (anticyclones) are caused by hot dry air descending on the land, and this is a characteristic of the climate of much of central Europe during the summer. The weather is settled and windless, the sky cloudless. High pressure blocks the penetration of the low-pressure weather systems (depressions) that follow the Gulf Stream to the coast of north-western Europe. We thus see, as shown in the weather chart of Figure 61.2 recorded in early October 2004, a familiar pattern associated with a particularly severe hurricane season in the USA and Caribbean islands.

**Figure 61.2  Weather chart of the British Isles, Europe and the North Atlantic, 4 October 2004 [3].**

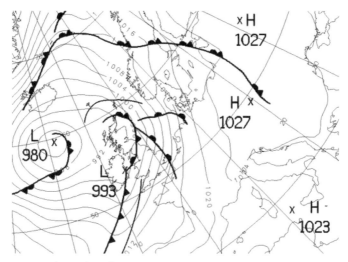

*Crown © 2004, adapted with permission.*

We can see the depressions (L) that are generated over the warm waters of the Gulf Stream and exert their major influence over the western British Isles. The anticyclones (H) to the east ensure that the depressions cannot penetrate into central Europe. After they have dropped most of their rain over the UK, they continue north to Scandinavia. The wet cloudy weather associated with the depressions exert an influence for just a short distance into continental Europe. This pattern explains why cloud cover is much greater over Ireland, western Scotland, Wales and the north-west of England, leading to much less sunlight penetration.

We can see the same pattern in the weather chart for 7 January 2005 (Figure 61.3). The depression from the Atlantic drifting across the north-west of the British Isles created gales of 100 m.p.h., but with relatively warm air at 11°C. There was heavy rainfall leading to floods in Cumbria; a ferry from Northern Ireland was blown ashore in south-west Scotland; 20 000 people had to be evacuated from their homes in Carlisle because of floods; 70 000 people of that city had their electricity supply interrupted for several days because power lines were blown down. At the same time the weather was mixed but windy in south-east England. Web-cams from the alpine ski resorts showed clear blue skies with no wind and the alpine air was dry and cool (about –4°C) with little or no influence of the Gulf Stream.

**Figure 61.3 Weather chart of the British Isles, Europe and the North Atlantic, 7 January 2005 [3].**

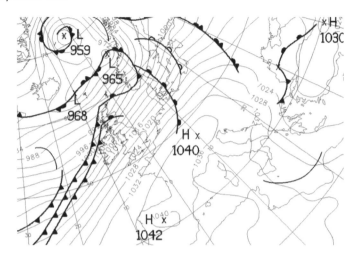

*Crown © 2004, adapted with permission.*

The main origin of the dry high-pressure air over Europe is the Tibetan plateau, a huge mass of rock at more than 4 km above sea level. Its effects on the climate of the northern hemisphere (the Raymo Uplift hypothesis) has been described well in the *New Scientist* by freelance journalist David Patterson [4], reviewing the work of Maureen Raymo (Research Professor, Department of Earth Sciences, University of Boston, USA), William Ruddiman (Professor, Environmental Sciences Department, University of Virginia, USA) and Philip Froelich (Professor of Oceanography, Florida State University, USA) [5]. Under virtually constant sun exposure with little protection from the atmosphere and none from cloud, the Tibetan plateau becomes extremely hot, as is the air that rises from it. As this process intensifies in the summer, the rising mass of hot air sucks in moist air from the warm Indian Ocean and creates the summer monsoon in India, south of the Himalayas. The hot air rising off the Tibetan plateau is then influenced by the rotation of the earth, descending to the west of Tibet. The hot dry air thus creates high pressure and a semi-desert across central Asia, extending towards Europe. This air brings the settled warm summer weather with clear skies for most of the time over continental Europe, and occasionally over the British Isles.

We saw in Figures 26.1 and 26.2 the sunshine data from Myerscough in central Lancashire, UK, located midway between Blackburn and Preston. It shows the paucity of sunshine in north-western England. Even in June

2002 (an average June) there were only 9 days with more than 6 hours of sunshine; on 8 days there were fewer than 2 hours of sunshine. This is a month in which the sun rises at about 5.00 am and sets at about 9.00 pm, that is 16 hours of daylight per day. We saw that in December 2002 there were only 8 days with more than 2 hours of sunshine, out of 8 hours when the sun is above the horizon.

These sunshine records indicate an unusual amount of cloud cover. In the UK we generally accept that our climate is the norm but in reality the climate is extremely unusual for populated areas; the vast majority of the world populations experiences much less cloud and much more sunshine. There are some general rules that arise generated from observation. It is well known from around the world that where the sea is cold, there is a desert on land. This is seen in the south-western and western parts of Australia, the western parts of south Africa and the coast of Chile. On the other hand, where the sea is warm, there is a great deal of evaporation and there tends to be a great deal of rain. It is the warm air rising from warm water through a background of colder air that produces low atmospheric pressure, cloud formation and rainfall. We can see this in tropical areas with rainforest, such as Malaysia and Indonesia. However, in the tropics the elevation of the sun ensures adequate sunlight penetration through the cloud. The UK is unusual for a location so far from the equator in having a supply of warm tropical water in the form of the Gulf Stream.

The unstable climate of the UK is responsible for the poor exposure of its population to the sun, a high susceptibility to a number of diseases, and consequently a higher burden of illness and higher mortality compared with other European countries. The UK is at the meeting point of warm moist air generated by the Gulf Stream and cold Arctic air found at such a northern location at about 50 degrees north of the equator. The continental mainland of Europe is protected by hot dry air generated in Tibet, which blocks the Atlantic low-pressure systems and ensures many more days with clear skies and plenty of sunshine.

# 62
# MODEL OF DISEASE AND ENVIRONMENT

M y concern is with susceptibility to disease and how this relates to its cause. I am particularly concerned with a population group that is at an unusual risk of ill-health and living in north-western Europe. Within this location, I am particularly concerned with the socio-economically disadvantaged and immigrants from South Asia, Africa and the Caribbean. We have seen that victim-blaming, diet and the traditional views of faulty lifestyle do not provide a coherent explanation. The evidence indicates that the answers are to be found in the interactions between genetically determined skin pigmentation, cultural traditions of skin cover, climatic factors of sunlight exposure and ever-present micro-organisms awaiting the opportunity to inflict disease.

It is an advantage and an indicator of understanding that these interactions can be represented in a diagrammatic format. We must start with the disease, and as an example I will use coronary heart disease. It became the major disease of western Europe and North America during the 20th century and the epidemic seems to be developing in Asia in the 21st century. We have seen the likelihood that it is caused by a micro-organism, initiating an inflammatory process that leads to the disease (see Chapter 44 and Figure 62.1).

**Figure 62.1  Role of micro-organisms.**

(Micro-organism) ⟶ Coronary heart disease

*Inflammation*

We have also seen that the inflammatory process is under the influence of  by vitamin D, which inhibits the development of the disease (Figure 62.2).

**Figure 62.2  The inflammatory process.**

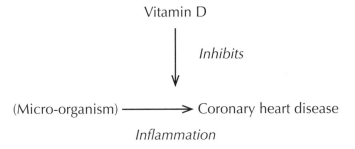

Vitamin D synthesis from 7-dehydrocholesterol depends on energy from the ultraviolet component of sunlight, and this is increased in areas close to the equator, at a high altitude and with air free of particulate pollution (Figure 62.3). In addition to these climatic factors, which are outside the control of individuals, sun exposure is reduced by clothing, indoor living and long hours of indoor work. The biological effectiveness of sunlight is reduced by skin pigmentation.

**Figure 62.3 Vitamin D synthesis.**

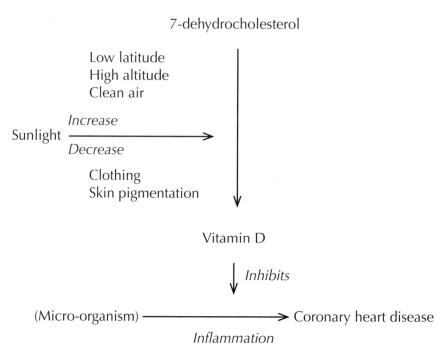

We have seen that the concentration of cholesterol in the blood stream, also derived from 7-dehydrocholesterol, increases in the absence of sunshine, particularly in the winter and in countries away from the equator. Although the relationship between cholesterol and coronary heart disease is not as strong as conventional wisdom maintains, the experience of familial hypercholesterolaemia at the present time lends support to the assertion that cholesterol can be an accelerating factor.

Coronary heart disease is closely associated with respiratory infection and chronic lung disease. The respiratory tract is likely to be the source of the causative infection, and perhaps the way by which cigarette smoking accelerates coronary heart disease and leads to earlier death.

We have seen that statin medication has an effect on cholesterol synthesis but the effect on coronary heart disease is independent of this. Through unknown mechanisms it modulates the inflammatory process in a way that is beneficial. Aspirin is an anti-inflammatory drug that has a beneficial effect, but this is thought to be mediated by a reduction in platelet stickiness and thus a reduction in blood clotting (Figure 62.4).

**Figure 62.4 A summary of processes.**

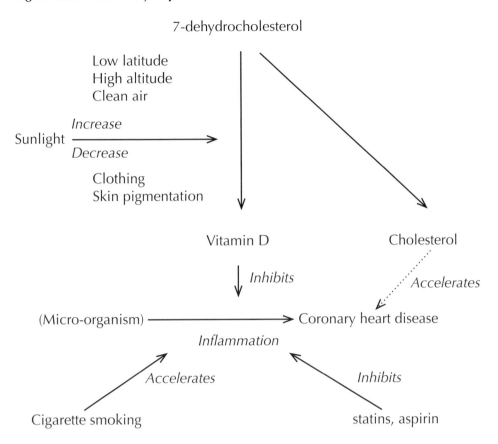

Figure 62.4 summarises the processes described in this book. It is a model that shows the interactions between the environment and human population. It is important to look at illness in this way, looking at the big picture and not just a small component, important though that component may be.

The model uses coronary heart disease. We have already seen that we can also apply it to other manifestations of atherosclerotic disease, stroke and peripheral vascular disease. We can tentatively apply it to the metabolic syndrome and certain aspects of diabetes. There are other conditions that might also interact with the environment but in which understanding is not so well developed. We can make the model less specific (Figure 62.5).

**Figure 62.5  A simplified model.**

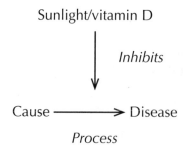

We will now look at other applications of this model. Many will show the cause to be elusive although possibly microbial, but the process, the pathology, will usually involve inflammation.

# PART 11

# PROTECTION BY THE SUN AGAINST CANCERS AND OTHER DISEASES

# 63
# PROTECTION AGAINST CANCER BY VITAMIN D AND SUNLIGHT

C ancer at the present time in Europe and North America is clearly regarded as a major public health problem, with cancers in various forms being responsible for about a quarter of all deaths. As deaths from stroke and coronary heart disease have declined in recent years, cancer deaths inevitably take their place. The ultimate public health objective is for everyone to die from old age, a reasonable ambition, but specific diseases remain common. Warfare, accidents and natural disasters are never far away.

Although the causes of cancer are generally unknown, susceptibility does vary and there are some geographical variations. A little-known study carried out in 1941 in the USA and Canada found an interesting geographical pattern [1]. The cancer death rate among residents of cities located at latitudes between 30° and 50° north was about twice that of cities further south at between 10° and 30°. In the most northern cities, at latitudes between 50° and 60°, the cancer death rate was two and a half times that of the most southern cities. The data are shown in Figure 63.1.

Figure 63.1 Relative risk of cancer deaths in North America [1].

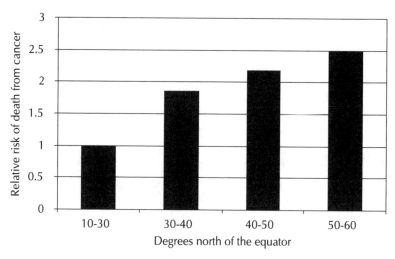

The author of this study was Frank Apperly, a pathologist from the Medical College of Virginia, USA, who was stimulated by work in the 1930s that indicated an inverse relationship between skin cancer and total cancer rates [2]. Apperly demonstrated a clear geographical pattern of cancer deaths and he was also the first to suggest that sunshine might be protective against cancer through stimulation of immunity. He proposed that sunlight would aid what is generally known as immunosurveillance, the process by which the body protects itself against foreign proteins and abnormal cells, including the destruction and removal of cancer cells. Apperly's ideas were very accurate, as demonstrated by more recent research.

William B. Grant is an independent researcher who has looked at geographical variations in cancer mortality at many locations in the USA, and in particular detail at the ultraviolet (UVB) light exposure of these locations [3]. He obtained the cancer data from the Atlas of Cancer Mortality, which can be viewed on-line from the National Institutes of Health, Bethesda, Maryland, USA [4]. He obtained the ultraviolet light data (also available on-line) from a satellite instrument called the Total Ozone Mapping Spectrometer (TOMS) [5]. He also accessed data from ground-based ultraviolet light detection stations [6].

Grant studied the data applying to men and women, white and black, and found that the following cancers are associated with low exposure to ultraviolet light: bladder, breast, colon, kidney, non-Hodgkin's lymphoma, oesophagus, ovary, prostate, rectum, stomach and uterus. Scattergraphs (which I have not reproduced here) showed significant negative correlations, indicating that the greater the UVB exposure, the lower the incidence of cancers.

He also looked at death rates from skin cancer and found that there was no correlation with UVB exposure. There was thus no indication of protection by ultraviolet light but similarly there was no indication that ultraviolet light causes fatal skin cancer. More of this later.

The geography of cancer of the prostate in the USA has an increasing incidence with distance from the equator, suggesting a protective effect of sunshine [7]. The incidence of prostate cancer is associated particularly with what the authors of the report called the epidemiological index, which is based on latitude, altitude and average cloud cover, all determining the ultraviolet light reaching ground level. Ultraviolet exposure is much greater in western states than eastern states. The authors noted an increased incidence of prostate cancer in the counties of the eastern states, with a decreasing incidence to the west. This is the same as we have seen with coronary heart disease and it is probably the result of altitude of residence, a high altitude being protective because of the greater ultraviolet light exposure of the population. The study included a regression analysis of 3073 counties. The highest incidence of prostate cancer was in central Wyoming and the lowest incidence was in southern Texas.

The association between prostate cancer and insufficiency of ultraviolet light has been investigated in the UK by a group from the North Staffordshire Hospital and Keele University [8]. Exposure to ultraviolet light was assessed rather than measured in 210 patients with cancer of the prostate and in 155 controls. The results were demonstrated by subdividing the patients with prostate cancer into four groups according to the level of ultraviolet exposure, group1 having the lowest and group 4 the highest, as shown in Figure 63.2.

**Figure 63.2  Relationship between prostate cancer and ultraviolet light exposure [8].**

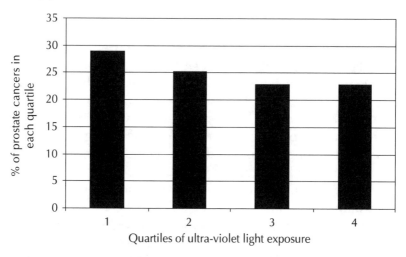

Quartiles of ultra-violet light exposure

*© 2001, adapted from* The Lancet *with permission from Elsevier.*

The greater the exposure to ultraviolet light, the smaller the risk of prostate cancer; 29% of the cancers occurred in the 25% with the lowest ultraviolet light exposure, and 22.9% of the cancers occurred in the 25% with the highest exposure. Ultraviolet light appears to provide protection against prostate cancer.

Throughout this book I have emphasised that sunlight insufficiency creates susceptibility to disease, rather than causing disease, other than osteomalacia and rickets, the direct results of vitamin D deficiency. High levels of sunshine exposure will give a relative protection against cancer rather than absolute protection. We have seen that coronary heart disease occurs earlier in susceptible people because of insufficient exposure to the sun, especially in South Asians.

In the study from Staffordshire, the authors also looked at the age of diagnosis of prostate cancer [8]. We can see in Figure 63.3 that the 25% with the lowest exposure to ultraviolet light (quartile 1) were particularly disadvantaged compared with the remaining 75%, with a relatively young age of onset of prostate cancer. Although the development of a potentially fatal disease is undesirable at any age, the age of onset is of great importance.

**Figure 63.3 Age at diagnosis of prostate cancer and ultraviolet exposure [8].**

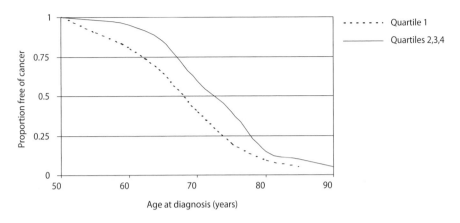

In this study, all of the patients with prostate cancer developed the disease after the age of 50 years, and so at that age all were disease-free. In the quartile with the lowest exposure to ultraviolet light, the cancer developed at a median age of 67.7 years, compared with 72.1 years in the other quartiles with greater exposure. Clearly there was a relative susceptibility to prostate cancer in those with low exposure to sunlight.

Although death from old age is perhaps ideal, some form of disease is more or less inevitable. A purpose of medicine and public health is to diminish and delay disease as much as possible, the compression of morbidity that we noted at the beginning of this book. Sunlight helps us to achieve it.

The body is constantly trying to defend itself against disease and the sun helps through vitamin D and its widespread metabolic effects. A good defence system might in theory protect the body absolutely against disease, but this is unusual and a delay of disease until late in life is what most of us hope for. An alternative is for the disease process to be as slow as possible. To survive for 5 years after a diagnosis of cancer is thought to be preferable to surviving for 3 years, and an improved 5-year survival is the usual measure of success of cancer treatments, rather than absolute cure.

In addition to geographical variations in cancer incidence there are geographical variations in cancer survival; data are available from the England and Wales Cancer Registry, established in 1962. Five-year survival figures from all cancers within the regions of England and Wales are shown in Table 63.1 [9].

**Table 63.1  Five-year age-adjusted survival (%) for all cancers [9]**

|                    | Males | Females |
|--------------------|-------|---------|
| Oxford             | 34.0  | 45.8    |
| Wales              | 33.7  | 46.0    |
| North-east Thames  | 34.0  | 45.2    |
| North-west Thames  | 33.4  | 45.3    |
| Wessex             | 33.4  | 45.2    |
| South-west England | 33.5  | 45.1    |
| East Anglia        | 32.9  | 44.1    |
| West Midlands      | 31.7  | 45.5    |
| South-west Thames  | 30.4  | 43.4    |
| Trent              | 30.1  | 43.7    |
| South-east Thames  | 28.0  | 39.6    |
| Mersey             | 27.1  | 41.3    |
| North              | 27.1  | 40.2    |
| North-west England | 25.8  | 40.1    |
| Yorkshire          | 25.8  | 38.8    |

Thirty-four per cent of men resident in the Oxford region will survive for 5 years following a diagnosis of cancer, compared with 25.8% in the north-west of England and Yorkshire. The findings are thus similar to what we have seen with coronary heart disease. With certain exceptions we see a general pattern, with the southern regions showing a much better cancer survival at 5 years compared with regions in the north of England. Figure 63.4 goes on to show survival curves from stomach cancer, comparing the north-west Thames region with north-western England for men. The survival curves for women are similar but with slightly better survival rate.

**Figure 63.4  Survival in men from stomach cancer [9].**

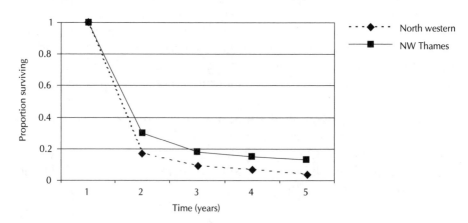

As before, we see a disadvantage to living in the north-west of England, probably because of the low levels of sunshine. The outcome from stomach cancer is poor for all, but survival is about twice as good in north-west Thames compared with north-west England. Comparable survival rates can be seen for bladder cancer, but with overall higher survival rates.

Colon cancer has a similar outcome [10]. We can see in Figure 63.5 once again a significantly better survival in the south of England compared with the north.

**Figure 63.5  Colon cancer: 5-year survival rates 1994–96 [10].**

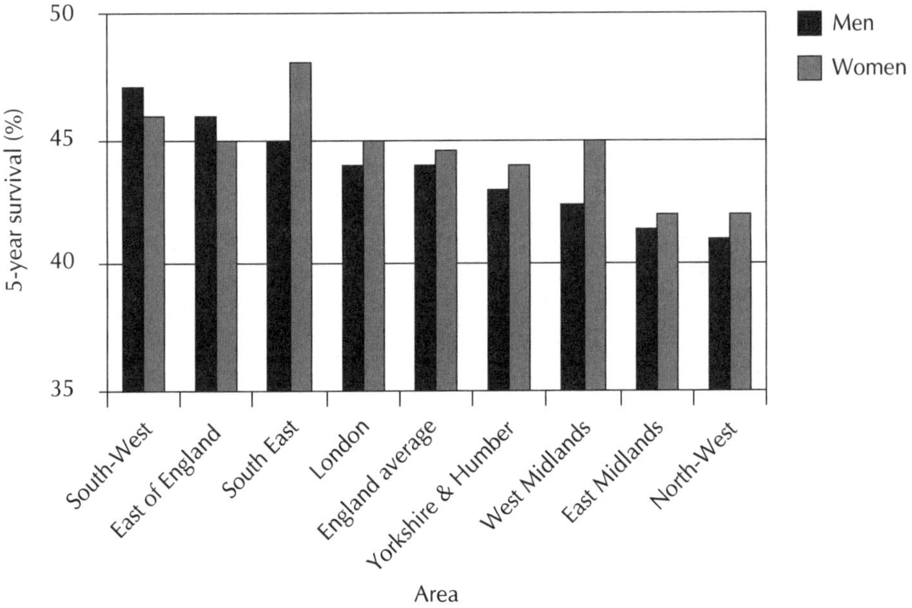

*Crown © 1999, adapted with permission.*

There might be a tendency to blame inferior medical services in the north-west of England, and there are certainly fewer doctors per thousand population than in London. But there is an overall pattern that suggests the climate is to blame. Sunlight exposure might help the body's defence mechanisms against cancer.

The study by Michel Coleman and colleagues from the London School of Hygiene and Tropical Medicine, UK [10], went on to look at social deprivation and found a progressively deteriorating 5-year survival from the most affluent to least affluent. Figure 63.6 shows the survival results for all cancers combined for men. Similar results occur in women, but with a slightly better overall survival rate.

**Figure 63.6 Cancer survival (men) related to social deprivation category [10].**

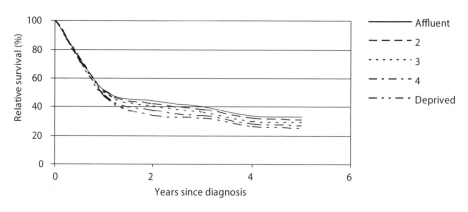

The poor health outcome of the socio-economically deprived is something that we have already seen, and it is a general principle of human health in northern Europe and North America. It applies to more than cancer, and so we must look for explanations not in a particular cancer and its treatment but in the nature of socio-economic deprivation.

This important and comprehensive review of cancer survival also compares the UK with other countries [10]. In this study, the UK is represented by England and Wales combined, and Scotland. The 5-year survival for UK citizens is worse for lung, breast, prostate and colon cancer compared with the European and USA averages, shown in Figure 63.7.

**Figure 63.7  Five-year survival from cancer [10]. E&W, England and Wales.**

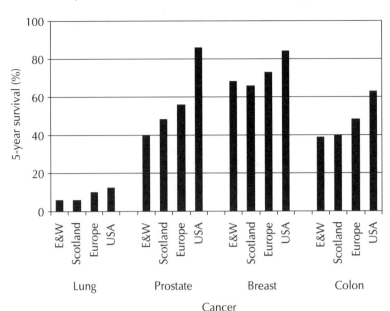

We can see that the survival from these cancers is significantly worse in the UK. This is similar to the other health disadvantages of the UK that we have seen in earlier chapters. These cancers are common and have been related to low levels of exposure to ultraviolet light.

A study to investigate why certain people develop cancer of the colon was undertaken by the USA Veterans Administration Co-operative Study Group [11]; 3121 asymptomatic people between the ages of 50 and 75 years were investigated by colonoscopy. Because of the nature of the organisation (medical services for war veterans), 96.8% of the study group members were male; 329 participants were found to have cancer of the colon, and the investigation was to try to determine the factors in life that might be responsible for the development of the cancer. Diet was investigated in some detail. Those who consumed beef, pork or lamb as a main dish five or more times per week had a slightly increased relative risk of cancer, and those with a high fibre intake were at a slightly reduced risk. Cigarette smoking and alcohol consumption were associated with an increased risk of cancer, as was increasing age.

But vitamin D consumption emerged as the major protective factor, as judged by dietary assessment. The contribution of vitamin D from sunlight exposure was not taken into consideration and blood levels of vitamin D were not measured. The numbers of cancers were calculated for each quintile of vitamin D intake, and the results are shown in Figure 63.8.

**Figure 63.8  Colon cancers and vitamin D intake [11].**

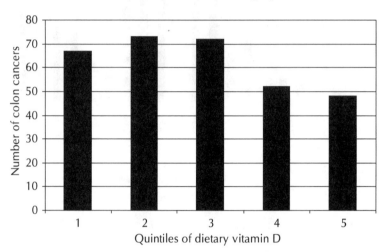

We can see that more colon cancers occurred in those with a low intake of vitamin D (quintiles 1, 2, 3) than in those with a high intake. The two lowest quintiles of vitamin D consumption represent 140 cancers and the two highest quintiles 100 cancers. This indicates a 40% increase in colon cancer risk in those consuming little vitamin D, significantly greater than other factors studied.

Dietary supplements of vitamin D might offer some protection against colon cancer, but this can only be a hypothesis. It would need to be put to the test of a randomised clinical trial before a definite conclusion could be drawn.

We return to Europe for an assessment of the outcome of colon cancer by 11 centres participating in the EUROCARE study [12]. We see once again that the UK centres are below average and, together with Cracow, Poland, have the worst survival, shown in Figure 63.9.

**Figure 63.9 Survival from colon cancer in Europe [12].**

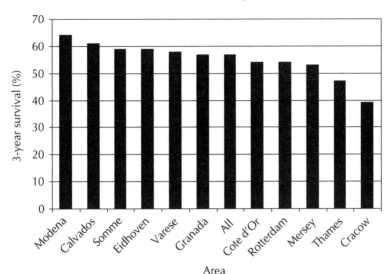

*Adapted with permission from the British Medical Journal Publishing Group.*

The authors comment that the best survival in Modena, Italy, is also found for other cancers and that it 'may be due to better medical care in this area of Italy'. This conclusion is the result of looking only at the small picture of the cancer data, not looking at the overall health advantages of the Italian population. Although the population of Modena might be blessed by outstanding medical services, there must be at least the suspicion that we are seeing another example of the health benefits of the Mediterranean sun.

We have already noted that vitamin D appears to delay the onset of cancer, to reduce its incidence, to slow down its progress and to improve surgical outcomes. We see the same in this study. Not only were outcomes poor in the English groups but the cancers were more frequently at a more advanced stage at the time of diagnosis. Although this could be blamed on poor medical and surgical services in England, without supportive evidence, it could also be that the biology of the cancers is more aggressive because of an insufficiency of vitamin D.

*Epidemiological studies reveal a protective role for 1,25(OH)$_2$ vitamin D (D$_3$) [calcitriol] against colorectal cancer. D$_3$ has been proposed for use as a therapeutic agent in colorectal carcinoma. [13]*

So states a group from the University of Birmingham, UK, who go on to demonstrate the presence of vitamin D receptors (VDRs) in 22 colon cancers and in normal colon mucosa specimens. This lends biological plausibility to the suggestion that vitamin D might be relevant to the development and outcome of colon cancer.

An earlier study from the Royal Postgraduate Medical School, London, UK, had undertaken an *in vitro* assessment of the effect of vitamin D on active human rectal mucosa and polyp specimens, and on cultured colorectal cancer cells [14]. It was found that 'Vitamin D and its metabolites inhibit proliferation in normal and pre-malignant rectal epithelium and suppress growth in a colorectal cancer line'. The evidence for a protective role of sunlight and vitamin D against cancer is becoming stronger.

There are important observations on the effect of vitamin D (as calcitriol) on the development of experimental cancer in animal models and cell lines. The majority show that vitamin D has a significant inhibitory effect on the development of cancer. The papers are of a very technical nature but are reviewed well by Helmut Reichel, Phillip Koeffler and Anthony Norman from the University of California, Riverside and Los Angeles, USA [15].

Disease patterns change over a period of time and this sometimes provides a clue to causation. Two changes that have been taking place during the past 30 years concern the incidence of cancer of the stomach and cancer of the oesophagus in Europe and North America. This has been documented in the UK by the National Cancer Intelligence Unit, looking at all cancer registrations for England and Wales between 1971 and 1999, reported by a group from Cambridge [16]. It demonstrates that the incidence of gastric cancer in men has fallen from 31.8 to 18.8 per 100 000 (expressed as the European age-standardised ratio; ESR). This is a dramatic reduction in a form of cancer that has traditionally involved mainly the lower part of the stomach, the gastric antrum.

During the same time, there has been a very significant increase in the incidence of cancer of the oesophagus, from 7.7 to 13 per 100 000. The reason for this change is not known but it is quite alarming as this new form of cancer of the oesophagus (histologically adenocarcinoma) is generally highly malignant with early metastases, occurring at a relatively young age and with a very poor outlook.

The geographical distribution of adenocarcinoma of the oesophagus is also extremely interesting. Misra and colleagues went on to look at the incidence in different countries, although data were available from only a few [17]. However, they identified that Scotland has the highest recorded incidence of oesophageal cancer in the world, and England and Northern Ireland have the next highest incidence. This is shown in Figure 63.10 and the pattern is now familiar to us.

**Figure 63.10 Cumulative life-time risk of developing adenocarcinoma of the oesophagus [17].**

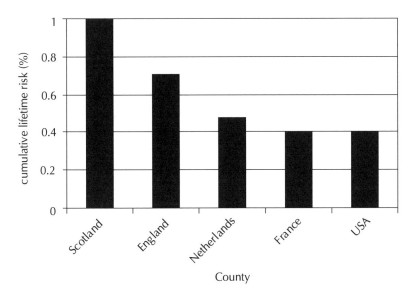

*Adapted with permission from the British Medical Journal Publishing Group.*

The cumulative life-time risk for an adult Scottish male developing cancer (adenocarcinoma) of the oesophagus by the age of 79 years is 1% and the risk for an English male is 0.71%. These compare with 0.48% for a male in Holland, 0.4% in France and 0.4% in the USA. The source of these data is the *Cancer in Five Continents* Volume VIII Database, which takes data from 252 cancer registers world-wide and is compiled by the International Association of Cancer Registries (IACR) [18]. The data in this study were from the years 1993–97.

In considering coronary heart disease, we looked at data that identified a distinct latitude relationship as evidence of the protective value of the sun, and we can do the same thing in respect of cancer. There is a view that not all cancers are associated with insufficiency of vitamin D but the common cancers of the breast and colon are associated. Table 63.2 shows mortality rates from breast and colon cancer in European nations [18].

**Table 63.2 Breast and colon cancer deaths in Europe [18].**
Death rates per 100 000 population and latitude.

| Country | Latitude | Breast | Colon |
|---|---|---|---|
| Greece | 39 | 15.1 | 5.2 |
| Spain | 40 | 15.0 | 7.8 |
| Italy | 42 | 20.4 | 10.5 |
| France | 46 | 19.0 | 11.2 |
| Switzerland | 47 | 24.9 | 12.2 |
| Austria | 47 | 22.0 | 15.2 |
| Belgium | 50 | 25.6 | 15.2 |
| Germany | 51 | 21.9 | 15.5 |
| Netherlands | 52 | 25.8 | 14.7 |
| England and Wales | 52 | 29.0 | 15.3 |
| Republic of Ireland | 53 | 25.7 | 16.6 |
| Northern Ireland | 54 | 26.9 | 16.4 |

The familiar pattern emerges. The lowest incidence rates are in Greece, Italy and Spain. The highest rates are in the British Isles, with an incidence of colon cancer three times higher than in Greece and Spain. Not only that, but we find a very strong association between both cancers and latitude, as shown in Figure 63.11.

**Figure 63.11 Deaths from cancer related to latitude [18].**

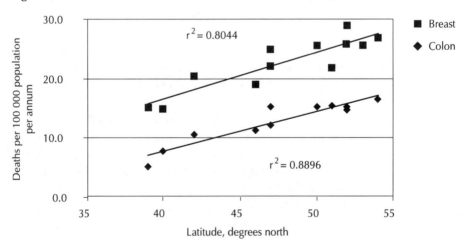

We can see $R^2 = 0.8044$ for breast cancer and $R^2 = 0.8896$ for colon cancer. These denote very powerful associations with latitude, very strong evidence for sunlight and vitamin D playing an important protective role.

Another clue regarding the protection offered by vitamin D against breast and colon cancers comes from studies of night-shift workers. Evidence is from the Harvard Nurses' Health Study, which we will meet again in looking at diseases of the nervous system; 78 586 nurses were followed and it was noted that breast and colon cancer incidence rates were up to 35% higher in those who worked regular night-shifts [19,20]. Although it has been suggested that artificial light during the night might increase cancer risk [21], there is no biological plausibility to this and I suggest that less exposure to the sun with reduced vitamin D synthesis gives greater susceptibility.

A report appeared in *The Times* on St George's Day 2005 entitled 'Sunlight Cancer Cure'. It was based on the results of a study presented to the 96th Annual Meeting of the American Association for Cancer Research [22]. A team from the Harvard School of Public Health, the Massachusetts General Hospital, the Dana-Farbar Cancer Institute and the Brigham and Women's Hospital, Boston, USA, investigated 456 people with early-stage lung cancer who had undergone surgery. Those in whom the diagnosis and operation took place in the summer, spring and autumn had a 5-year survival significantly greater than those in whom the operation was performed in the winter, as shown in Figure 63.12.

**Figure 63.12  Effect of season and vitamin D on outcome of lung cancer [22].**

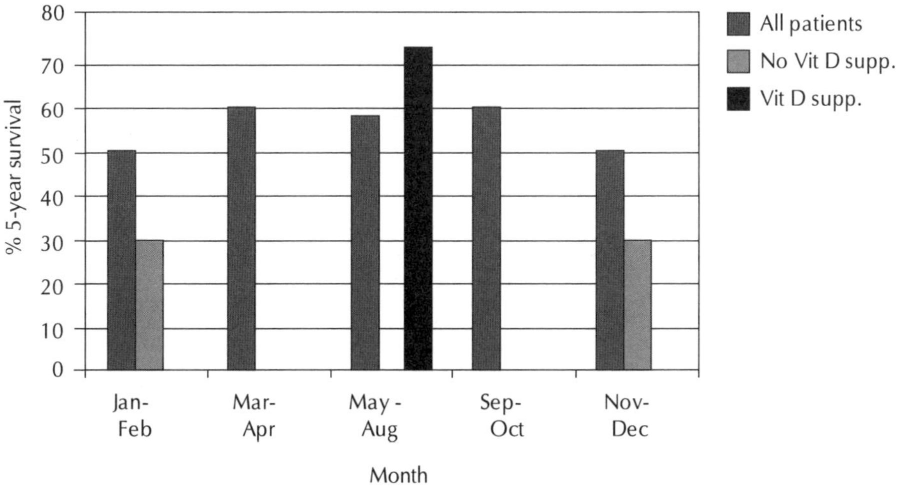

529

The authors interpreted this as a beneficial effect of sunshine and they therefore took their research a step further. They identified as far as possible the dietary intake of vitamin D, recording whether or not the subjects took vitamin D supplements. The results are also shown in Figure 63.12. The worst 5-year survival, 29%, was in those who took no vitamin D supplement and had treatment in the winter. The best 5-year survival, 72% was in those who took vitamin D supplements and had treatment in the summer. The combined benefit of sunlight and dietary vitamin D was associated with more than twice the 5-year survival rate. A randomised controlled trial would be more conclusive of the benefits of vitamin D in patients with lung cancer.

There are important similarities between the patterns of coronary heart disease and cancer. Both are common in the north of England compared with the south, and in the UK compared with most of Europe and the USA. Both affect the socio-economically disadvantaged more than the affluent. Both are associated with latitude, with incidence increasing with distance of residence from the equator. An interesting departure is that in middle-aged men, whilst the incidence of coronary heart disease increases slightly with increasing blood cholesterol, the incidence of cancer decreases, as shown in Figure 63.13. The data are taken from the Renfrew and Paisley study in Glasgow, UK [23].

**Figure 63.13  Cancer and coronary heart disease (CHD) [23].**

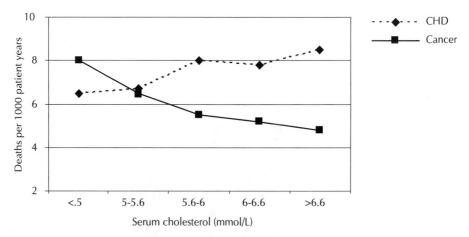

It can be seen that in this study the advantage of a high serum cholesterol in cancer protection (three deaths per 1000 patient years) is greater than the increased risk of death from coronary heart disease (two per 1000). The association between cancer and low serum cholesterol is well-recognised but the nature of the relationship is not clear. For example, a survey of colon cancer and serum cholesterol was published in 1974 [24], the authors being some of the leading epidemiology researchers in the UK and the USA, including Geoffrey Rose from St Mary's Hospital Medical School, London, UK, Henry Blackburn and Ancel Keys from the University of Minnesota, USA, William B. Kannel from the Framingham study, Massachusetts, USA, Ogesby Paul from the Northwestern Memorial Hospital, Chicago, USA, and Jeremiah Stammler the Northwestern University, Chicago, USA. They noted an association between colon cancer and coronary heart disease, data being taken from the World Health Organization (WHO) mortality tables, 8th revision, in 1969 [25]. They presented the association as a scattergraph, shown in Figure 63.14; it is a fairly strong association, with $R^2 = 0.5839$.

**Figure 63.14  Deaths from coronary heart disease (CHD) and colon cancer [24].**

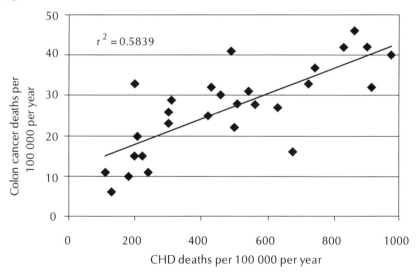

© 1974, adapted from The Lancet with permission from Elsevier.

The authors interpreted this as a common cause effect, not considering common susceptibility; in keeping with the diet–cholesterol–heart hypothesis they proposed a diet–cholesterol–colon cancer hypothesis. Because they expected dietary fat to be the cause of both coronary heart disease and colon cancer, their investigation was to look at serum cholesterol as a predictive factor in people who developed colon cancer compared with those who did not. Their data source was six studies of the epidemiology of cholesterol and coronary heart disease: Whitehall [26], Seven Countries [27], Framingham [28], Western Electric Company [29], Chicago Gas Company [30] and Minnesota businessmen [31]. They were able to obtain details of the causes of death of the subjects over a time period of 10 or more years and identify those who died from colon cancer. The initial mean serum cholesterol of the subgroup was compared with the majority who did not die from colon cancer. The results are shown in Figure 63.15.

**Figure 63.15  Blood cholesterol and colon cancer [24].**

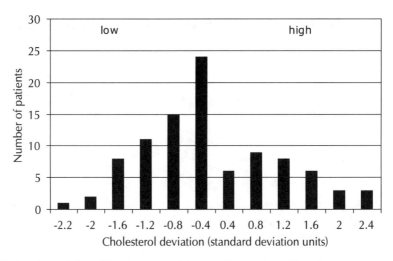

We can see the distribution of initial serum cholesterol levels in those who subsequently died from colon cancer, expressed relative to the total from the six studies. The units are those of standard deviation, which means how far they are from zero, the arithmetic mean or average. In a normal distribution, such as we have seen for serum cholesterol in population samples, about 90% are between −2 and +2, and any outside this range can be judged to be significantly abnormal. It is quite a useful way of expressing normality (as opposed to perfection) and it can be applied to a wide range of parameters, for example height, weight, IQ, blood glucose, blood pressure, etc. The usefulness of a single unit of measurement is obvious.

Returning to the study of Rose *et al.* [24], we can see that the distribution in Figure 63.15 shows a definite skew to the left, to a lower range of serum cholesterol than would be expected. The authors reported that 'initial blood cholesterol levels of those who subsequently developed colon cancer were surprisingly lower than the expected values'.

This study is an example of what Thomas Kuhn called normal research [32]. The authors were looking for what they expected, 'white swans' (see Chapter 50), and when they did not find one they simply moved on. What they did not realise is that they had found an anomaly, an unexpected 'black swan'. Here was an opportunity to move into research that increases knowledge, but they failed to do so. It shows not only lack of objectivity but also the overwhelming captivation of the diet–cholesterol–disease hypothesis, to which they clung.

If Rose and colleagues proposed a high serum cholesterol to be a fundamental truth concerning the development of coronary heart disease, they should equally have regarded a low serum cholesterol to be a fundamental truth concerning cancer, especially as the association is more general, applying not only to young and middle-aged men. Cholesterol scientists work very hard to sustain the diet–cholesterol–heart hypothesis but their time would probably be spent more constructively investigating the clear relationship between cancer and pre-existing low serum cholesterol.

I have suggested that cholesterol must have a physiological role, which appears to be defensive. We will remember from Chapter 43 that high serum cholesterol is protective against HIV infection and that low serum cholesterol is a predictor of several other infections, poor outcome after surgery and major illness. Perhaps this is the case with cancer, low serum cholesterol being an indicator that defence processes are becoming overwhelmed or are not making an adequate response. I have indicated that natural defence against cancer is thought to be mediated by immunosurveillance and this is how the benefit of vitamin D has been explained.

It is known that people on immunosuppressive therapy have a higher than expected incidence of cancer. There is something in the body that predisposes to cancer, presumably poor immune competence, as shown by the observation that a person who has had one cancer is at increased risk of another, a different form of cancer.

*It was in 1863 that Rudolf Virchow noted leucocytes [white blood cells] in neoplastic tissues and made a connection between inflammation and cancer. He suggested that the 'lympho-reticular infiltrate' reflected the origin of cancer at sites of chronic inflammation. Over the past ten years our understanding of the inflammatory micro-environment of malignant tissues has supported Virchow's hypothesis, and the links between cancer and inflammation are starting to have implications for prevention and treatment. [33]*

We are now entering a complex subject involving the inflammatory process and its relationship with cancer, but it is extremely well reviewed by Professor Fran Balkwill of the ICRF Translational Oncology Laboratory, St Bartholomew's and Royal London School of Medicine and Dentistry, UK, and Professor Alberto Mantovani of the Department of Immunology and Cell Biology, Milan State University, Italy [33]. They list a number of cancers that develop at sites of inflammation, often with a microbial cause. These include oesophagus, stomach, colon, liver, pancreas, breast, lung, pleura, bladder and uterine cervix. The fundamental issue is whether an inflammatory reaction becomes completed, with remodelling and restoration of normal tissue structure, or whether the inflammatory process continues, perhaps with malignant change. The key cell is the macrophage that is found in inflammation. It is also found in malignant tissue, where it is called the tumour-associated macrophage (TAM). When appropriately activated, TAMs can kill tumour cells but may also induce tumour-cell proliferation and factors that encourage invasion of tissue and metastasis. The dual potential of TAMs is called the 'macrophage balance hypothesis' [34], which is far from fully understood. It is possible that vitamin D plays its role here, determining the activity of TAMs and thus the outcome of inflammation, whether it is completed with tissue restoration under the influence of transforming growth factor (TGF-β), whether the inflammatory process continues (auto-immune or immune-mediated disease) or whether malignant change develops. Harold F. Dvorak, Mallinckrodt Professor of Pathology at the Harvard Medical School, USA, first introduced this idea, provocatively expressed as 'Tumors: wounds that do not heal' [35].

The similarities between infections and cancers are greater than their differences, especially when we consider chronic infections rather than acute infections that can overwhelm and kill within a matter of days. Before the antibiotic era, tuberculosis of the lung behaved in a very similar way to lung cancer, even with the development of tumours called tuberculomas. Late syphilis was also characterised by tumour development in a metastatic pattern, in this case called gummas. Perhaps the main difference between infections and cancers is that infections respond to a group of chemicals that are called antibiotics, if derived from other living organisms, or anti-microbial compounds, which include synthetic medicines. We do not know how many cancers will be found to have a microbial cause. It came as some surprise to the media when in October 2005 it was announced that immunisation against a virus protected against cancer of the cervix uteri [36]. It was suggested that a viral cause of cancer was exceptional, but this is not the case. For example, the B and C hepatitis viruses can cause both inflammation and cancer, in these cases some of the most common cancers in the world.

Figure 63.16 shows a model of how inflammation and cancer are related, with an indication of where the protective effect of vitamin D might occur.

**Figure 63.16 A model of the relationship between inflammation and cancer**

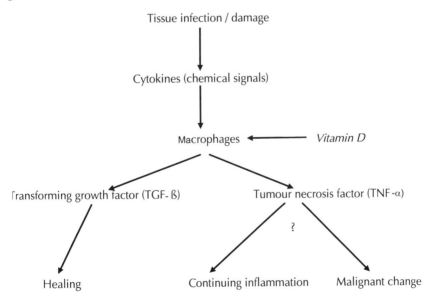

A further conundrum emerged from a 10-year follow-up of the 4S study into the clinical effects of simvastatin [37]. Subjects treated with simvastatin had a reduced incidence of cancer compared with the control group. The initial cohorts were 2221 subjects allocated to receive simvastatin and 2223 to receive placebo. A reduced incidence of cancer in the simvastatin group became noticeable after 5 years. At 10 years there were 227 cancers and 85 cancer deaths in the simvastatin group, compared with 248 cancers and 100 cancer deaths in the placebo group. It is interesting, therefore, to note that not only were there fewer cancers among those receiving simvastatin (91.5% of the placebo group) but the mortality of cancer was disproportionately lower (85%). The cancers that showed a significant reduction were colorectal, lung and prostate, and we have already seen that these tend to be more common with worse survival in places with low levels of sunlight. Figure 63.17 shows the 4S data in more detail.

**Figure 63.17  Cancer incidence at 10 years and simvastatin [37].**

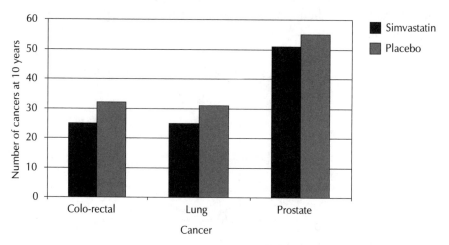

© 2004, adapted from The Lancet with permission from Elsevier.

This line of research was taken a stage further at the Molecular Epidemiology of Colorectal Cancer Unit in Israel, reporting in the *New England Journal of Medicine* in the early summer of 2005 [38]. The study assessed 1953 patients diagnosed between 1998 and 2004 as having colorectal (colon or rectum) cancer, and compared them with 2015 matched controls. It was found that 6.1% of those diagnosed with colorectal cancer were taking statin medications before the diagnosis was made. This compared with 11.6% of the controls, a very significant difference, shown in Figure 63.18. The incidence of colorectal cancer was thus only half of what would be expected, indicating a possible protective role of statins. In both groups of patients statins were being taken to treat hypercholesterolaemia or coronary heart disease.

**Figure 63.18 Statin use and colorectal cancer [38].**

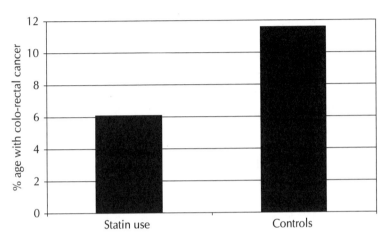

The conundrum, or what we might call the Israel cancer paradox, is this. Why is it that a therapeutic reduction of serum cholesterol by statin therapy is associated with a much-reduced risk of colorectal cancer, when we know that colon cancer is associated with low serum cholesterol? The answer is becoming clear: the varied beneficial effects of statin therapy are unrelated to the cholesterol-lowering property. A reduction of serum cholesterol cannot be expected to reduce cancer risk; there must be a direct effect of statin therapy, just as in the reduction of cardiovascular risk. We have seen several unexpected effects of statin therapy and we will shortly be seeing more. It is such anomalies that lead to productive research.

Two studies presented at the British Society of Gastro-enterology at its spring meeting in 2006 reported effects on oesophageal cancer. The first, from the University of East Anglia, indicated that simvastatin, lovastatin and pravastatin *in vitro* inhibit the proliferation of oesophageal cancer cells [39]. The second, also from the same hospital and university, reported that, in an animal model, fish oils inhibited what are thought to be malignant processes in oesophageal cancer [40].

There are similarities between cancer and other diseases whose incidence and outcome are modulated by vitamin D and sunlight. The causes of most cancers are not recognised but several are known to be caused by a virus, for example primary liver cell cancer, cancer of the cervix uteri and Burkitt's lymphoma (the most rapidly progressive of all cancers). It has been suspected for many years that breast cancer might be caused by a micro-organism, based on considerations such as family clustering (constitutional) and geographical variation, with an increase of risk when moving from a low risk to a high risk location. There is also the parallel of the mouse mammary tumour virus, and using polymerase chain reaction (PCR) techniques variants of this virus have been detected in human breast cancer by many laboratories. This has recently been reviewed, with the evidence-based suggestion that the domestic cat might transmit the virus from mice to human beings [41]. We can therefore see the way in which vitamin D might be protective, enhancing immunosurveillance against cancer-inducing micro-organisms.

It has become clear that the sun is of great and extensive importance for human health, and this includes relative protection against several common cancers. We need to look beyond coronary heart disease and cancer at further possibilities, although they are not as well researched as those that we have already seen.

# 64
# CROHN'S DISEASE

At the end of the previous chapter we touched upon the relationships between cancer, malignant processes and inflammation. It looks as though macrophage function holds the key, and Crohn's disease provides another example of this.

Crohn's disease is an inflammatory disease of the gastro-intestinal tract and the major symptoms are abdominal pain, diarrhoea and weight loss. Blood tests show inflammatory markers to be present, for example elevation of the erythrocyte sedimentation rate (ESR) and C-reactive protein (CRP) that we have already seen. Barium x-rays can show the extent of the disease and fibre-optic endoscopy helps in obtaining tissue for microscopic examination.

The history of the understanding of Crohn's disease has been recorded [1] but the disease was first clearly described by Oppenheimer, Ginzberg and Crohn in 1932 [2]. It would have been called Oppenheimer's disease after the major author, but he selflessly allowed the names of the authors of the paper to be presented in alphabetical order. The term Crohn's disease came into popular usage at a later date: the authors of the paper used the term regional enteritis to draw attention to its patchy distribution within the intestine. This term was considered to be inadequate when it was realised that the extent of the disease could include the anus, stomach and mouth; I look after one patient with Crohn's disease of the face.

The similarity between Crohn's disease and tuberculosis of the intestine has always been recognised. Both are chronic long-term diseases, both are inflammatory and both tend to occur in the terminal part of the ileum, the distal small intestine and the caecum. Both exhibit microscopic inflammatory features called granulomas. Both can form cold abscesses, unlike the hot abscesses associated with usual bacterial infections.

I first came across Crohn's disease when I was a medical student at the beginning of my first ward attachment in 1963. The patient concerned was Rebecca, a girl of 18 years, and the experience of her fatal illness had a great effect on me.

Rebecca developed the characteristic symptoms of Crohn's disease: weight loss, abdominal pain and diarrhoea. She developed an abscess in the mesentery, the sheet of tissue that attaches the long, mobile and folded intestine to a short section of the posterior abdominal wall. At the time the treatment of Crohn's disease was mainly surgical and resection of diseased intestine was heroic by today's standard practice. In order to remove the Crohn's abscess, the surgeon had to remove the intestine that was attached by that section of mesentery. I was present at the operation, which I remember vividly. This surgical resection left her with too little intestine to sustain life, and intravenous nutrition had not been developed at that time. She died about 2 weeks after the operation.

We are all aware that cancers generally give rise to weight loss, general ill-health, sometimes pain, a rapid decline and early death if treatment is not successful. This pattern of clinical presentation and downhill course was characteristic of tuberculosis (consumption) in earlier times. The point is that a microbial disease can have what is effectively a malignant course, with the behaviour of the disease very similar to that of cancer. In both conditions, and in untreated Crohn's disease, the patient becomes 'consumed' by the malignant nature of what becomes a fatal illness.

Tuberculosis and Crohn's disease are similar to cancer in that both diseases invade adjacent tissues, breaking down fibrous and other tissue barriers. They can spread locally from one organ to another, in Crohn's disease from the intestine into the bladder, or from one part of the intestine into another, or from the intestine to the skin. It is thought that this invasion is achieved to a large extent by the inflammatory protein tumour necrosis factor (TNF-$\alpha$), which is produced by activated macrophages. This is another feature shared with cancer. Medications to inhibit TNF-$\alpha$ have been used with limited success in the treatment of Crohn's disease, and also rheumatoid arthritis, another chronic inflammatory disease.

However, anti-TNF-$\alpha$ medications (which are given by intravenous infusion) can cause dormant tuberculosis to become active. This returns us to the macrophage balance hypothesis, that TNF-$\alpha$ has defensive properties but its activity in the inflammatory process can sometimes make the disease worse. There is a lot more about this to be understood, and I would refer to the excellent review by Fergus Shanahan, Professor of Medicine at the University of Cork, Ireland [3].

Cancers not only spread locally, the process of invasion, but they can also spread via lymphatic channels to regional lymph glands and distant organs. This is the way in which metastases, secondary tumours, develop. The same thing can happen with tuberculosis. The involvement of regional lymph glands is usual and the disease can spread to distant organs, such as liver and brain. Such distant lesions of tuberculosis are not called metastases but miliary lesions. Tuberculosis when widespread in this way is called 'miliary' and at this stage it is rapidly fatal if untreated, and sometimes treatment fails to halt the progress of the disease.

Crohn's disease can also spread to regional lymph nodes, as described some time ago by Kenneth Heaton and his colleagues at the Bristol Royal Infirmary, UK [4], but it does not appear to spread to distant organs. The purpose of Heaton's paper was to draw attention to the similarity between Crohn's disease and tuberculosis, indicating that lymph gland spread was not necessarily a distinguishing feature of tuberculosis.

The distinction between the two conditions is difficult, and perhaps Crohn's disease only became defined when tuberculosis was well into decline [5]. We have seen that in recent years tuberculosis has remained relatively common in South Asians living in the UK. When a white UK patient develops an illness of weight loss, abdominal pain and diarrhoea with positive inflammatory markers, Crohn's disease is suspected and the diagnosis is accepted if barium x-rays show features of regional enteritis. If, on the other hand, the patient is South Asian then a diagnosis of intestinal tuberculosis is likely to be made on the basis of preconceived probability. What is not generally appreciated is that Crohn's disease occurs in South Asians in the UK and its incidence in children of South Asian parents is higher than in the white population [6,7].

We have seen a number of geographical variations of disease that have indicated susceptibility of people living at a considerable distance from the equator, suggesting protection by the sun. Crohn's disease is a rare condition compared with coronary heart disease and cancer. Research into its distribution is limited and it is not sufficiently important for WHO to collect data. Specific epidemiological studies have found the incidence of Crohn's disease to be highest in north-west Europe, especially in the UK and Scandinavia.

In a study of a semi-rural area of north-west Greece with 157 214 inhabitants, only five cases of Crohn's disease were diagnosed between 1982 and 1991, an incidence rate of about 0.3 per 100 000 per annum [8]. In contrast, during the same time period the incidence in Stockholm County, Sweden, was about 15 times higher, at 4.7 per 100 000 per annum [9], shown in Figure 64.1.

541

Figure 64.1 Crohn's disease in Greece and Sweden [8,9].

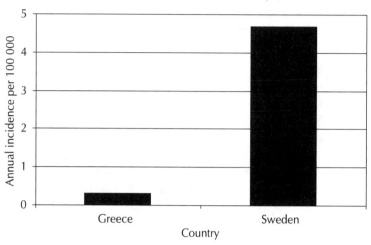

We can immediately recognise a familiar pattern, seen with coronary heart disease, respiratory disease and certain cancers. Is lack of sunlight and consequent vitamin D deficiency the reason for the susceptibility of the population of north-west Europe to Crohn's disease?

We have noted that fish-oil supplements comprise the only dietary manipulation that has consistently been found to help people with coronary heart disease. Its vitamin D content is likely to be the active ingredient but other fatty acids might contribute. It is interesting to note that fish-oil supplements are also helpful in the treatment of Crohn's disease [10]. Before looking at this paper, however, it is important to understand the clinical pattern of Crohn's disease. In the present era, in which treatment is effective but does not truly cure, the course of the illness is variable; the patient will experience times of remission, when the symptoms have settled without the disease having been necessarily cured in the long term. Then there are times of relapse, when the disease becomes active again and a further course of treatment is given. The purpose of treatment is to end a relapse and induce a remission for as long as possible.

The study undertaken by Andrea Belluzzi and his colleagues from the University of Bologna and the S. Giovanni Battista Hospital, Turin, Italy, was a randomised controlled clinical trial of fish-oil supplements, with 39 patients in the treatment group and 39 in the control group, all with Crohn's disease. The patients were all in remission from the disease at the time of enrolment into the trial and the outcome measure was the occurrence of a relapse. Eleven of the patients receiving fish-oil supplements suffered relapses, compared with 27 controls (Figure 64.2). There was thus a significant benefit from fish-oil supplements, perhaps, but not definitely, mediated by vitamin D.

**Figure 64.2  Occurrence of relapses of Crohn's disease [10].**

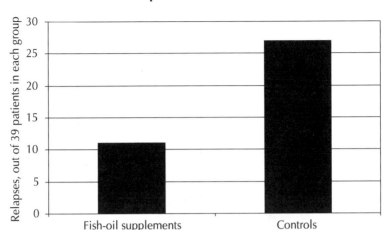

We noted earlier that children might develop rickets despite adequate exposure to sunlight and with normal vitamin D levels in the blood. The key to understanding this conundrum was the identification of abnormal VDRs, which are inherited on chromosome 12. Mutations (also called genetic variation or genetic polymorphism, depending on frequency) can be passed on to the next generation and they are not uncommon. In the presence of abnormal VDRs, vitamin D as calcitriol is relatively inactive because its tissue receptors will not allow it to 'dock' and therefore it is unable to activate biochemical processes within the cells. We have seen in Chapter 10 that people with VDR mutations are particularly susceptible to tuberculosis [11].

They are also susceptible to Crohn's disease, demonstrated in a study from Oxford, UK, and this probably explains some of the genetic risk for Crohn's disease [12]. The genetic details of the paper are highly specialised and complex to the average reader such as myself. However, the main result is that VDR mutations in the homozygote state were found in 53 out of 245 patients with Crohn's disease (22%), compared with 20 out of 164 controls (12%). The frequency was the same in normal controls and patients with ulcerative colitis, a different form of inflammatory disease restricted to the large intestine and not vitamin D dependent (Figure 64.3).

**Figure 64.3  Frequency of VDR mutations [12].**

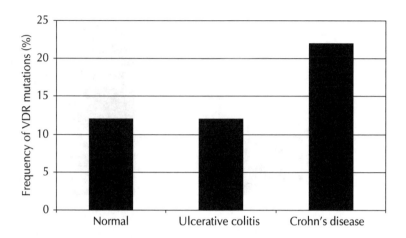

*Adapted with permission from the British Medical Journal Publishing Group.*

There is thus an identified and understood genetic factor that leads to susceptibility to Crohn's disease. The authors comment that the immunoregulatory effects of vitamin D are complicated and the precise mechanisms and interactions with other regulators of the immune/inflammatory response are not yet clear [12].

A more recent study from Los Angeles, USA, takes the vitamin D and Crohn's disease story a stage further [13]. The results are once again not easy to interpret, but the study identified low levels of calcidiol in patients with Crohn's disease; remember that calcidiol is the indicator of vitamin D from sunlight or diet.

This observation would fit in with vitamin D insufficiency causing susceptibility to Crohn's disease. However, some of the patients had increased levels of calcitriol, the most active form of vitamin D synthesised by the addition of a hydroxyl (-OH) group in position 1 of the a ring of the calcidiol molecule, as explained in Chapter 16. This process takes place under the influence of the enzyme 1α-hydroxylase, known to be active in the kidneys. However, the authors [13] quote work that indicates that this enzyme can be produced by macrophages, which might explain their findings. The important thing is that it emphasises the importance of vitamin D in controlling the inflammatory process. The study made no mention of VDR genotypes and it is possible that mutations were present, allowing calcitriol levels to increase without any metabolic effect.

The genetics of the VDR provides an explanation for the inheritance of Crohn's disease but there is another interesting aspect to the familial clustering. A study from northern France and Belgium determined that Crohn's disease occurs subsequent to marriage to sufferers from Crohn's disease more often than would be expected [14]. This clearly indicates an environmental and transmissible non-genetic familial factor, very suggestive of a micro-organism.

The pathological similarity between Crohn's disease and tuberculosis suggests that they might have a very similar cause. Whereas tuberculosis is caused by the micro-organism *Mycobacterium tuberculosis*, as determined by Robert Koch (see Chapter 8), the cause of Crohn's disease is not quite so clear. The chief contender is *Mycobacterium avium* subspecies *paratuberculosis*, a long name that is abbreviated to MAP. Most of the work to develop this line of research has been undertaken by Professor John Hermon-Taylor at St George's Hospital Medical School, London, UK [15,16]. There are those who are very sceptical and protest that MAP as a cause of Crohn's disease cannot be accepted because 'it has not been proven' [17]. This objection fails to acknowledge the meaning of proof, as we discussed in Chapter 49. MAP as the cause of Crohn's disease is the best concept that we have at the present time, and in the absence of an alternative plausible hypothesis it should be accepted as the paradigm. A more plausible concept might appear in the future and then the paradigm would change. The alternative is to remain in the pre-paradigm era, as defined by Thomas Kuhn [18].

Using PCR technology to amplify its DNA, MAP has been detected in diseased intestinal tissue taken from 65% of a group of patients with Crohn's disease but in only 12.5% of normal controls and 4.3% of patients with ulcerative colitis [15]. The extreme sensitivity of PCR means that tiny and clinically insignificant amounts of DNA can be detected and this will be the reason for the higher detection rates in normal controls in other studies.

Further support for a causal role for MAP in Crohn's disease comes from more recent work from Orlando and Gainsville in Florida, USA [19]. Viable DNA from MAP was detected in the blood of 50% of patients with Crohn's disease, 22% with ulcerative colitis and in none of the normal controls.

The problem is that Koch's postulates, the foundation of proof in microbial disease, are simply not applicable to Crohn's disease [20,21]. Unlike *Mycobacterium tuberculosis*, MAP cannot be grown in the laboratory and it cannot be transmitted to a laboratory animal. There are, however, natural animal hosts for MAP, namely the ruminants – goats, sheep and cattle. Although MAP has been identified only fairly recently, its effect on ruminants has been known since the early 20th century as Johne's disease [22].

It is thought that MAP is acquired from cows' milk in childhood and that it lies dormant as spheroplasts, creating disease only rarely, particularly when tissue and immunological defences are low. The overall load of the infecting agent is also likely to be important. The village of Blockley in Gloucestershire, UK, has a population of only 200 but the prevalence of Crohn's disease was found to be 12%, almost 10 times the expected 1.8% [23]. Johne's disease was found to be very common in the local cows and sheep, and a single spring supplying the village and farms with water was suggested as a common source of infection with, at the time, an unknown micro-organism. Although it appears that human beings acquire the causative organism of Crohn's disease from cows or other ruminants, perhaps the infection can also travel in the other direction.

Alan has spent his life farming in the beautiful valley of the River Hodder, to the north of Clitheroe in Lancashire, UK. As we saw earlier, this is an area where only grass can be expected to grow to agricultural maturity, and so Alan's farm was concerned with livestock, mainly beef cattle. Alan developed Crohn's disease in 1985, at the age of 45 years, and he settled down quite well on medical treatment with no need for surgery. As is usual with Crohn's disease, he has been in remission for most of the time but occasionally he has a relapse, the major symptom of which is diarrhoea. This necessitates ready access to a toilet, something that can disrupt work depending on the type of employment. A farmer cannot really take time off work and toilets are not readily available outside the house. There is, however, solitude and so, if Alan is 'caught short', he must rely on the toilet facilities that nature supplies.

In December 2001 a calf was born on Alan's farm and it needed a great deal of attention in its first few days. Alan provided the necessary care but it was during an occasion of relapse of his disease (it was also mid-winter); his urgent diarrhoea meant that he had to use the barn in which he was working for toilet purposes. The calf developed very well initially but at about 1 year of age it became sick with weight loss and diarrhoea. Alan called in the vet, who was uncertain of the nature of the illness. Alan had been seeing me regularly in the outpatient clinic for several years and I had taken the opportunity to explain to him as much about Crohn's disease as I knew. I had told him of the Johne's disease connection and so he wondered if this might be the cause of the calf's illness. He suggested this to the vet, who was quite surprised as he had never seen Johne's disease, which is very rare. Before long the calf deteriorated and died, and an autopsy was performed as part of government regulation. The vet telephoned Alan to say that that he had been absolutely correct: the calf had suffered from Johne's disease, which was the cause of its death. The only possible local source of infection was Alan. Is this the first example of human to animal transmission?

Access to tissue is much easier in animals with Johne's disease than human beings with Crohn's disease and a great deal of work has been undertaken in veterinary schools regarding its cause. It is here that MAP was first identified.

*Mycobacterium avium* is the bird strain of tuberculosis but it can occur in humans. Like its subspecies *paratuberculosis*, it is of much lower pathogenicity (virulence) than *Mycobacterium tuberculosis* and causes disease only in immunocompromised people. Inflammatory disease caused by *Mycobacterium avium* is seen relatively frequently in patients with AIDS, and it is here that treatment regimes have been developed, with a combination of the anti-microbial medications rifabutin and clarithromycin. Following its success in AIDS sufferers, it has been used for the treatment of Crohn's disease, pioneered by John Hermon-Taylor but also by others, and I have used it quite extensively in my clinical practice. About 50% of sufferers respond well to a prolonged course that might extend over a few years. The bacterium grows only very slowly, and eradication can never be assured.

Most illnesses that we have looked at have a maximal incidence in the winter, at a time when vitamin D synthesis is at its lowest and when a body's reserves will have become exhausted. The same phenomenon applies to Crohn's disease. A study from Vancouver Hospital, Canada, looked at 592 relapses of Crohn's disease during a total of 10 693 months of follow-up of 193 patients [24]. The highest relapse rate occurred in January and the lowest rates were in the summer. The authors commented that 'The cause of the peak is unknown, however, seasonal or exogenous factors may be involved'. The role of sunlight was not mentioned.

Crohn's disease is almost certainly caused by a micro-organism, probably MAP. Susceptibility is a result of poor immunocompetence resulting from vitamin D insufficiency or the inheritance of VDR polymorphisms. The tissue destruction has great similarities to a malignant process and TNF-$\alpha$ produced by macrophages plays a key role.

I have indicated that Crohn's disease is similar to several other conditions that we have encountered in that it is a chronic inflammatory disease. It has often been classified as auto-immune, meaning that the inflammatory process continues over many years rather than becoming completed with resolution of the disease. I have also indicated that susceptibility to

Crohn's disease, as with coronary heart disease and other conditions, is the result of an inadequate immune response. This can have a variety of reasons but I have emphasised the importance of vitamin D insufficiency, vitamin D being essential for full immune competence.

This understanding of the fundamental basis of Crohn's disease is given strong support by an extremely interesting and detailed study undertaken by Professor Anthony Segal and colleagues at the Department of Medicine, University College, London, UK, published in *The Lancet* in 2006 [25]. A series of experiments performed on a small number of patients with Crohn's disease indicated defective acute inflammation in the rectum, ileum and skin, compared with reactions in healthy individuals. This was demonstrated by poor accumulation of neutrophils (white cells) at sites of injury. The study also identified defective macrophage function and we have seen how this is important in the inflammatory response and how vitamin D has a positive effect on the macrophage.

Segal and colleagues indicated that the cause of Crohn's disease is not known with any conclusion, meaning that it is not known with certainty. They generally support the microbial hypothesis but they suggest that, rather than a specific micro-organism, the cause might be the total bacterial load within the caecum, which overwhelms the body defences of susceptible individuals. This would lead to Crohn's disease, which would be particularly likely to occur at this site. This is similar to the 'dirty chicken' hypothesis in respect of coronary heart disease [26], again accepting a microbial cause but as a large bacterial load rather than a specific micro-organism. However, the transmission of Crohn's disease that we have seen would suggest a specific micro-organism, even if not yet identified with certainty.

The defective immune response identified by Segal and colleagues appears to be in part, but by no means totally, the result of specific and identifiable genetic factors with an inheritance of the impaired immune response. Unfortunately the study did not investigate vitamin D status nor, in particular, vitamin D polymorphism, which we have already seen has a major influence on susceptibility to Crohn's disease. The important message of the paper is that it is important to separate susceptibility from cause. Even if the cause cannot be identified, certain susceptibility factors can be identified at the molecular level and hopefully influenced by treatment. Furthermore, the study confirms that impaired immunity is a major factor in the development of Crohn's disease.

Segal and colleagues indicate that present-day treatments are designed to suppress the inflammatory response, which reduces the clinical manifestations of the disease, but this approach cannot be expected to cure it. If we are looking for curative treatment, then we must look for something that stimulates the immune response rather than suppresses it. We cannot at present reverse genetic factors but we can certainly reverse the acquired impairment of immune activity that results from insufficiency of vitamin D, hence the beneficial effect of fish oils. Heliotherapy in Crohn's disease has not yet been attempted but we have seen that there is an advantage to living in Greece rather than in north-west Europe.

A further attempt to understand Crohn's disease appeared as a review paper early in 2007, and once again looked at defective immunity, especially genetically determined processes [27]. There was no mention of vitamin D as important in immunity, and no report of the high prevalence of VDR mutations in Crohn's disease. The value and role of vitamin D in human health is seriously unrecognised.

I have given a lot of attention to Crohn's disease as it a major part of my clinical work. It is interesting because it is a disease without an accepted cause, much like tuberculosis and syphilis were in the mid-19th century. The standard of debate is hampered by the limitations of microbial technology, an intrinsic inability to apply Koch's postulates, and a poor understanding of the concept of proof. It involves complex inflammatory pathways that are incompletely understood, but most of all it is vitamin D dependent and this is generally not acknowledged.

# 65

# THE SUN, VITAMIN D AND DISEASES OF THE NERVOUS SYSTEM

In recent years there has been a great deal of interest in seasonal affective disorder (SAD). Most people appear to be unhappy or depressed during the winter months which, it could be said, is hardly surprising. The short days and long nights, the almost constant grey skies and frequent rain characterise the winter of the British Isles in particular. The associated low mood is generally accepted and is assumed to be psychological. But if seasonal affective disorder is real, could it perhaps be mediated by low vitamin D synthesis in the winter? We have noted that vitamin D as calcitriol has widespread effects on metabolism. It is possible that certain brain functions might also be vitamin D dependent but this does not appear to have been the subject of detailed research.

A clue, however, lies in schizophrenia, the development of which is related to prenatal factors; it is well-recognised that a child born in the winter and spring is more likely to develop schizophrenia than a child born in the autumn [1]. This observation is noted in Europe and Australia but not in Singapore, a location on the equator that has no seasons [2].

We cannot be certain of the reason for this, although the suggestion has been made that it is the result of the effects of maternal influenza during the winter. This could damage the brain of the developing foetus, especially in city-dwellers and the socio-economically deprived, who are particularly at risk of both influenza and schizophrenia [3].

Whether or not this suggestion is true, it shows that thinking is taking place concerning the possibility of micro-organisms causing chronic and disabling neurological disease. Such thoughts were prompted by the mysterious appearance of the disabling conditions encephalitis lethargica and post-encephalitic Parkinson's disease that followed immediately after the 1918 pandemic of influenza and are thought to be a result of it [4,5].

It has also been suggested that Borna disease virus might be responsible for human depression and other mental illnesses [6]. Borna is a town close to Leipzig in Germany, where 2000 horses of the Prussian cavalry died in 1885 in a mysterious epidemic. The disease has recently been recognised as being caused by a virus that now bears the name of the town. A review of the relationship between Borna disease virus and human neurological disease appeared in the *Quarterly Journal of Medicine*; the overall opinion is that the link remains controversial without a consistent association [7].

Depression is associated with the metabolic syndrome that we looked at in Chapter 57. A study from Finland has found a positive correlation between depression and insulin resistance; patients with more severe depression had greater levels of insulin resistance, whether or not diabetes had been diagnosed [8]. This suggests a metabolic connection; perhaps like SAD it is linked by vitamin D insufficiency, rather than the explanation being psychological.

However, although chronic brain disorders could be caused by viruses acquired during gestation or after birth, the relationship between schizophrenia and birth in the spring conforms to the maternal factor that we have already seen. Gestation during the summer months enables the developing foetus to acquire adequate vitamin D, which is essential for development of the brain. Gestation during the winter means that the baby acquires insufficient vitamin D from its mother before birth; vitamin D stores in the mother reach a minimum in April, the month in which vitamin D synthesis can begin in temperate latitudes. Low amounts of vitamin D transferred to the foetus might have a detrimental effect on subsequent brain development and function. There is recent concern that a baby born at less than 25 weeks gestation and surviving has a high risk of poor brain development [9]. Perhaps this could be the result of insufficient supplies of vitamin D.

We have seen that the excess of respiratory infections in the winter is the result of vitamin D insufficiency, and the question is whether this has a direct or indirect effect in creating susceptibility to schizophrenia. The alternative models are shown in Figure 65.1.

**Figure 65.1 Models of the relationship between vitamin D and schizophrenia.**

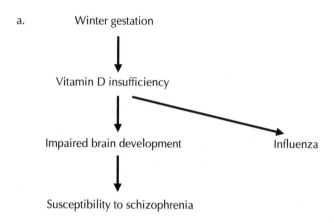

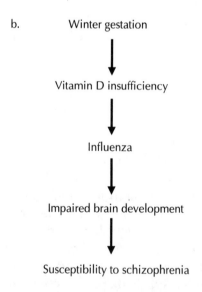

In both of these models, the factor linking winter gestation and spring birth with excess risk of schizophrenia is vitamin D insufficiency, and here must be an opportunity for preventative measures. We know that vitamin D has a beneficial effect on brain development and I would suggest that model (a) is more likely to be correct, and influenza need not be on the causative pathway.

A direct link between vitamin D insufficiency and schizophrenia is suggested by schizophrenia being more common in Afro-Caribbean people in the UK, a fact that has never been satisfactorily explained. Although this is a very complex topic concerning the interactions of biology, culture and upbringing, it has probably not been suggested that a contributing factor could be vitamin D insufficiency resulting from skin pigmentation.

Several observations suggest that multiple sclerosis might be vitamin D sensitive, including its geography, which is very similar to that of coronary heart disease. Multiple sclerosis is a rare disease but especially so in communities that live close to the equator. The world's highest incidence is in north-west Europe, especially in Scotland and particularly in Orkney and Shetland; this observation has led to the suggestion of a latitude effect, which is most obvious in high prevalence areas such as Europe [10]. An increased susceptibility to multiple sclerosis in locations such as Europe north of the Alps, with relatively little sunlight, is suggestive of a protective effect from vitamin D, as we have seen with other diseases.

Then there is seasonality. It has been reported that the incidence of multiple sclerosis is highest in the winter, once again suggesting protection by the sun and vitamin D [11]. A meta-analysis undertaken in Sweden by pooling data from previous studies indicated that the incidence of multiple sclerosis is highest in the spring. This is similar to the findings in tuberculosis that we saw earlier. It is interpreted as vitamin D dependent, the body stores being maximal in early winter as the result of the summer sun but exhausted by the spring before significant vitamin D synthesis has re-started.

The seasonal variation of activity of disease has also been demonstrated with magnetic resonance imaging (MRI), a modality that has been of value in helping the understanding and diagnosis of multiple sclerosis [12]. In this study from Amsterdam, the Netherlands, there were clear seasonal fluctuations in the size of the lesions within the brain (called plaques), which were larger in the winter. There was no seasonal variation in the number of plaques. The authors observed a corresponding seasonal variation of cellular inflammatory markers and they believed that these findings represented an environmental trigger to the disease, obviously one that is related to season.

I mentioned in Chapter 59 that particulate atmospheric pollution blocks ultraviolet radiation, reduces vitamin D synthesis and thereby increases susceptibility of the population to coronary heart disease in particular. It is noted in a study from Finland that the risk of relapse of multiple sclerosis increases four-fold at times when particulate air pollution is highest [13].

The authors suggest that the mediation is by increasing susceptibility to transmissible infections, a possibility that we will consider shortly.

A study from Tasmania looked at links between sun exposure and multiple sclerosis in the following way. They investigated 136 patients with multiple sclerosis and 272 matched community controls, assessing exposure to the sun when aged between 6 and 15 years. They found that with summer sun exposure averaging 2–3 hours or more per day there was a decreased risk of multiple sclerosis, at only 31% of those without such sun exposure [14].

A long-term study of nurses has been undertaken in Harvard, USA; 92 253 were followed-up between 1980 and 2000 and 95 310 between 1991 and 2001 [15]. During follow-up, 173 developed multiple sclerosis. At entry into the study a careful diet history was taken for each nurse and was updated at regular intervals. Based on this the subjects were grouped into five groups according to their vitamin D intake. The relative risk of developing multiple sclerosis in the quintile with the highest intake was only two-thirds that of the lowest quintile (Figure 65.2).

**Figure 65.2  Relative risk of developing multiple sclerosis [15].**

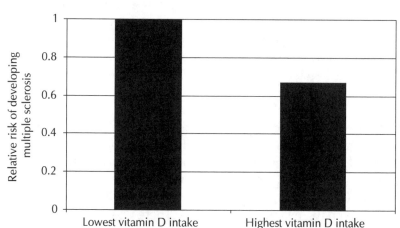

This part of the study supported a protective role of vitamin D against the risk of developing multiple sclerosis, something that does not appear to have been widely publicised. The study also recorded the nurses who were taking vitamin D supplements, but this would be on their own initiative rather than part of a clinical experimental trial. Those taking a supplement of vitamin D of 400 international units (IU) per day had just over half the incidence of multiple sclerosis compared with those taking no supplement (Figure 65.3).

**Figure 65.3  Relative risk of developing multiple sclerosis with vitamin D supplement [15].**

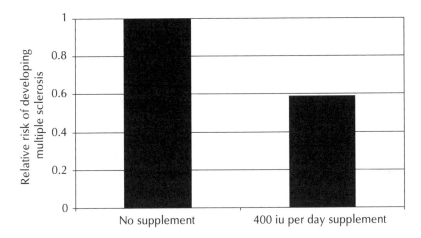

A more recent study from the USA investigated more than 7 million US military personnel, who had had blood samples stored when on active duty [16]. These samples were analysed for vitamin D as calcidiol and the incidence of subsequent multiple sclerosis recorded. The subjects were divided into quartiles in respect of blood vitamin D levels. It can be seen in Figure 65.4 that those with the lowest levels of vitamin D had the highest incidence of multiple sclerosis, and those in the highest quartile had the lowest incidence. This applied only to those with white skin. The subjects with black skin had overall significantly lower blood levels of vitamin D but no variation in incidence of multiple sclerosis. The vitamin D levels were probably not high enough to offer protection.

**Figure 65.4 Vitamin D and risk of multiple sclerosis [16].**

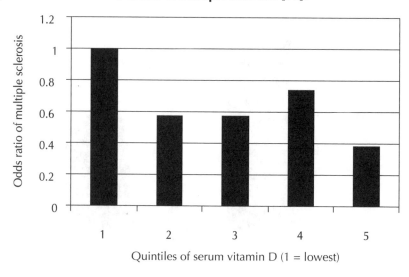

Quintiles of serum vitamin D (1 = lowest)

Important evidence suggesting a role of vitamin D in protection against multiple sclerosis comes from observations linking month of birth with risk of developing the disease [17]. The study indicates that birth in November leads to the lowest risk and birth in May leads to the highest risk, shown in Figure 65.5, which also shows the months in which vitamin D is synthesised at these latitudes. The study is based on pooled data from Canada, UK, Denmark and Sweden, involving a total of 45 045 people with multiple sclerosis.

**Figure 65.5 Vitamin D and risk of multiple sclerosis [17].**

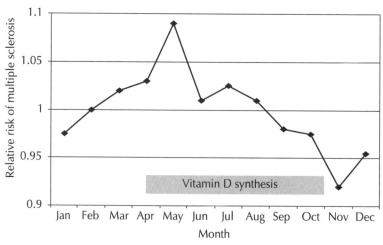

*Adapted with permission from the British Medical Journal Publishing Group*

Obviously a birth in April follows a winter gestation and a birth in November follows a summer gestation. The pattern with multiple sclerosis is a very similar to that we noted with schizophrenia, and we have also seen the same pattern of month of birth determining the risk of developing diabetes. The interpretation must lie in a general feature of seasonal variation and not in the specifics of multiple sclerosis or other diseases. The main way in which season interacts with human metabolism is through sun exposure and vitamin D synthesis.

The influence of season of birth on risk of multiple sclerosis was shown in an earlier study from the USA, which also showed a similar pattern for Alzheimer's disease, amyotrophic lateral sclerosis (motor neurone disease), epilepsy, cerebral palsy, mental retardation and congenital malformations of the central nervous system. The risk of development of epilepsy appeared to have the most consistent pattern, with a particularly low risk following birth in September, with multiple sclerosis and motor neurone disease showing an excess of births in the spring [18]. These observations emphasise the importance of vitamin D in development of the brain, in addition to the immune system and the skeleton.

Transmission of vitamin D from mother to foetus is maximal during the summer months, hence the better outcome of birth in September, October and November. This indicates a maternal factor, seen in coronary heart disease and in the metabolic syndrome. It is also seen in multiple sclerosis, identified through an increased risk for siblings who shared a mother compared with those who shared a father (Figure 65.6) [19,20].

**Figure 65.6  Risk of developing multiple sclerosis [19].**

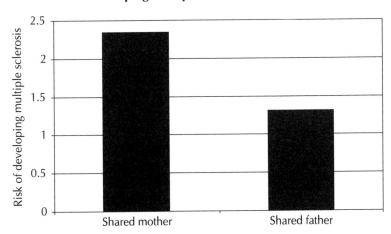

© 2004, adapted from The Lancet with permission from Elsevier.

The point is that a genetic disease would receive an equal contribution from mother and father; an excess inheritance from the mother usually indicates non-genetic inheritance, the maternal factor. An exception to this rule is the inheritance of mitochondrial disorders. Mitochondria are the energy-producing structures within the cell, found outside the nucleus and thus in the cytoplasm. All cytoplasm is inherited from the mother, including the mitochondria and the DNA that they contain. However, it has recently been noted that spermatozoa contain a tiny component of mitochondria that can be passed to the child and there is a single case report of this transmitting inherited disease [21]. Mitochondrial disorders are rare but inheritance by the maternal route is a very important feature.

The family clustering of multiple sclerosis has been recognised for many years, but whether this is caused by genetic or environmental factors has remained uncertain. This study [21] indicates a maternal factor that in theory could be mitochondrial inheritance but could also be the result of intra-uterine factors. The additional evidence of seasonality points towards the latter and suggests protection by vitamin D.

The cause of multiple sclerosis is not known. Conventional wisdom calls it an auto-immune disease, meaning that immune phenomena (and thereby inflammation) form a major part of the disease process. However, auto-immunity can only be a mechanism and not a cause and so understanding is obviously very limited. One of the problems is the inaccessibility of the central nervous system for biopsy specimens to improve understanding.

The inflammatory nature of multiple sclerosis, its seasonality and geography and the presence of a maternal factor indicate a model similar to that of coronary heart disease. It also shows clustering in isolated communities, suggesting an environmental cause that could be a micro-organism. The highest incidence in the world at present, as the result of a local epidemic, is in the villages of Kirkholm and Leswalt on the western shore of Loch Ryan in south-west Scotland. The local population has concerns about the cause being the presence of tributyltin, a chemical previously used in the protection of ships' hulls, but there are no suggestions from elsewhere of this having a part to play in the development of multiple sclerosis [22].

There have been several epidemics of multiple sclerosis in the isolated community of 45 000 people living in the Faeroe Islands, in the North Atlantic Ocean. Multiple sclerosis was unknown there until the first epidemic of 21 cases in 1943, and there have been subsequent epidemics of 10, 10 and 13 cases. At 62° north of the equator, the location makes the population highly susceptibility to multiple sclerosis, but the trigger factor is thought to be the introduction of an unknown micro-organism into the population by British troops who occupied the islands in 1941 [23].

Like coronary heart disease, the onset of clinical manifestations of multiple sclerosis is often preceded by respiratory infections, more frequently than would be expected by chance. This has led Subramaniam Sriram and colleagues at Vanderbilt University, Tennessee, USA, to focus on *Chlamydia pneumoniae*. They identified *Chlamydia pneumoniae* in the cerebrospinal fluid (CSF) in 64% of 37 patients with multiple sclerosis but in only 11% of controls [24]. When DNA testing was used, 97% of the patients with multiple sclerosis showed a positive result compared with 18% of controls.

An increased incidence of preceding glandular fever has led to the investigation of the Epstein–Barr virus (also the cause of Burkitt's lymphoma), but with no overall conclusion [25]. There is also the suggestion that multiple sclerosis might be cause by a spirochaete (as syphilis is) that gains entry to the brain through the sphenoidal sinus, behind the nose [26]. Such ideas are important but at present inconclusive.

Many other people have looked for a causative micro-organism but none has been found consistently. Another recent example has been a retrovirus detected in the blood in all patients with multiple sclerosis in Sardinia but only rarely in healthy blood donors who acted as controls [27]. However, there is no general agreement and at present no therapeutic antiviral treatment.

The recognition of multiple sclerosis being driven by an inflammatory process, and parallels with coronary heart disease, has led to the successful use of statin drugs for its treatment. In a multi-centre study in the USA, 30 patients with remitting–relapsing multiple sclerosis were treated with simvastatin in a high dose of 80 mg daily for 6 months [28]. There was a considerable improvement shown by MRI scans, with a 44% reduction in the number of brain lesions and a 41% reduction in their total size (volume). As with coronary heart disease, the benefit is independent of effects on cholesterol, and the precise mechanisms of the action of statin drugs in the inflammatory process need to be clarified. The authors suggest that statins induce the T-helper (inflammatory) cells produce anti-inflammatory rather than pro-inflammatory enzymes (cytokines). This is interesting because vitamin D also influences T-lymphocyte function.

There is a preventative opportunity to reduce susceptibility to multiple sclerosis by vitamin D supplements or increasing exposure to the sun, but this requires a public health initiative that acknowledges the importance of the sun in human health. At the present time this is not possible: public health information tells us that the sun is dangerous and that sun exposure must be avoided. Where does such an idea come from and is it true?

# 66

# RHEUMATIC AND
# AUTO-IMMUNE DISORDERS

There has been a long tradition of an illness called rheumatism, ill-defined in pathological terms but self-diagnosed by the population with quite a high level of confidence. It implies muscular pains in various parts of the body, with minor rather than major disability and a nuisance rather than a danger. It has characteristically been a feature of middle age onwards, in the poor rather than the rich and in those with unsatisfactory and usually damp housing. There is a feeling that it has been more common in the north of England than the south and that it is worse in the winter than the summer, particularly when there is wet weather, meaning not only rain and damp but also low atmospheric pressure, cloud cover and an absence of sunshine. Exposure to the sun has always been thought to be helpful and fish oils have been taken as empirical treatment. We hear of it much less now than 50 years ago but there might have been a change of terminology. The patterns identified lead to at least a suspicion that sunlight and vitamin D might be protective but, in the absence of any pathological studies and clinical trials, this is obviously conjectural. It is possible that some sufferers of rheumatism had osteomalacia at a time when investigations were not as readily available as at present.

Rheumatic fever was common in the UK until about 50 years ago. It affects the joints, heart and kidneys, also with early skin manifestations, but the important feature is the initiating event of a streptococcal infection in the throat. It is possible that the decline of the condition has been the result of a mutation of the bacteria into a less virulent form, but the disease still occurs in poor countries. An alternative view is that a decline of the throat infection has been caused by widespread use of antibiotics, without the organism being able to mutate into resistant strains. Another view is that the immunocompetence of the population has improved, and I have suggested that this might be because of a combination of improved diet, more holidays abroad and a major reduction of atmospheric pollution, leading to increased exposure of the population to the sun.

There are still many types of musculoskeletal disorder and many of them can be viewed as degenerative, with joints wearing out under the repeated strain of extreme exercise, damage and excessive body weight. This applies particularly to the knees, hips and lumbar spine. There are, however, many inflammatory diseases of joints, various patterns of inflammatory polyarthritis.

The main inflammatory joint disease that we know is rheumatoid arthritis, a disease affecting a wide range of joints, most obviously the hands. It is a serious and very disabling inflammatory disease that can have manifestations in parts of the body other than the joints. In particular, it can be associated with disease of the skin, eyes and lungs.

The inflammatory aspects of the disease are shown by inflammatory markers in the blood, in particular elevated ESR and CRP. There are other manifestations of inflammatory activity, including an over-expression of cytokines derived from macrophages, including TNF-$\alpha$. There are also a number of positive tissue antibodies found in the blood, the main one of which is rheumatoid factor, which is positive in sero-positive rheumatoid arthritis and negative in sero-negative rheumatoid arthritis. These various factors are expressions of the disease and its activity, rather than causative.

An associated disease is lupus, also called systemic lupus erythematosus (SLE). This is a systemic disease, meaning that it affects a wide range of organs. In particular the arteries are inflamed and this can produce manifestations in, for example, the brain. The joints can be inflamed, as in rheumatoid arthritis, skin rashes occur and the most life-threatening aspect of the disease is glomerulonephritis (immune-mediated disease of the kidneys). Once again, the inflammatory markers ESR and CRP are elevated in the blood. The hallmark of the disease is the presence of anti-nuclear antibodies in the blood, and it is the presence of such antibodies that has led to lupus and related diseases being referred to as auto-immune.

Another rather more restricted variant of inflammatory joint disease is polymyalgia rheumatica (PMR), which is characterised by pain and stiffness around the shoulders and the hips in particular, with quite severe disability, occurring mainly in elderly people. The ESR is usually very high. An associated disease is temporal arteritis, an inflammatory disease of the arteries that manifests mainly in the head, causing headaches and possible loss of vision or stroke, following occlusion of important arteries. Temporal arteritis and polymyalgia rheumatica may co-exist and they appear to be associated.

A related disease is systemic sclerosis, in which various tissues of the body become hardened with a subsequent lack of mobility. It can affect the skin (scleroderma), particularly the fingertips and the mouth, but internal structures can also be affected. It is a disease affecting collagen, which makes up the supporting structure of the tissues. It is thought that the primary abnormality is in the small blood vessels and, in particular, the endothelium, the cells that line the blood vessels.

We can thus see a fairly wide spectrum of diseases that all have something in common but the causes of which are completely unknown. It is possible that the distinction between them is artificial but each is diagnosed on the basis of its own clinical pattern, rather than causation.

All these diseases are disabling but they do not tend to be fatal and therefore there are no good international studies demonstrating its geography. WHO almost always collects statistics only for fatal diseases; the rheumatic/auto-immune diseases are not included. There are, however, some indications that the conditions are more common in northern Europe and north America [1], suggesting a similar geographical pattern to the various ones that we have already seen. There is also evidence that rheumatoid arthritis, more common in women than men, reached a peak incidence in about 1970 and has been declining thereafter [2]. It thus has a similar time relationship as the epidemic of coronary heart disease.

The pathological process of coronary heart disease commences in the endothelium, the lining of the arteries, and it is suggested that at least scleroderma has the same basis. There is also evidence from Sweden and Canada that malignancy is more common in patients with scleroderma than in the general population, about twice the incidence, particularly for lung cancer [3,4]. This indicates that there is probably a common susceptibility factor, and we have seen in the example of lung cancer that this is vitamin D insufficiency.

A study of 143 women with rheumatoid arthritis in Finland investigated the relationship between the disease and vitamin D [5]; 16% of the women had serum calcidiol concentrations below the limit at which vitamin D-deficient osteomalacia would be diagnosed. During the winter, 73% of the women had levels of calcitriol below the seasonally adjusted normal range and the lowest levels were in patients with a very active form of the disease. It became clear, therefore, that there was a disturbance in vitamin D metabolism in patients with rheumatoid arthritis, and the low levels of calcidiol in particular indicated a low intake or synthesis of vitamin D.

A study from the Friedrich-Schiller University of Jena, Germany, looked at various inflammatory markers in patients with rheumatoid arthritis, including CRP, ESR and three interleukins (cytokines) [6]. The markers were all negatively associated with blood levels of vitamin D, measured as both calcidiol and calcitriol. In other words, the lower the level of vitamin D, the higher the level of inflammatory markers and vice versa. This could be interpreted as vitamin D having a suppressant effect on rheumatoid arthritis, but in this study there was no time sequence that would have made this more clear. The alternative view, and the one taken by the authors of the paper, is that the inflammatory component of rheumatoid arthritis 'down-regulated' vitamin D. By this, they mean that the inflammatory process suppresses calcidiol in an undetermined way and also suppresses its conversion into calcitriol. The purpose of the study was to investigate the development of poor bone quality in patients with rheumatoid arthritis, and this was considered to be the result of low vitamin D levels in the blood. The message that we can take from the study is that vitamin D insufficiency is associated with greater inflammatory activity in rheumatoid arthritis.

The vitamin D insufficiency and rheumatoid arthritis association has been taken a stage further. A study from Budapest, Hungary, investigated the effect of vitamin D treatment in 19 patients already established as having rheumatoid arthritis and on standard therapy [7]. Vitamin D was given for 3 months as an additional treatment, in the form of the commercial preparation alpha-calcidiol, 2 mcg daily. Nine of the 19 patients reported a complete remission of symptoms and the effect was felt to be satisfactory in a further eight. Only two patients experienced no improvement. Inflammatory markers also improved. The average ESR dropped from 42 to 18 mm/h (a 43% reduction) and the average CRP from 11.07 to 5.8 mg/100 mL (52% reduction), as shown in Figure 66.1.

**Figure 66.1 The effect of vitamin D on inflammatory markers in rheumatoid arthritis [7].**

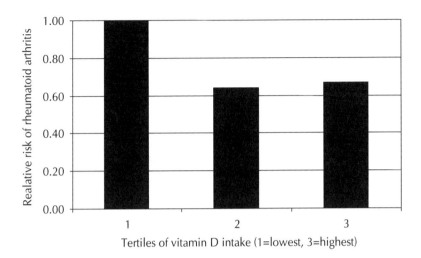

Tertiles of vitamin D intake (1=lowest, 3=highest)

These improvements were quite dramatic for a treatment for which untoward effects were neither expected nor experienced. The study was not randomised or controlled. It was what might be called a preliminary study, the sort that, if showing a benefit, would lead to a much larger randomised controlled trial. Such a clinical trial might be in progress at present but, if so, results have not yet been published.

There are thus indications that sunshine and vitamin D might be protective against rheumatoid arthritis and associated diseases. Much of the evidence from laboratory studies has been assembled by Margherita Cantora and Brett Mahon of the Pennsylvania State University, USA [8]. They have reviewed a great deal of research that has demonstrated a high level of inflammatory activity in rheumatoid arthritis and auto-immune diseases, particularly with over-active T lymphocytes. These inflammatory cells contain abundant VDRs and can be inhibited by sufficient amounts of vitamin D [9,10]. Anne-Louise Ponsonby and colleagues from the Royal Children's Hospital, Melbourne, Australia, have reviewed the epidemiological evidence indicating that ultraviolet radiation is protective against auto-immune diseases [11] and we have already seen much of this evidence.

We should not forget that atorvastatin has been shown to be beneficial in patients with rheumatoid arthritis [12]. This cannot be explained by conventional wisdom, but once again we can see a similarity between the protective effect of vitamin D and the protective effects of statin drugs.

We will explore this further in the final chapter.

We see once again the accumulation of evidence but the conservatism of the scientific community. The diseases are described in terms of pathological phenomena rather than cause, and that seems to be acceptable. It requires a certain pragmatism to move on to identify environmental trigger factors and protective factors. How much evidence is necessary to demonstrate a protective role for vitamin D for it to receive general acceptance?

Although these diseases have no identifiable cause, they are regarded as auto-immune disorders because of the inflammatory factors and the mediation of the disease seems to be through immune mechanisms. However, auto-immunity can only be a mechanism rather than a cause; it is never quite clear at what stage the immune manifestations occur in relation to the unknown trigger factor. 'Auto-immune diseases' often exhibit arteritis, an inflammatory process in the arteries, which can lead to closure of the arteries and infarction of tissue. Exactly the same thing occurs in coronary heart disease, except that the inflammatory process is not quite the same and it is associated with the accumulation of a great deal of cholesterol. Swelling is a characteristic part of an inflammatory reaction, and will inevitably produce what are called 'space-occupying effects' when in the brain (abscess, gumma, tuberculoma), and obstruction in a hollow organ, not only an artery but also the intestine in Crohn's disease and the throat in childhood tonsillitis.

Like so many diseases that we have looked at, there has long been a suggestion that rheumatoid arthritis might be caused by a micro-organism. The main one studied has been the Epstein–Barr virus, which also causes glandular fever and Burkitt's lymphoma, but no conclusion has been reached. However, the epidemiology and the clustering of cases of rheumatoid arthritis make a microbial causation attractive. It can be appreciated, therefore, that there are a lot of parallels between rheumatoid disorders and many other conditions that we have seen, and also the possibility of increased susceptibility in the presence of insufficiency of vitamin D.

# 67
# IS THE SUN DANGEROUS?

Much of what I have presented might come as a surprise: the message is that the sun is of immense benefit to human health, but we are repeatedly told through the media that the sun is dangerous and is to be avoided. The Cancer Research Council of the UK issues many public warnings that the sun is dangerous and that a major way to avoid cancer is to avoid the sun [1]. How is it that such apparently official advice is not supported by evidence and is in such contrast to the information presented in this book? In fact a Cancer Research Council UK publication [2] indicates that ultraviolet light is of very little importance in causing cancer in the UK, and this can be seen clearly in Figure 67.1. We have seen that there is good evidence that the sun protects against some of the major cancers, especially tobacco-induced lung cancer (see Chapter 40), but this was not considered.

**Figure 67.1 Environmental and behavioural factors and cancer in the UK [1].**

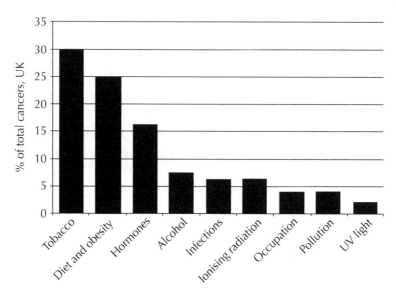

The nature of official information is a subject in itself but can perhaps be summarised in four ways. First, it is self-perpetuating, as even in the face of conflicting evidence few experts feel able to admit to being wrong. Second, experts increasingly become attracted into media posts and become detached from their research or academic base. Third, there is a huge industrial following behind ideas and, after considerable investment, a change of ideas would not be welcome. Fourth, a new feature is that official information becomes even more official by becoming part of government policy, controlled by people who inevitably have little idea of the truth. But the doubt must remain: is there evidence that the sun is as dangerous as public health announcements indicate?

Our skin is of great importance. We have seen its role as an endocrine organ, synthesising with the help of sunlight a pre-hormone called vitamin D or cholecalciferol. This is clearly vital to human health, but of course every solution creates its own problem. Do the disadvantages of sun exposure exceed the obvious advantages?

The immediate disadvantage of sunlight is sunburn, which is painful and unpleasant. It is also unnecessary; the sun must be treated with respect. The body has its own defence mechanisms in that skin synthesises the pigment melanin in response to sunlight. Melanin absorbs ultraviolet light and thereby prevents its penetration to deeper levels of the skin and prevents burn. This takes time, and so exposure of white skin to the sun should be a gradual process, allowing a tan to build up through melanin production. This happens automatically during the spring and early summer in outdoor workers but indoor workers must control their sun exposure carefully. We have seen the development of heliotherapy in alpine tuberculosis treatment centres. Sun exposure was prescribed very carefully, just like any other medical therapy, with exposure, extent and duration being increased gradually to prevent burning [3].

Artificial sun-blocks can be applied as creams, performing a similar function as melanin but reducing the production of melanin. There is a great deal of ignorance about such creams; when a sunny day is expected in the summer I hear on the radio advice to use 'suntan creams'. This is a misnomer: they should be called sun protection creams. The ideal is to reduce sun exposure to a minimum if this is possible and then increase the exposure time gradually as a tan develops. When this is not possible and when extreme sun exposure on a pale skin will be inevitable, sun-block creams will be essential to prevent burn. This will be important in exposed locations, especially on mountains, where the high altitude increases the amount of ultraviolet energy reaching the skin.

Evolution determined that fair-haired, pale-skinned people, a tiny minority of the world population, were confined to north-west Europe: Scandinavia, north Germany and the British Isles. The 20th century in particular has seen migrations of people to places where their skin colour is a disadvantage; white-skinned people may now live close to the equator in northern Australia, and dark-skinned people may live close to the Arctic in Scotland. We have seen the disadvantages of dark-skinned people living where the sun is low is the sky and where there is a great deal of cloud cover. What are the disadvantages of white-skinned people living close to the equator?

We are warned of skin cancer but again there is a great deal of ignorance. The term skin cancer is best avoided as it lumps together two entirely different conditions that must not be confused.

The most common cancers occurring on the skin are the basal cell and squamous cell carcinomas. These can be considered together and they occur on exposed parts of the skin, almost entirely on non-pigmented skin. It is accepted that the cause is sun acting on pale skin that has little protection by pigment, and they are seen almost exclusively on the face and scalp. They are much less common in people with genetically determined skin pigmentation and they are seen less often in people who acquire skin pigmentation as a tan. It is very interesting to note an observation made in the US Navy in the 1930s that sailors had an increased incidence of (non-melanoma) skin cancers but correspondingly a reduced incidence of internal cancers compared with population of the USA [4,5].

569

The dangers of cancer in general are in the ability of the tumour to invade across tissue planes into adjacent organs and to metastasise to distant locations. Basal cell and squamous cell carcinomas can invade locally, causing tissue destruction, but this is a slow process and the tumours can be removed easily when just a few millimetres in diameter. If they are allowed to become large the surgical removal must be more extensive, leaving an unsightly scar or needing plastic surgical repair. These cancers do not usually metastasise, although squamous cell carcinomas can do if left untreated. They affect almost entirely people older than 60 years and they are not life-threatening.

The other form of cancer affecting the skin is the malignant melanoma, a very different and very serious condition. It is not common, about 3000 new cases in the UK each year [6] and, even though treatment might initially appear successful, delayed death may occur because of the appearance of late metastases. It is often suggested that malignant melanoma is the result of damage done to the skin by the sun, but the evidence is far from clear [7].

Basal cell and squamous cell carcinomas occur on exposed parts of the skin, parts that might have been damaged by the sun. But this is not the pattern of malignant melanoma, most occurring on hidden parts of the skin. The distribution is shown in Table 67.1; it does not support a causative role for sunlight exposure.

**Table 67.1 Sites of malignant melanoma [6]**

|  | % |
| --- | --- |
| Leg | 45.1 |
| Trunk | 18.5 |
| Arm | 14.4 |
| Face | 11.6 |
| Scalp and neck | 3.9 |
| Ear | 1.2 |
| Eye and eyelid | 1.1 |
| Lip | 0.3 |
| Other | 3.9 |

*Crown © 1995, adapted with permission.*

We can see the effect of socio-economic deprivation expressing itself again in survival after the diagnosis of malignant melanoma. During 1981–85, the 5-year survival of the affluent was 13% greater than that of the poor [8]. The survival of all groups has been improved by chemotherapy and the advantage of the affluent has fallen to 8% since 1985. This is shown in Figure 67.2. Please note that this figure illustrates just the relative survivals of the two socio-economic groups at two different times: it does not compare in absolute terms one time period with another.

**Figure 67.2  Socio-economic status and survival from malignant melanoma [8].**

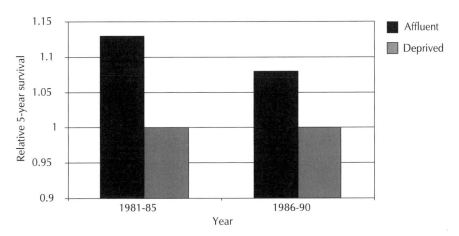

*Crown © 1999, adapted with permission.*

Fair skins are undoubtedly more susceptible to the development of malignant melanoma and there are indications that sunlight exposure might be significant, especially if there is a history of sunburn. Occasional or irregular exposure to the sun appears to increase risk whereas regular exposure to the sun appears to be protective: malignant melanoma is less common in outdoor workers than indoor workers [9]. This is suggested by a study of the incidence of malignant melanoma on various occupational groups in the US navy [10].

Although occasional sun exposure of the fair skin might increase risk, the distribution of malignant melanoma in Table 67.1 suggests that the effect might somehow be systemic, acting on the body in general, rather than local. Continual exposure to the sun appears to be protective and this is likely to be because of the development of pigmentation, a tan, and the anti-cancer properties of vitamin D that we have already seen.

There might be a balance in play, the damage from sun exposure being counteracted by vitamin D synthesis and melanin production. Thus just occasional sun exposure will tip the balance in favour of malignant melanoma whereas more frequent sun exposure will give protection.

Malignant melanoma is a relatively uncommon form of cancer in the UK, with just more than 3000 new cases per year [6]. In 1995, 697 men and 198 women died from this cancer and the risk is considered to be very low, at about 1 per 10 000 [11,12]. The relative risks of major cancers can be seen in Table 67.2 and Figure 67.3.

**Table 67.2  Cancers in England and Wales (annual mean 1986–91) [6]**

| | |
|---|---|
| Lung | 29 215 |
| Breast | 23 548 |
| Colon | 13 696 |
| Prostate | 10 382 |
| Bladder | 9864 |
| Rectum | 8878 |
| Stomach | 8717 |
| Non-Hodgkin's lymphoma | 4744 |
| Pancreas | 4563 |
| Ovary | 4248 |
| Oesophagus | 4146 |
| Cervix | 3822 |
| All leukaemias | 3551 |
| Uterus | 3302 |
| Melanoma of skin | 3188 |
| Kidney | 3034 |
| Brain | 2400 |
| Multiple myeloma | 2106 |
| Larynx | 1757 |
| Chronic lymphoid leukaemia | 1265 |
| Acute myeloid leukaemia | 1125 |
| Testis | 1116 |
| Hodgkin's disease | 1004 |
| Gall-bladder | 997 |
| Vagina and vulva | 932 |
| Connective tissue | 825 |
| Oral cavity | 739 |
| Liver | 733 |
| Thyroid | 717 |
| Pleura | 641 |
| Chronic myeloid leukaemia | 579 |
| Tongue | 556 |

**Table 67.2  Cancers in England and Wales (annual mean 1986–91) [6]**
*(Continued)*

| | |
|---|---:|
| Eye | 347 |
| Nasal cavities, sinuses | 342 |
| Bone | 326 |
| Oropharynx | 324 |
| Hypopharynx | 322 |
| Salivary glands | 309 |
| Small intestine | 298 |
| Penis | 265 |
| Lip | 229 |
| Acute lymphoid leukaemia | 224 |
| Nasopharynx | 155 |
| Adrenal | 65 |
| Monocytic leukaemia | 62 |
| Pituitary | 45 |
| Spinal cord | 39 |
| Thymus | 33 |
| All cancers | 156 520 |

*Crown © 1995, adapted with permission.*

# Figure 67.3 Cancers in adults in England and Wales, 1986–91 [6].

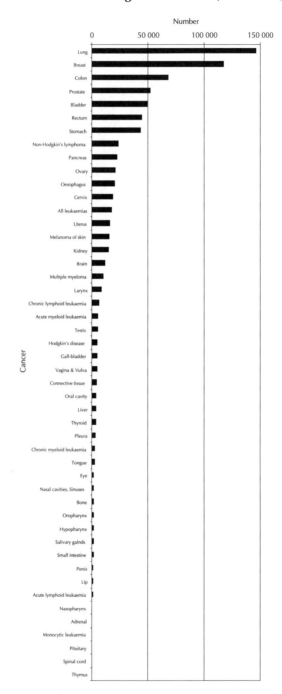

The incidence of malignant melanoma has increased in recent decades, particularly so in Queensland, Australia, which now has the highest incidence of malignant melanoma in the world. There is undoubtedly a very high level of sun exposure in this tropical location and there has been a public health initiative to control ultraviolet damage with the use of sunscreens and clothing. These are firmly part of public health policy in Australia. An interesting and thoughtful paper has recently been published by Johan Moan and colleagues from the Institute for Cancer Research and the Department of Physics, University of Oslo, Norway, and the Brookhaven National Laboratory, Upton, USA [13]. It addresses the 'controversy as to whether increased sun exposure to Western populations would prolong or shorten lifetime expectancy, result in fewer or more cancer deaths, and, in general, lead to health benefits or risks'. The authors noted that in Norway malignant melanoma rates increased by a factor of 6 between 1960 and 1990 while the prognosis improved during the same period (when chemotherapy had not advanced to its present standards). Since 1990, the incidence has remained constant and decreased in the age group <50 years but the prognosis has not improved further (despite advances in chemotherapy). They confirm the findings of others that the incidence of malignant melanoma is much higher in Australia and New Zealand than in Norway, Sweden, Denmark and the UK (Figure 67.4) but death rates are lower (Figure 67.5). We can see that the incidence of malignant melanoma in men in Australia is seven times that men in the UK but the death rate is half. The conclusion of the group is that 'increased sun exposure may lead to improved cancer prognosis and, possibly, give more positive that adverse health effects'. The cancer incidence data used by Moan and colleagues is taken from *Cancer Incidence in Five Continents* [14].

We must remember that incidence defined as the diagnosis rate is dependent on patient and doctor behaviour, whereas death is much more absolute and reliable. This is relevant when we look at changes in the apparent incidence of melanoma.

## Figure 67.4 Diagnosis rate of malignant melanoma [14]

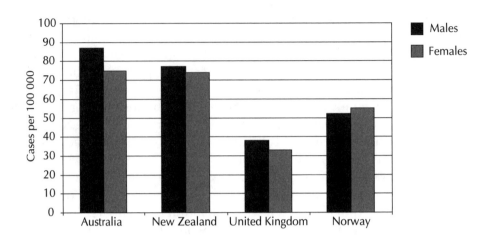

## Figure 67.5 Death rate from malignant melanoma [14]

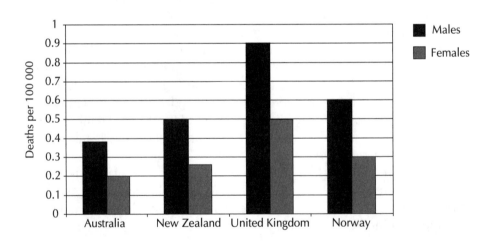

In Chapter 63 we saw the work of Grant, who studied the relationship of many cancers to ultraviolet light exposure at ground level. His observation was that, while several cancers had a lower death rate with high levels of ultraviolet light, there was no effect in respect of malignant melanoma [15]. It appears, therefore, that the sun might increase the incidence but at the same time reduce the chance of dying from melanoma.

The incidence of malignant melanoma in children and adolescents in Europe is not what might be expected: the highest incidence is in the UK, particularly in the north of the UK (Figure 67.6) [16]. This observation indicates that we must be open-minded about the relationship between the sun and malignant melanoma.

**Figure 67.6 Incidence of malignant melanoma in children and adolescents [16].**

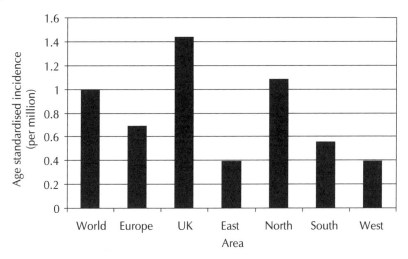

Although the reported incidence of malignant melanoma has increased by a factor of 2.5 during the past 15 years, the death rate has remained unchanged. This could indicate the excellence of current medical treatment, but some observers feel that this is not the only explanation. The biopsy rate of skin lesions suspected of being malignant melanoma has also increased by a factor of 2.5, leading to suspicions that the increased incidence is apparent rather than real [17]. The authors of this study remind us that there is a great deal of pressure on doctors, and dermatologists in particular, to diagnose malignant melanoma as early as possible, but early diagnosis is associated with a greater error rate. Erring on the side of caution, uncertainty by the pathologist will lead to a diagnosis a diagnosis of malignant melanoma, with removal of the lesion 'to be on the safe side'. The increase in incidence is of non-invasive lesions; until recently, when malignancy is in doubt a biopsy and removal may have been undertaken. The details can be seen in Figure 67.7, indicating that the incidence of late-stage cancer matches the mortality rate. Dermatologists used differentiate between benign melanoma and malignant melanoma. There is now a tendency to simply use the term 'melanoma', upgrading what would previously be considered to be benign and thereby increasing the incidence of what we consider to be malignant. This is an example how a change in the behaviour of doctors can have a significant impact on health statistics.

**Figure 67.7  Incidence of malignant melanoma [17].**

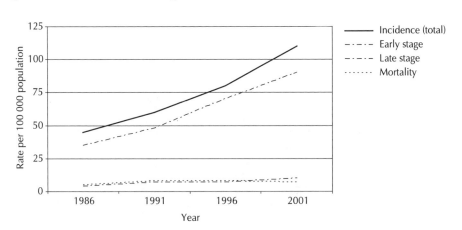

*Adapted with permission from the British Medical Journal Publishing Group.*

Vitamin D has been shown to have inhibitory effects on cell proliferation, and this provides laboratory support for the epidemiological evidence of its protective role against certain cancers. It has been shown to be true for malignant melanoma cells [18]. Sun-block creams probably reduce vitamin D synthesis in the skin and this might be a factor in the failure to prevent malignant melanoma [19].

Inflammation and malignancy are closely related, and protection against both processes appears to be provided by high levels of immunity. Although this can be a function of the sun and vitamin D, immuno-enhancement can be provided in another way that has been recognised for some time. A recent study from Germany and the UK demonstrated a reduced risk of malignant melanoma as a result of vaccination against smallpox with vaccinia or against tuberculosis with BCG, these immunisations stimulating immunity within the body [20]. The paper went on to review the possible role of retroviruses as a causative factor of malignant melanoma. There is thus a general model of a causative micro-organism, the development of inflammation and malignancy, and protection by immune-enhancing processes including immunisation and the sun.

Any damaging effect of the sun is clearly negligible compared with the benefits, but it is important to control exposure to the sun and avoid sunburn. Even so, the study of the protective effects of vitamin D against multiple sclerosis indicated that actinic change, non-malignant sun damage to the fair skin, was associated with a particularly low risk of the disease [21]. Dermatologists acknowledge one role for ultraviolet light, and that is as treatment for the skin disease psoriasis. Ultraviolet light treatment is now used extensively and effectively as PUVA treatment [22].

The SunSmart campaign in the UK is based on the public health campaign in Queensland, Australia. It has been reviewed critically in an excellent document 'Sunlight Robbery' [23], in which freelance medical researcher and writer Oliver Gillie, based in London, UK, claims that 'Health benefits of sunlight are denied by public health policy in the UK'. He emphasises that a sunlight policy in a tropical location at 27° south should not be transferred to the edge of the arctic at, for example, Aberdeen, 57° north.

Protection of the skin and the maintenance of a perfect and untanned white skin is the aim of SunSmart, driven by its dermatology advisers. The health benefits of the sun are not acknowledged and it is particularly sad that dermatologists, specialists in the skin, appear to have no regard for its important physiological functions. They see the skin as being a site of disease, and not an important and metabolically active organ that is able, with the help of the sun, to protect internal organs and minimise disease.

Oliver Gillie draws attention to the Consensus Statement by the UK Skin Cancer Prevention Working Party that 'There is no such thing as a healthy tan'. This is fed into the SunSmart campaign. It is clearly wrong and misleading: the tan is the way in which the body protects itself against the damaging effects of the sun, and it should be encouraged. After the health benefits of clean air and the historical recognition of the importance of ultraviolet light, it is both sad and worrying to see children today playing outside wearing hats and extensive clothing and smeared with total sun-block creams.

SunSmart appears to take the view that all the inhabitants of the UK are white, with delicate skins easily burned by the sun. It will have been apparent from the Prologue onwards that I have a particular concern with the extraordinary burden of illness and disease of the South Asian, African and Caribbean immigrants into the UK. I have identified the problems, and the evidence that these are mediated by vitamin D insufficiency is overwhelming. SunSmart pays no heed to the importance of sun exposure in those with pigmented skins, in the same way that it fails to recognise the importance of physiological skin pigmentation in those with pale skins.

The medical advice for SunSmart comes from the British Association of Dermatologists. This represents specialists in diseases of the skin who have no continuing experience of the many diseases to which susceptibility is increased by inadequate exposure to the sun. There is a great burden of illness and premature death in the UK that could be reduced by additional sunlight exposure, as long as caution is taken to avoid sunburn.

Perhaps this blinkered attitude of British dermatologists can be countered by the recently-published conclusion of a group from the USA [24]: *'The lowest quartile of 25(OH)D [calcidiol] level (<17.8ng/ml) is independently associated with all-cause mortality in the general population'.*

It is quite clear that all-cause deaths from all causes, coronary heart disease, cancer and infectious diseases are all higher for those with the lowest blood levels of vitamin D.

**Figure 67.8 Association between death rate and calcidiol level (sample size 31 331) [24]**

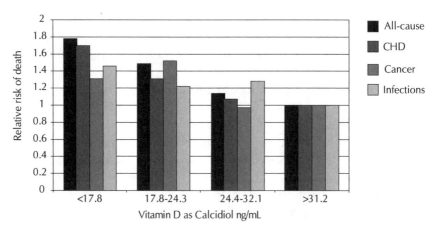

580

# PART 12

# EPILOGUE
# VITAMIN D AND STATINS

# 68
# VITAMIN D AND STATINS

The official line in the UK is that the influence of the sun on health is damaging, based on the SunSmart campaign with endorsement by the government, dermatologists and cancer prevention groups. We can see that the advice to avoid exposure to the sun is misguided and is totally the opposite of the Italian tradition, *dove non va il sole, va il medico* (where the sun does not go, the doctor goes). SunSmart appears to take the view that all the inhabitants of the UK are white, with delicate skins easily burned by the sun.

But the medical advice for SunSmart came from the British Association of Dermatologists. These specialists in diseases of the skin see only a small picture, just one piece of the puzzle that I have attempted to complete. They have no continuing experience of the many diseases to which susceptibility is increased by inadequate exposure to the sun. I hope that I have been able to paint a bigger and more complete picture, indicating that the sun through vitamin D is of great importance in maintaining human health.

There is a significant burden of illness and premature death in the UK that could be reduced by additional sunlight exposure. We have seen a number of diseases with a high incidence in the north-west of England, Scotland and Ireland compared with the south-east of England, in the British Isles compared with southern Europe, in the socio-economically deprived compared with the affluent, and in South Asians compared with the indigenous white-skinned population.

There is an opportunity to improve health by increasing the exposure of the UK population to the sun, in particular its vulnerable subgroups. But the feasibility of this is doubtful, especially if the official line is that the sun is dangerous. Much research needs to be undertaken and there is no reason why this should not happen. In reality, most of the research money in the UK provided by the government through the Medical Research Council funds research institutions. A great deal of money is provided by pharmaceutical companies as part of their research and development functions. As there would be no obvious commercial benefit, funding research into therapeutic sun exposure would need to be funded through the Medical Research Council, using government money as part of its public health responsibility.

An alternative to prescribed exposure to the sun would be vitamin D supplements by mouth or injection, and we have seen the effectiveness of these in the prevention of multiple sclerosis and the suppression of cancer. The problem is that the appropriate dose of vitamin D is not really known and prescribed doses tend to be cautious. The Chief Medical Officer of the National Health Service (NHS) acknowledged in his *Update* in the summer of 2005 that rickets is re-emerging in the UK [1]. He informs us that fair-skinned people should be able to obtain enough vitamin D from casual exposure to the sun but that this may not be the case in high-risk groups such as South Asian and African-Caribbean women and children and other groups who cover their skin extensively for cultural reasons. He continues:

*As a safety net, in order to avoid deficiency, the Committee on Medical Aspects of Food and Nutrition Policy and the Scientific Advisory Committee on Nutrition recommend dietary vitamin D supplements for pregnant and nursing mothers of 10 micrograms [400 units]/day and 7 micrograms [280 units]/day for children under five years of age. Vitamin D supplements of 10 micrograms [400 units]/day are also recommended for older people to maintain good bone health and to reduce the risk of fractures.*

This at least indicates that vitamin D is still regarded as important, but only in respect of bone disease: rickets and osteomalacia. It has been known since about 1980 that vitamin D has an action in the functioning of the immune system [2] but this is still not generally acknowledged. Although older people are encouraged by the Chief Medical Officer through his advisory committees to receive dietary supplements of vitamin D (not increased exposure to the sun), the purpose is to prevent bone fractures. The vast majority of bone fractures in elderly people are caused by osteoporosis, a lack of osteoid, and not a failure of the ossification process that is controlled by vitamin D. It has been determined recently that vitamin D is of benefit in the prevention of bone fractures only when (rarely) there is osteomalacia. It is not effective in osteoporosis [3].

There is a danger of too much vitamin D (hypervitaminosis D) in people who inadvertently receive excessive dietary supplements, especially in people with poor exposure to sunlight. It is not possible to develop hypervitaminosis D from exposure to the sun. The ideal level of vitamin D in the blood is above 30 ng/mL. A level below 10 is likely to result in bone disease, osteomalacia or rickets but it is thought that above 30 ng/mL is necessary for the full health benefit of vitamin D [4].

The ideal health promotion measure would be to improve the climate of the UK, or improve the wealth of the poorest members of society to allow them to have better houses, better access to the outdoors and holidays in the sun. Neither is plausible. Alternatively, and for South Asians in particular, there would need to be diet supplements of vitamin D, as cultural behaviour is unlikely to change. The major problem facing those who advise vitamin D supplements is how to manage the possible development of too much vitamin D without continual blood monitoring. There has been an effort to develop variations of the vitamin D molecule to enable vitamin D activity without producing hypercalcaemia [5]. Perhaps this is an example of 'pharmacophobia', the fear of medications leading to people not being appropriately treated. The size of the problem of hypervitaminosis D should not be exaggerated: it is exceptionally rare. We must not forget that hypervitaminosis does not occur with adequate exposure to the sun. In this respect a dietary/pharmaceutical approach to vitamin D supplementation must be considered to be of secondary importance to increasing exposure to the sun, even for immigrant groups with inherited skin pigmentation. However, pharmaceutical companies in particular have been searching for a compound that acts like vitamin D but without the effects on calcium metabolism, and many possibilities have emerged. A thorough and very technically detailed review has been provided by Sunil Nagpal and colleagues from Eli Lilly [5]. It illustrates a wide range of molecules that activate vitamin D receptors without having undesirable effects. It is possible that a different one has been found by accident.

The primary metabolic role of vitamin D is bone development; the primary metabolic role of statins is the reduction of serum cholesterol concentration. Both have other effects discovered subsequently. These secondary effects are in fact of great importance, and in the case of statins it would appear that the primary role of cholesterol reduction is of the least importance. As we touched upon in Chapter 28, statins also have an unexpected beneficial effect on bone. A long-term study of post-menopausal osteoporosis in 1003 women in Chingford, UK, found that the 31 who were taking statins had a greater bone density than comparable women not taking statins [6]. Bone histology was not part of the study and so we do not know the precise effect of the statins, whether it was correcting undetected osteomalacia or improving osteoporosis. More research is necessary and no doubt is in progress.

The interesting and most exciting phenomenon is that vitamin D and statins appear to share several functions: they are of benefit in coronary heart disease, in the very short term as well as in the long term; they both have an action in the prevention of diabetes; they both reduce the incidence of colorectal cancer; they both benefit multiple sclerosis; they both benefit rheumatoid arthritis; they both have an immune-enhancing function. Although vitamin D has a preventative effect on breast cancer and relapses of Crohn's disease, we do not yet know whether statins also have these effects.

Two further beneficial effects of statin therapy were added at the end of 2005. It was reported to the meeting of the American Heart Association in Dallas, Texas, USA, that pravastatin increases the production of stem cells in heart muscle [7]. Stem cells are the fundamental cells of the body and they can differentiate into a variety of specialised cells; this is how the embryo develops. The study (from the University of Buffalo, New York, USA) also demonstrated that pravastatin promoted the differentiation of stem cells into heart muscle cells (myocytes). The clinical benefit was an improvement in the function of the heart and an improvement of blood flow within the coronary arteries. This is clearly a finding of great importance, albeit in an animal model.

There is a similar effect from vitamin D, but not an exact parallel; the appropriate research has almost certainly not been undertaken. We saw in Chapter 38 (Figure 38.12) that low levels of vitamin D are found in patients with poor heart function [8]. We have also seen that an important part of tissue repair is the activity of metaloproteinases, and these are dependent on vitamin D activity. It appears that both statins and vitamin D have an important role in the repair and restoration of damaged tissue.

2006 saw the publication of an important clinical experiment involving the treatment of 108 patients known to have heart failure because of conditions other than coronary heart disease [9]. Half were randomised to receive atorvastatin 20 mg per day and the others were controls receiving a placebo. As judged by echocardiography appearances, the ejection fraction (a measure of the strength of the heart muscle) improved in the treated group but not in the placebo group (Figure 68.1) [9]. There was also a reduction of TNF in those treated with atorvastatin (24.3 versus 34.5 in controls) and these findings are in keeping with the beneficial effects of vitamin D.

**Figure 68.1 Effect of atorvastatin in heart failure [9].**

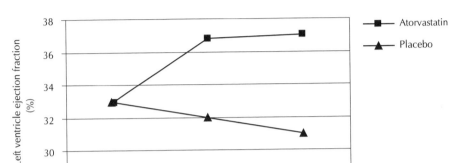

Later in 2006 there was a report of 24 598 adults diagnosed with heart failure [10]. During an average of 2.4 years of follow-up, those who received statin therapy had an obvious advantage, with a mortality of 14.5 per 100 person years, age adjusted, compared with 25.3 in those not receiving statins [10]. The admission rate to hospital for heart failure was 21.9 in those receiving statin therapy compared with 31.1 in those without statins (once again rate per 100 person years, age adjusted). The benefit of statins in heart failure is clear, but statins are still regarded as a treatment of high blood cholesterol.

The *New Scientist* reported on 12 November 2005 that 'It just gets better … Is there anything that statins can't do?' [11]. The story was that Alcino Silva and colleagues from the University of California, Los Angeles, USA, were investigating the inherited disease neurofibromatosis type 1 [12]. It is caused by a mutation of the *NF1* gene and one of the clinical features is learning difficulties. The same mutation can occur in mice, so there is an animal model for research. The study reported that the learning-related behaviour of mice with this mutation improved by 30% when they were given lovastatin. We thus see an affect of statins on brain function and perhaps development. We have already seen that sunshine and vitamin D have such an effect.

It was recognised early on that children with rickets are sickly and prone to infections. This was the first clue to the immune-enhancing effects of vitamin D. We have seen that respiratory infections in particular are more likely to occur in the winter, and this is explained by a reduction in vitamin D synthesis. Research published early in 2006 indicated that, in a study of 173 410 patients aged more than 65 years with cardiovascular disease, those who received statin therapy had a lower rate of infections during follow-up of more than 2 years [13]. The rate was 71.2 infection events per 10 000 person years in the treatment group compared with 88 in the controls. This is another example of the similarities of action of statins and vitamin D. It is also a further example of the paradoxical effect of statins: they reduce serum cholesterol but we have also seen that high serum cholesterol is associated with a reduced risk of infection. The cholesterol-lowering effect of statins is irrelevant to their widespread benefits.

In early 2007 it was reported from a meta-analysis that statins lower blood pressure, like other effects this being independent of serum cholesterol changes [14]. We have already seen that blood pressure is lower in the winter and this is presumably the result of less vitamin D synthesis [15]. The list of comparable effects of vitamin D and statins is shown in Table 68.1.

**Table 68.1 The effects of vitamin D and statins**

|                        | Vitamin D  | Statins    |
| ---------------------- | ---------- | ---------- |
| Bone                   | Active     | Active     |
| Cholesterol            | Active     | Active     |
| Coronary heart disease | Active     | Active     |
| Diabetes               | Active     | Active     |
| Colorectal cancer      | Active     | Active     |
| Breast cancer          | Active     | Not known  |
| Lung cancer            | Active     | Active     |
| Multiple sclerosis     | Active     | Active     |
| Crohn's disease        | Active     | Not known  |
| Transplantation        | Not known  | Active     |
| Fertilisation success  | Active     | Not known  |
| Rheumatoid arthritis   | Active     | Active     |
| Tissue repair          | Active     | Active     |
| Heart failure          | Active     | Active     |
| Brain development      | Active     | Active     |
| Immunomodulating       | Active     | Active     |
| Infection control      | Active     | Active     |
| Hypertension           | Active     | Active     |

We have some understanding of vitamin D activity through the identification of vitamin D receptors, but we have little understanding of the various actions of statins, other than the HMG-coenzyme A reductase action that blocks cholesterol synthesis (see Chapter 27). The benefits of statin therapy have been noted only recently and extended research has barely begun.

We become accustomed to medications having undesirable side-effects, and pharmaceutical companies undertake a great deal of pre-launch research and post-marketing surveillance with a view to minimising danger to the population. What we are certainly not accustomed to is unexpected benefits of medications, and in particular the many benefits of statin therapy. In the various actions, for example the anti-infection effect [11], the prevention of colorectal cancer [16] and the Israel cancer paradox [17], statins must be switching on a defensive function, probably in cells involved in immune and inflammatory processes. This must be via the activation of cellular receptors setting in progress a cascade of intracellular and extracellular effects. In other words statins have a vitamin-like effect, either a new and previously unsuspected vitamin or an existing vitamin.

Because of the similarity of actions, it is most likely that at least some of the benefits of statins, if not all, are mediated through activation of vitamin D receptors in certain cells. In other words statins are vitamin D analogues, molecules with a different structure but having the same function and activating the same receptors.

This is obviously speculative, but research must start with the identification of an anomaly or a paradox, following which speculation must occur in order to influence a direction for the research. Research cannot occur in an intellectual vacuum. It is fundamental that we determine how statins work, how they activate defensive processes. This unexpected opportunity might result in a greater understanding of immunity and inflammation and, of greater importance, an understanding of the development of cancer and protective mechanisms.

Figure 68.2 shows a model in which vitamin D and cholesterol have the same metabolic precursors.

**Figure 68.2  A model showing the relationship between vitamin D and cholesterol.**

CoA = coenzyme A.

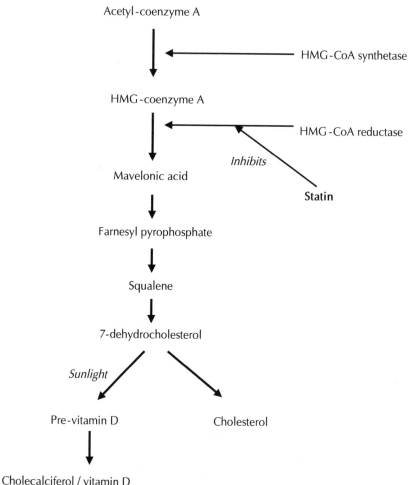

The most important statin paradox leads from this. In this metabolic process, acetyl-CoA, associated with the Krebs cycle, is transformed into HMG-CoA by the action of HMG-CoA synthetase. The next step is the removal of HMG-CoA by the action of the enzyme HMG-CoA reductase, leading to mavelonic acid in a series of further steps, some of which are shown in Figure 68.2, and the important molecule 7-dehydrocholesterol. In the presence of sunlight, 7-dehydrocholesterol in the skin is converted into vitamin D as cholecalciferol. In the absence of sunlight, in the skin in the winter and in the liver, 7-dehydrocholesterol is converted into cholesterol.

The paradox is this: as statins inhibit the synthesis of 7-dehydrocholesterol and thereby the synthesis of cholesterol, they will inevitably inhibit the synthesis of vitamin D. The conundrum is why have clinical features of vitamin D deficiency not been described in people taking satin therapy? The logical answer is that statins are analogues of vitamin D, and thus they perform the functions of vitamin D by activating vitamin D receptors (VDRs) directly.

The observation that statins reduce the risk of colorectal cancer is likely to lead to the widespread prescription of statins for this purpose, similar to their widespread prescription to reduce the risk of coronary heart disease and stroke. This approach would be much easier and might be much more effective than screening the adult population by colonoscopy, a proposal that is being activated at present. It could be, however, that the prescription of statins for this purpose is simply an expensive way of prescribing vitamin D supplements or increasing sunlight exposure. Statins as marketed by the original manufacturers cost about £1 per day, 20 p for generics, whereas the annual physiological dose of vitamin D, as 300 000 units of ergocalciferol, is £5.92.

I have mentioned in previous chapters that research into statin activity is impeded by the assumption that clinical activity is through cholesterol-lowering, itself an obsession and a delusion. Once the diet–cholesterol–heart theory is abandoned then research can move on to explore the details of the therapeutic potential of statins and the mysteries that will be uncovered. Pharmaceutical companies are responsible for a great deal of medical research but of course their financial investment needs to be realised through subsequent sale. This has an impact on what happens to the research data, of which they have copyright. A non-statin cholesterol-lowering drug called ezetimibe has recently been evaluated by Merck and Schering-Plough Pharmaceuticals. A study, called ENHANCE, has recently been conducted comparing simvastatin alone with simvastatin plus ezetimibe. It appears that the addition of ezetimibe brought about an additional lowering of cholesterol but no clinical benefit, in fact a worsening of carotid artery plaque progression [18]. This result was issued only after a USA congressional inquiry was set up to look into why the result had not been published 2 years after the study was completed. It provides further evidence that the benefit of statins is unrelated to cholesterol-lowering, a process that is not important.

This also shows how the medical and general public are subjected to publication bias: we are fed only the information that supports conventional wisdom and commercial interests. This has been commented on very cleverly by James Le Fanu, a retired general practitioner in London, UK

[19]. He used a Sherlock Holmes–Dr Watson dialogue to demonstrate that, in 'The Case of the Missing Data', 'details that could reasonably have been expected to appear in evidential text were absent'. I hope this book has gone some way in supplying the missing data in the complex story of the sun, vitamin D, cholesterol, coronary heart disease and disease resulting from micro-organisms.

Although considerations of statin medications are important, the main thrust of this book is to examine the benefits of sunlight and the harm done by its absence. There are immense public health ramifications in accepting that insufficient sun exposure is responsible for a high burden of disease. The present climate of victim-blaming could come to an end and effort could be concentrated on the socio-economic and ethnic groups most at risk. The government, with its responsibility for public health, would need to become much more active than simply persuading people to alter their lifestyles.

An early critic of the diet–cholesterol–heart hypothesis was Sir John McMichael, one of the great academic physicians of the second half of the 20th century, and formerly Professor of Medicine at the Royal Postgraduate Medical School attached to the Hammersmith Hospital, London, UK. He wrote of the diet–cholesterol–heart hypothesis in the *European Journal of Cardiology* in 1977 [20]:

> It is a sobering thought that our profession has allowed itself to be brainwashed by propaganda into a widespread acceptance of a fashion which can only be transient … It is not for us to advise governments to interfere with the nature of the fats we consume for a probability of no gain at all.

It is difficult to change a paradigm, especially one that is so strongly entrenched within society, even more now than when McMichael penned his thoughts 30 years ago. I hope that I have demonstrated the weaknesses of the existing paradigm and that I have shown that it is time to think again. We must recognise the importance of the sun in human health.

# REFERENCES

## Prologue

1.  Horner JS. Why me? *BMJ* 1990; 301: 1480–1481.
2.  Åsne Seierstad. *The Bookseller of Kabul*. Virago Press: London 2002.

## Introduction

1.  Kuhn TS. *The Structure of Scientific Revolutions*. University of Chicago Press: Chicago 1996.
2.  Butterfield H. *The Origins of Modern Science, 1300–1800*. Bell: London 1949.

## Chapter 1  The nature of disease

1.  Fries JF. Aging, natural death, and the compression of morbidity. *N Engl J Med* 1980; 303: 130–136.
2.  Fries JF, Green LW, Levine S. Health promotion and the compression of morbidity. *Lancet* 1989; 333: 481–483.
3.  Payer L. *Medicine and Culture: notions of health and sickness in Britain, the US, France and West Germany*. Victor Gollancz: London 1989.
4.  Hatt G. What is low blood pressure? *Lancet* 1992; 339: 1049.
5.  Mechanic D. The concept of illness behavior. *J Chronic Dis* 1961; 15: 189–194.
6.  Zborowski M. Cultural components in responses to pain. *J Social Issues* 1952; 8: 16–30.

7. Koos E. *The Health of Regionsville: what the people thought and did about it*. Columbia University Press: New York 1954.
8. Hopkins HH, Kapary NG. A flexible fibrescope using static scanning. *Nature (Lond)* 1954; 173: 39.
9. Webster C. *From Paracelsus to Newton: magic and the making of modern science*. Cambridge Press: Cambridge 1982.
10. Webster C. Paracelsus, and 500 years of encouraging scientific inquiry. *BMJ* 1993; 306: 597–598.

## Chapter 2 Disease patterns in the 18th and 19th centuries

1. Percival T. *Observations on the State of the Population of Manchester and Other Adjacent Places*. Manchester 1773.
2. Tröhler U. *To Improve the Evidence of Medicine. The 18th century British origins of a critical approach*. Royal College of Physicians of Edinburgh: Edinburgh 2000.
3. Heberden W. *Observations on the Increase and Decrease of Different Diseases*. T. Payne: London 1801.

## Chapter 3 The changing pattern of disease in the 20th century

1. Keynes JM. *The Economic Consequences of the Peace*. Macmillan: London 1919.
2. McKeown T. *The Role of Medicine: dream, mirage, or nemesis?* The Nuffield Provincial Hospital Trust: London 1976.

## Chapter 4 The causation of disease and individual susceptibility

1. Susser M. *Causal Thinking in the Health Sciences: concepts and strategies of epidemiology*. Oxford University Press: New York, London, Toronto 1973.
2. Farnham FR, Kennedy HG. Acute excited states and sudden death (editorial). *BMJ* 1997; 315: 1107–1108.
3. Carroll D, Ebrahim EB, Rahim S, *et al*. Admissions for myocardial infarction and World Cup football: database survey. *BMJ* 2003; 325: 1439–1442.
4. Kannel WB, McGee D, Gordon T. A general cardiovascular risk profile. The Framingham study. *Am J Cardiol* 1976; 38: 46–51.
5. Orchard TJ. Epidemiology in the 1980s: need for a change? *Lancet* 1980; 316: 845–846.

# Chapter 5 Possible causes of disease

1.  Stewart CP, Guthrie D, eds. *Lind's Treatise on Scurvy*. Edinburgh University Press: Edinburgh 1953.

# Chapter 6 Resistance to infection

1.  Yearsley KA, Ramadas AV, Gilby LJ, *et al*. Proton pump inhibitors as a risk factor for *Clostridium difficile* associated diarrhoea. *Gut* 2005; 54, Supple 11: Abstract 312.
2.  Ananthaswamy A. Infections explain why our blood groups differ. *New Scientist* 2004; 17 April: 15.

# Chapter 7 The seasonality of illness

1.  UK Office for National Statistics. *Deaths, by Months of Occurrence, in 2000, in England and Wales*. The Stationery Office: London 2001.
2.  Curwen M. Excess winter mortality: a British phenomenon? *Health Trends* 1990/91; 22: 169–175.
3.  Scragg R. Seasonal variation of mortality in Queensland. *Comm Health Stud* 1982; VI: 120–129.
4.  Crawford VLS, McCann M, Stout RW. Changes in seasonal deaths from myocardial infarction. *QJM* 2003; 96: 45–52.
5.  Gyllerup S, Lanke J, Lindholm LH, Schersten B. Cold climate is an important factor in explaining regional differences in coronary mortality even if serum cholesterol and other established risk factors are taken into account. *Scott Med J* 1993; 38: 169–172.
6.  Anderson TW, Lerache WH. Cold weather and myocardial infarction. *Lancet* 1970; 296: 291–296.
7.  Douglas A, Al-Sayer H, Rawles JM, Allan TM. Seasonality of disease in Kuwait. *Lancet* 1991; 337: 1393–1397.
8.  Wong CM, Ma S, Lam TH, Hedley AJ. Coronary artery disease varies seasonably in sub-tropics. *BMJ* 1999; 319: 1004.
9.  Douglas AS, Strachan DB, Maxwell JB. Seasonality of tuberculosis: respiratory diseases in the UK. *Thorax* 1996; 51: 944–946.
10. Thorpe LE, Frieden TR, Laserson KF, *et al*. Seasonality of tuberculosis: is it real and what does it tell us? *Lancet* 2004; 364: 1613–1614.
11. Brennan PJ, Greenburg G, Miall WE, Thompson SG. Seasonal variation in arterial blood pressure. *BMJ* 1982; 285: 919–923.
12. Woodhouse PR, Khaw K-T, Plummer M. Seasonal variation of blood pressure and its relationship to ambient temperature in an elderly population. *J Hypertension* 1993; 11: 1267–1274.

13. Hsu CH, Yang CS, Patel SR, Stevens MG. Calcium and vitamin D metabolism in spontaneously hypertensive rats. *Am J Physiol* 1987A; 253: F712– F718.
14. Krause R, Buhring M, Hopfenmuller W, *et al.* Ultraviolet B and blood pressure. *Lancet* 1998; 352: 709–710.
15. Appleby J. Winter mortality. *Health Service J* 2004; 29 January: 25.
16. Venning G. Recent developments in vitamin D deficiency and muscle weakness among elderly people. *BMJ* 2005; 330: 524–526.
17. Biscoff-Ferrari HA, Dawson-Hughes B, Willett WC, *et al.* Review: prophylactic use of vitamin D reduces falls in older people. *JAMA* 2004; 291: 1999–2006.
18. Rothwell PM, Staines A, Smail P, *et al.* Seasonality of birth of patients with childhood diabetes in Britain. *BMJ* 1996; 312: 1456–7.
19. Wood SJ, Quinn A, Kingsland CR, Lewis-Jones D. *Seasonality and the role of sunlight in assisted conception.* Presented to the Annual British Fertility Society Meeting: Cheltenham 2004.
20. Sher L. Seasonal variation in coronary heart disease and seasonal mood changes. *QJM* 2000; 93: 385–386.
21. Woodhouse PR, Khaw KT, Plummer M, *et al.* Seasonal variations of plasma fibrinogen and factor VII activity in the elderly: winter infections and death from cardiovascular disease. *Lancet* 1994; 343: 435–439.
22. Boulay F, Berthier F, Schoukroun G, *et al.* Seasonal variations in hospital admission for deep vein thrombosis and pulmonary embolism: analysis of discharge data. *BMJ* 2001; 323: 601–602.

## Chapter 8 Hepatitis, tuberculosis and syphilis

1. Kuhn TS. *The Structure of Scientific Revolutions.* University of Chicago Press: Chicago 1996.
2. Hayden D. *Pox.* Basic Books: New York 2003.

## Chapter 9 Peptic ulcer: a microbial disease

1. Marshall BJ, Warren JR. Unidentified curved bacilli in the stomach of patients with gastritis and peptic ulceration. *Lancet* 1984; 324: 1311–1314.
2. Brinton W. *On the Pathology, Symptoms and Treatment of Ulcer of the Stomach.* John Churchill: London 1857.
3. Illingworth CFW, Scott LDW, Jamieson RA. Acute perforated peptic ulcer: frequency and incidence in the west of Scotland. *BMJ* 1944; 2: 617–620.

4. Jamieson RA. Acute perforated peptic ulcer: frequency and incidence in the west of Scotland. *BMJ* 1955; 2: 222–227.
5. Hurst AF. New views on the pathology, diagnosis, and treatment of gastric and duodenal ulcer. *BMJ* 1920; 1: 559–563.
6. Doll R, Friedlander P, Pygott F. Dietetic treatment of peptic ulcer. *Lancet* 1956; 267: 5–9.
7. Fitzgerald FT. The tyranny of health. *N Engl J Med* 1994; 331: 196–198.
8. Langman MJS. *The Epidemiology of Chronic Digestive Disease.* Edward Arnold: London 1979; 22.
9. Parsonnet J, Friedman GD, Vandersteen DP, *et al. Helicobacter pylori* infection and the risk of gastric carcinoma. *N Engl J Med* 1991; 325: 1127–1131.
10. Yoemans ND, Kolt SD *Helicobacter heilmannii* (formerly *Gastrospirillum*): association with pig and human gastric pathology (Editorial). *Gastroenterology* 1996; 111: 244–259.

## Chapter 10 Tuberculosis and South Asian ethnicity

1. Medical Research Council Tuberculosis and Chest Diseases Unit. National survey of tuberculosis notifications in England and Wales 1978–9. *BMJ* 1980; 281: 895–898.
2. Finch PJ, Millard FJC, Maxwell JD. Risk of tuberculosis in immigrant Asians: culturally acquired immunodeficiency? *Thorax* 1991; 46: 1–5.
3. Strachan DP, Powell KJ, Thaker A, *et al.* Vegetarian diet as a risk factor for tuberculosis in immigrant south London Asians. *Thorax* 1995; 50: 175–180.
4. Wilkinson RJ, Llewelyn M, Toossi Z, *et al.* Influence of vitamin D deficiency and vitamin D receptor polymorphisms on tuberculosis among Gujarati Asians in west London. *Lancet* 2000; 355: 618–21.
5. UK Health Protection Agency. *Migrant Health: a baseline report.* Chapter 2, Tuberculosis. The Stationery Office: London 2006.

## Chapter 12 Glasgow, a microcosm of the industrial society

1. Henderson JB, Dunnigan MG, McIntosh WB, *et al.* The importance of limited exposure to ultraviolet radiation and dietary factors in the aetiology of Asian rickets: a risk factor model. *QJM* 1987; 63: 405–412.
2. British Heart Foundation. Statistics. *BMJ* 2001; 322: 694.

## Chapter 13 Belfast and Toulouse

1.  Tunstall-Pedoe H, Kuulasmaa K, Amouyel P, *et al.* Myocardial infarction and coronary deaths in the World Health Organization MONICA project. *Circulation* 1994; 90: 583–612.
2.  Evans AE, Ruidavets J-B, McCrum EE, *et al.* Autres pays, autres coeurs! Dietary patterns, risk factors and ischaemic heart disease in Belfast and Toulouse. *QJM* 1995; 88: 469–477.

## Chapter 14 Association as a clue to causation

1.  La Porte RE. Patterns of disease: diabetes and the rest – we should be investigating relations between diseases (Editorial). *BMJ* 1995; 310: 545–546.
2.  Muller CJB. Hiatus hernia, diverticula and gall stones: Saint's Triad. *S Afr Med J* 1948; 376–382.
3.  Phillips JA. Is Burkitt's lymphoma sexy enough? *Lancet* 2006; 368: 2251–2252.
4.  Burkitt DP. Related disease: related cause? *Lancet* 1969; 294: 1229–1232.

## Chapter 15 Rickets and the discovery of vitamin D

1.  Pasco JA, Henry MJ, Nicholson GC, *et al.* Vitamin D status of women in the Geelong osteoporosis study: association with diet and casual exposure to sunlight. *Med J Aust* 2001; 175: 401–405.
2.  Ferguson M. *A Study of Social and Economic Factors in the Causation of Rickets, with introductory historical survey by Leonard Findlay.* Special Report Series No. 20. Medical Research Council: London 1918.
3.  Hutchison HS, Shah SJ. The aetiology of rickets, early and late. *QJM* 1922; 15: 167–195.
4.  Dungan MG, Paton JPO, Hasse S, *et al.* Late rickets and osteomalacia in the Pakistani community in Glasgow. *Scott Med J* 1962; 7: 159.
5.  Mukamel MN, Weisman Y, Somech R, *et al.* Vitamin D deficiency and insufficiency in orthodox and non-orthodox Jewish mothers in Israel. *J Isr Med Assoc* 2001; 3: 419–421.
6.  Gloth M, Gundberg CM, Hollis BW, *et al.* Vitamin D deficiency in homebound elderly persons. *JAMA* 1995; 274: 1683–1686.
7.  Sato Y, Kikuyama M, Oizumi K. High prevalence of vitamin D deficiency and reduced bone mass in Parkinson's disease. *Neurology* 1997; 49: 1273–1278.

8.    Carvalho NF, Kenney RD, Carrington PH, Hall DE. Severe nutritional deficiencies in toddlers resulting from health food milk alternatives. *Paediatrics* 2001; 107: E46.

## Chapter 16 The biology of vitamin D

1.    Tsujimoto M. A highly saturated hydrocarbon in shark oil. *J Ind Eng Chem* 1916; 8: 889–896.
2.    Dusso AS, Brown AJ. Mechanism of vitamin D action and its regulation. *Am J Kidney Dis* 1998; 32: S13–S24.
3.    Fraser DR. The physiological economy of vitamin D. *Lancet* 1983; 321: 969–972.
4.    Iqbal SJ. Vitamin D metabolism and clinical aspects of measuring metabolites. *Ann Clin Biochem* 1994; 31: 109–124.
5.    Lo CW, Paris PW, MD, Holick MF. Indian and Pakistani immigrants have the same capacity as Caucasians to produce vitamin D in response to ultraviolet irradiation. *Am J Clin Nutr* 1986; 44: 683–685.
6.    Rashid A, Mohammed T, Stephens WP, *et al*. Vitamin D state of Asians living in Pakistan. *BMJ* 1983; 286: 182–184.
7.    Wharton B, Bishop N. Rickets. *Lancet* 2003; 362: 1389–1400.

## Chapter 17 Sunshine and tuberculosis

1.    Pennington C. Tuberculosis. In *Health Care as Social History: the Glasgow case*. Aberdeen University Press: Aberdeen 1982; 92.
2.    Hobday, R. *The Healing Sun: sunlight and health in the 21st century*. Findhorn Press: Forres 1999.
3.    Health Protection Agency. *Migrant Health: infectious diseases in non-UK born populations in England, Wales and Northern Ireland. A baseline report 2006*. The Stationery Office: London 2006. http://www.hpa.org.uk/publications/2006/migrant_health.
4.    Wharton B, Bishop N. Rickets. *Lancet* 2003; 362: 1389–1400.
5.    Wilkinson RJ, Llewelyn M, Toossi Z, *et al*. Influence of vitamin D deficiency and vitamin D receptor polymorphisms on tuberculosis among Gujarati Asians in west London: a case-control study. *Lancet* 2000; 355: 618–21.
6.    Davies PDO. A possible link between vitamin D deficiency and impaired host defence to *Mycobacterium tuberculosis*. *Tubercle* 1985; 66: 301–306.
7.    Yang S, Smith C, Prahl JM, *et al*. Vitamin D deficiency suppresses cell mediated immunity *in vitro*. *Arch Biochem Biophys* 1993; 303: 98–106.

8. Rook GAW. Activated macrophages in the immunopathology of tuberculosis. *Br Med Bull* 1988; 44: 661–623.
9. Wetherall D. Evolving with enemy of science. *New Scientist* 2003; 22 November.
10. Medical Research Council. Streptomycin treatment of pulmonary tuberculosis: a Medical Research Council investigation. *BMJ* 1948; ii: 764–782.
11. Ryan F. *Tuberculosis: the greatest story never told*. Swift: Bromsgrove 1992.

## Chapter 18 The emergence of coronary heart disease and its decline

1. Osler W. *Principles and Practice of Medicine*. Appleton: London 1912; 836.
2. Lian C. Le Diagnostic Clinique de l'Infarctus du Myocarde. *La Medicine* 1921: 450.
3. Johansson BW, Nicol P. A Swedish report on acute myocardial infarction in 1959. *BMJ* 1982; 284: 888–889.
4. MacKenzie J. *Diseases of the Heart*. Oxford University Press, Hodder & Stoughton: London 1908.
5. Stehbens WE. Appraisal of the epidemic rise of coronary heart disease and its decline. *Lancet* 1987; 329: 606–611.
6. Stehbens WE. The hypothetical epidemic of coronary heart disease and atherosclerosis. *Med Hypoth* 1995; 45: 449–454.
7. Painter NS, Burkitt DP. Diverticular disease of the colon: a deficiency disease of western civilisation. *BMJ* 1971; 1: 450–454.
8. Bland-Sutton J. Discussion on diverticulitis. *Proc Royal Soc Med Sect Surg* 1920; 13: 64–65.
9. Cleave TL, Campbell GD, Painter NS. *Diabetes, Coronary Thrombosis and the Saccharine Disease*, 2nd edn. Wright: Bristol 1969.
10. Editorial. Coronary deaths. *BMJ* 1971; 4: 64.
11. Gordon T, Kannel WG. Premature mortality from coronary heart disease. The Framingham study. *JAMA* 1971; 215: 1617–1625.
12. Florey C, Du V, Melia RJW, Darby SC. Changing mortality from ischaemic heart disease in Great Britain 1960–76. *BMJ* 1978; 1: 635–637.
13. Hampton JR. Falling mortality in coronary heart disease (editorial). *BMJ* 1982; 284: 1505–1506.
14. Stewart AW, Beaglehole R, Fraser GE, Sharpe DN. Trends in survival after myocardial infarction in New Zealand, 1974–81. *Lancet* 1984; 324: 444–446.

15. Stamler J. The marked decline in coronary heart disease mortality rates in the United States, 1968–1981; summary of findings and possible explanations. *Cardiology* 1985; 72: 11–22.
16. Beagleholme R. Medical management and the decline in mortality from coronary heart disease. *BMJ* 1986; 292: 33–35.
17. Tuomilehto J, Geboers JEF, Salonen JT, *et al*. Decline in cardiovascular mortality in North Karelia and other parts of Finland. *BMJ* 1986; 293: 1068–1071.
18. Salonen JT. Did the North Karelia project reduce coronary mortality? *Lancet* 1987; 330: 269.
19. Hopper JL, Pathik B, Hunt V, Cham WWC. Improved prognosis since 1969 of myocardial infarction treated in a coronary care unit: lack of relation in changes of severity. *BMJ* 1989; 299: 890–896.
20. National Institutes of Health. *National Conference on Health Research Principles, 3 and 4 October, 1978 : conference report*. Department of Health, Education, and Welfare, Public Health Service, National Institutes of Health: Bethesda: 1978.
21. Tunstall-Pedoe H, Kuulasmaa K, Amouyel P, *et al*. Myocardial infarction and coronary deaths in the World Health Organization MONICA project. *Circulation* 1994; 90: 582–612.
22. Rosamond WD, Chambless LE, Folsom AR, *et al*. Trends in the incidence of myocardial infarction and in mortality due to coronary heart disease, 1987 to 1994. *N Engl J Med* 1998; 339: 861–867.
23. UK Department of Health. *The National Service Framework for Coronary Heart Disease: winning the war on heart disease*. The Stationery Office: London 2004.
24. Unal B, Critchley JA, Capewell S. Explaining the decline in coronary heart disease mortality in England and Wales between 1981 and 2000. *Circulation* 2004; 109: 1101–1107.
25. Crawford VLS, McCann M, Stout RW Changes in seasonal deaths from myocardial infarction . *QJM* 2003; 96: 45–52.

## Chapter 19 The biology of coronary heart disease

1. Stary HC. Evolution and progression of atherosclerotic lesions in coronary arteries of children and young adults. *Arteriosclerosis* 1989; 99, Supple1: 1–32.
2. Bertomeu A, García-Vidal O, Farré X, *et al*. Preclinical coronary atherosclerosis in a population with low incidence of myocardial infarction: cross sectional autopsy study. *BMJ* 2003; 327: 591–592.
3. Fuster V, Badimon L, Badimon JJ, Chesebro JH. The pathogenesis of coronary artery disease and the acute coronary syndromes. *N Engl J Med* 1992; 326: 242–250.

4.    Michinson MJ, Ball RY. Macrophages and atherogenesis. *Lancet* 1987: 330: 146–148.

## Chapter 20 The causation of coronary heart disease

1.    Hopkins PN, Williams RR. A survey of 246 suggested coronary risk factors. *Atherosclerosis* 1981; 40: 1–52.
2.    Ouyang P, Michos ED, Karas RH. Hormone replacement therapy and the cardiovascular system: lessons learned and unanswered questions. *J Am Coll Cardiol* 2006; 47: 1741–1753.
3.    Ford ES, Freedman DS, Byers T. Baldness and ischaemic heart disease in a national sample of men. *Am J Epidemiol* 1996; 143: 651–657.
4.    Lutgendorf SK, Russell D, Ullrich P, *et al.* Religious participation, interleukin-6, and mortality in older adults. *Health Psychol* 2004; 23: 465–475.
5.    Walker AR. The epidemiology of ischaemic heart disease in the different ethnic populations in Johannesburg. *S Afr Med J* 1980; 57: 748–752.
6.    Rayman MP. Dietary selenium: time to act (editorial). *BMJ* 1997; 314: 387.
7.    Ravnskov U. Is atherosclerosis caused by a high cholesterol? *QJM* 2002; 95: 397–403.
8.    Kuhn TS. *The Structure of Scientific Revolutions.* University of Chicago Press: Chicago 1996.
9.    Fitzgerald FT. The tyranny of health. *N Engl J Med* 1994; 331: 196–198.

## Chapter 21 Psychological factors and coronary heart disease

1.    Angell M. Disease as a reflection of the psyche. *N Engl J Med* 1985; 312: 1570–1572.
2.    Townsend P, Davidson N. *Inequalities in Health.* Pelican Books: London 1988.
3.    Department of Health and Social Security. *Inequalities in Health: report of a research working group.* Department of Health and Social Security: London 1980.
4.    Bass C, Wade C. Type A behaviour: not specifically pathogenic? *Lancet* 1982; 320: 1147–1149.
5.    Bortner RW. A short rating scale as a potential measure of pattern A behaviour. *J Chron Dis* 1967; 20: 525–533.
6.    Case RB, Heller SS, Case NB, Moss AJ, Multicenter Post-Infarction Research Group. Type A behavior and survival after acute myocardial infarction. *N Engl J Med* 1985; 312: 737–741.

7.  Johnston DW, Cook DG, Shaper AG. Type A behaviour and ischaemic heart disease in middle aged British men. *BMJ* 1987; 295: 86–89.
8.  Ragland DR, Brand RJ. Type A behavior and mortality from coronary heart disease. *N Engl J Med* 1988; 318: 65–69.
9.  Mitchell JRA. Hearts and minds. *BMJ* 1984; 289: 1557–1558.
10. Arnott EM. The changing aetiology of heart disease. *BMJ* 1954; 2: 887–891.
11. Hinkle LE, Whitney LH, Lehman EW. Occupation, education and coronary heart disease. *Science* 1968; 161: 238–246.
12. Yan LL, Liu K, Daviglus ML, *et al.* Education, 15-year risk factor progression, and coronary artery calcium in young adulthood and early middle age. *JAMA* 2006; 295: 1793–1800.
13. Carroll D, Ebrahim EB, Rahim S, *et al.* Admissions for myocardial infarction and World Cup football: database survey. *BMJ* 2003; 325: 1439–1442.
14. Schattner A. The emotional dimension and the biological paradigm of illness: time for a change. *QJM* 2003; 96: 617–621.
15. Holick MF. *The UV Advantage.* Simon & Schuster: London 2004.
16. Strandberg TE, Pyörälä K, Cook TJ, *et al.* Mortality and incidence of cancer during 10-year follow-up of the Scandinavian Simvastatin Survival Study (4S). *Lancet* 2004; 364: 771–777.
17. Marmot M. *Status Syndrome: how your social standing directly affects your health and life expectancy.* Bloomsbury Publishing: London 2004.
18. Webster C. *From Paracelsus to Newton: magic and the making of modern science.* Cambridge Press: Cambridge 1982.
19. Tracey K. The monster within. *New Scientist* 2005; 2 April: 38–41.

## Chapter 22 Diet and coronary heart disease

1.  Stary HC. Evolution and progression of atherosclerotic lesions in coronary arteries of children and young adults. *Arteriosclerosis* 1989; 99, Supple 1: 1–32.
2.  Keys A. Seven countries: a multivariate analysis of death and coronary heart disease. Harvard University Press: Cambridge 1980.
3.  Cade JE, Barker DJP, Margetts BM, Morris JA. Diet and inequalities in health in three English towns. *BMJ* 1988; 296: 1359–1362.
4.  Morris JN, Marr JW, Clayton DG. Diet and heart: a postscript. *BMJ* 1977; 2: 1307–1314.
5.  He K, Merchant A, Rimm EB, *et al.* Dietary fat intake and risk of stroke in male US healthcare professionals: 14 year prospective cohort study. *BMJ* 2003; 327: 777–781.

6. Ascherio A, Rimm EB, Giovannucci EL, *et al.* Dietary fat and risk of coronary heart disease in men: cohort follow up study in the United States. *BMJ* 1996; 313: 84–90.
7. Yudkin J. Diet and coronary thrombosis: hypothesis and fact. *Lancet* 1957; 270: 155–162.
8. Yudkin J. Dietary fat and dietary sugar in relation to ischaemic heart disease and diabetes. *Lancet* 1964; 284: 4–5.
9. Yudkin J, Roddy J. Levels of dietary sucrose in patients with occlusive atherosclerotic disease. *Lancet* 1964; 284: 6–8.
10. Elwood PC, Waters WE, Moore S, Sweetnam P. Sucrose consumption and ischaemic heart disease in the community. *Lancet* 1970; 295: 1014–1016.
11. Cleave TL, Campbell GD, Painter NS. *Diabetes, Coronary Thrombosis and the Saccharine Disease.* 2nd edn. Wright: Bristol 1969.
12. Rendle Short, J. The causation of appendicitis. *Br J Surg* 1920; 8: 171–188.
13. Kromhout D, Bosschieter EB, de Lezenne Coulander C. Dietary fibre and 10-year mortality from coronary heart disease, cancer, and all causes. The Zutphen study. *Lancet* 1982; 320: 518–522.
14. Heaton KW, Pomare EW. Effect of bran on blood lipids and calcium. *Lancet* 1974; 303: 49–50.
15. Vanharanta M, Voutilainen S, Lakka TA, *et al.* Risk of acute coronary events according to serum concentrations of enterolactone: a prospective population-based case-control study. *Lancet* 1999; 354: 2112–2115.
16. Hooper L, Summerbell CD, Higgins JPT, *et al.* Dietary fat intake and prevention of cardiovascular disease: systematic review. *BMJ* 2001; 322: 757–763.
17. Bang HO, Dyerberg J, Sinclair HM. The composition of the Eskimo food in north western Greenland. *Am J Clin Nutr* 1980; 33: 2657–2661.
18. Kromhout D, Bosschieter EB, Coulander C de L. The inverse relation between fish consumption and 20-year mortality from coronary heart disease. *N Engl J Med* 1985; 312: 1205–1209.
19. Hu FB, Bronner L, Willett WC, *et al.* Fish and omega-e fatty acid intake and risk of coronary heart disease in women. *JAMA* 2002; 287: 1815–1821.
20. Ramsay LE, Yeo WW, Jackson PR. Dietary reduction of serum cholesterol concentration: time to think again. *BMJ* 1991; 303: 953–957.

21. Burr ML, Fehily AM, Gilbert JF, *et al*. Effects of changes in fat, fish, and fibre intakes on death and myocardial reinfarction: diet and reinfarction trial (DART). *Lancet* 1989; 3342: 757–761.

22. Ravnskov U. Diet–heart hypothesis is wishful thinking. *BMJ* 2002; 324: 238.

23. Ravnskov U. The questionable role of saturated and poly-unsaturated fatty acids in cardiovascular disease. *J Clin Epidem* 1998; 51: 443–460.

24. Singh RB, Rastogi SS, Verma R, *et al*. Randomised controlled trial of cardioprotective diet in patients with recent myocardial infarction: results of one year follow up. *BMJ* 1992; 304: 1015–1019.

25. Singh RB, Dubnov G, Niaz MA, *et al*. Effect of an Indo-Mediterranean diet on progression of coronary artery disease in high risk patients (Indo-Mediterranean Diet Heart Study): a randomised single-blind trial. *Lancet* 2002; 360: 1455–1461.

26. Hu FB. The Mediterranean diet and mortality: olive oil and beyond. *N Engl J Med* 2003; 348: 2595–2596.

27. White C (ed.). Suspected research fraud: difficulties at getting at the truth. *BMJ* 2005; 331: 281–288.

28. Editorial. Expression of concern: Indo-Mediterranean Diet Heart Study. *Lancet* 2005; 366: 354–356.

29. Soman CR. Indo-Mediterranean diet and progression of coronary artery disease. *Lancet* 2005: 366: 365–366.

## Chapter 23 The Leningrad paradox

1. Sparén P, Vågerö D, Shestov D B, *et al*. Long term mortality after severe starvation during the siege of Leningrad: prospective cohort study. *BMJ* 2004; 328:11–14.

## Chapter 24 Cholesterol and coronary heart disease

1. Martin MJ, Hulley SB, Browner WS, Kuller LH, Wentworth D. Serum cholesterol, blood pressure, and mortality: implications from a cohort of 361,662 men. *Lancet* 1986; 328: 933–936.

2. National Institutes of Health. Consensus conference on lowering blood cholesterol to prevent heart disease. *JAMA* 1985; 253: 2080–2086.

3. Rose G, Shipley M. Plasma cholesterol concentration and death from coronary heart disease: 10 year results of the Whitehall study. *BMJ* 1986; 293: 306–307.

4.   NHS Centre for Reviews and Dissemination. *Effective Health Care Bull* 1998; 4: 1.

5.   Lande KE, Sperry WM. Human atherosclerosis in relation to the cholesterol content of the blood serum. *Arch Path* 1936; 22: 301–12.

6.   Ravnskov U. Is atherosclerosis caused by high cholesterol? *QJM* 2002; 95: 397–403.

7.   Sijbrands EJG, Westendorp RGJ, Defesche JC, *et al*. Mortality over two centuries in a large pedigree with familial hypercholesterolaemia: family tree mortality study. *BMJ* 2001; 322: 119–123.

8.   Longo M, Crosigman IA, Battezzati PM, *et al*. Hyperlipidaemic state and cardiovascular risk in primary biliary cirrhosis. *Gut* 2002; 51: 265–269.

9.   Kannel WB, Castelli WP, Gordon T. Cholesterol in the prediction of atherosclerotic disease. New perspectives based on the Framingham study. *Ann Int Med* 1979; 90: 85–91.

10.  Pekkanen J, Linn S, Heiss G *et al*. Ten-year mortality from cardiovascular disease in relation to cholesterol level among men with and without preexisting cardiovascular disease. *N Engl J Med* 1990; 322: 1700–1707.

11.  Rossouw JE, Lewis B, Rifkind BM. The value of lowering cholesterol after myocardial infarction. *N Engl J Med* 1990; 323: 1112–1119.

12.  Ahrens EH. The management of hyperlipidaemia: whether rather than how. *Ann Int Med* 1976; 85: 87–93.

## Chapter 25 The metabolism of cholesterol

1.   Miller GJ, Miller NE. Plasma high-density-lipoprotein concentration and development of ischaemic heart disease. *Lancet* 1975; 1: 16–19.

2.   Martin MJ, Hulley SB, Browner WS, *et al*. Serum cholesterol, blood pressure, and mortality: implications from a cohort of 361,662 men. *Lancet* 1986; 328: 933–936.

3.   Rose G, Shipley M. Plasma cholesterol concentration and death from coronary heart disease: 10 year results of the Whitehall study. *BMJ* 1986; 293: 306–307.

4.   Durrington P. Dyslipidaemia (seminar). *Lancet* 2003; 362:717–731.

5.   Salonen JT. Liver damage and protective effect of high density lipoprotein cholesterol. *BMJ* 2003; 327: 1082–1083.

# Chapter 26 Seasonal variation of vitamin D and cholesterol

1.    Stamp TCB, Round JN. Seasonal changes in human plasma levels of 25-hydroxyvitamin D. *Nature* 1974; 247:563–565.
2.    Webb AR, Kline L, Holick MS. Influence of season and latitude on the cutaneous synthesis of vitamin D3: exposure to winter sunlight in Boston and Edmonton will not promote vitamin D3 synthesis in human skin. *J Clin Endocrinol Metab* 1988; 67: 373–378.
3.    Grimes DS. *The effect of sunshine on blood cholesterol, its relationship to vitamin D metabolism, and implications for the pathogenesis of coronary heart disease*. MD Thesis. University of Manchester: Manchester 1993.
4.    Grimes DS, Hindle E, Dyer T. Sunlight, cholesterol and coronary heart disease. *QJM* 1996; 89: 579–589.
5.    Scragg R. Seasonality of cardiovascular disease mortality and the possible protective effect of ultra-violet radiation. *Int J Epidemiol* 1981; 10: 337–341.
6.    Scragg R, Jackson R, Holdaway IM, *et al.* Myocardial infarction is inversely associated with plasma 25-hydroxyvitamin D3 levels: a community-based study. *Int J Epidemiol* 1990; 19: 559–563.
7.    Miettinen M, Turpeinen O, Karvonen MJ, *et al.* Effect of diet on coronary heart disease mortality. *Lancet* 1973; 302: 1266–1267.
8.    Paloheimo J. Seasonal variation of serum lipids in healthy men. *Ann Med Exp Biol Fenn* 1961; 39, Supple 8: 1–88.
9.    Ripley RM. Overview: seasonal variations on cholesterol. *Prevent Med* 1981; 10: 655–659.
10.   Miettinen TA. Diurnal variation of cholesterol precursors squalene and methyl sterols in human plasma lipoproteins. *J Lipid Res* 1982; 23: 466–473.
11.   Jones PJH, Schoeller DA. Evidence for diurnal periodicity in human cholesterol synthesis. *J Lipid Res* 1990; 31: 677–73.
12.   Gordon DJ, Trost DC, Hyde J, *et al.* Seasonal cholesterol cycles: the Lipid Research Clinic's Coronary Primary Prevention Trial placebo group. *Circulation* 1987; 76: 1224–1231.
13.   Robinson D, Beven A, Hinohara S, Takahashi T. Seasonal variation in serum cholesterol levels: evidence from UK and Japan. *Atherosclerosis* 1992; 95: 15–24.
14.   UK Office for National Statistics. *General Household Survey*. The Stationery Office: London 1991; 66–69.
15.   Gordon DJ, Hyde J, Trost DC, *et al.* Cyclic seasonal variation in plasma lipid and lipoprotein levels: the Lipid Research Clinic's Coronary Primary Prevention Trial placebo group. *J Clin Epidem* 1988; 41: 679–689.

# Chapter 27 Cholesterol-lowering therapies

1. Martin MJ, Hulley SB, Browner WS *et al.* Serum cholesterol, blood pressure, and mortality: implications from a cohort of 361,662 men. *Lancet* 1986; 328: 933–936.
2. Rose G, Shipley M. Plasma cholesterol concentration and death from coronary heart disease: 10 year results of the Whitehall study. *BMJ* 1986; 293: 306–307.
3. Hooper L, Summerbell CD, Higgins JPT, *et al.* Dietary fat intake and prevention of cardiovascular disease: systematic review. *BMJ* 2001; 322: 757–763.
4. Kristiansen IS, Eggen AE, Thelle DS. Cost effectiveness of incremental programmes for lowering serum cholesterol concentration: is individual intervention worth while? *BMJ* 1991; 302: 1119–1122.
5. Burr ML, Fehily AM, Gilbert JF, *et al.* Effects of changes in fat, fish, and fibre intakes on death and myocardial reinfarction: diet and reinfarction trial (DART). *Lancet* 1989; 3342: 757–761.
6. Bateson MC, Maclean D, Ross PE, Bouchier IAD. Comparison of biliary lipid secretion in non-obese cholesterol gallstone patients with normal, young, male volunteers. *Digestive Disease and Science* 1978; 23: 623–628.
7. Committee of Principal Investigators. A co-operative trial in the prevention of ischaemic heart disease using clofibrate. *Br Heart J* 1978; 40: 1069–1118.
8. Committee of Principal Investigators. WHO co-operative trial on primary prevention of ischaemic heart disease using clofibrate to lower serum cholesterol: mortality follow-up. *Lancet* 1980; 2: 379–385.
9. Yudkin JS. How can we best prolong life? Benefits of coronary risk factor reduction in non-diabetic and diabetic subjects. *BMJ* 1993; 306: 1313–1318.
10. Scandinavian Simvastatin Survival Study Group. Randomised controlled trial of cholesterol lowering in 4444 patients with coronary heart disease: the Scandinavian Simvastatin Survival Study (4S). *Lancet* 1994; 344: 1383–1389.
11. Shepherd J, Cobbe SM, Ford I, *et al.*, for the West of Scotland Coronary Prevention Study Group. Prevention of coronary heart disease with pravastatin in men with hypercholesterolaemia. *N Engl J Med* 1995; 333: 1301–1307.

12. Sacks FM, Pfeffer MA, Moye L, *et al.*, for the Cholesterol and Recurrent Events Trial Investigators. The effects of pravastatin on coronary events after myocardial infarction in patients with average cholesterol levels. *N Engl J Med* 1996; 335: 1001–1009.

13. Pitt B, Waters D, Brown WV, *et al.*, for the Atorvastatin versus Revascularisation Treatment Investigators. Aggressive lipid-lowering therapy compared with angioplasty in stable coronary artery disease. *N Engl J Med* 1999; 341: 70–76.

14. Smilde TJ, van Wissen S, Wollersheim H, *et al.* Effect of aggressive versus conventional lipid lowering on atherosclerosis progression in familial hypercholesterolaemia (ASAP): a prospective, randomised, double-blind trial. *Lancet* 2001; 357: 557–581.

15. Heart Protection Study Collaborative Group. Effects of cholesterol-lowering with simvastatin on stroke and other major vascular events in 20 536 people with cerebrovascular disease or other high-risk conditions. *Lancet* 2004; 363: 757–767.

16. Oliver MF. Doubts about preventing coronary heart disease. *BMJ* 1992; 304: 393–394.

17. Oliver MF. Statins prevent coronary heart disease. *Lancet* 1995; 346 1378–1379.

18. Byrne CD, Wild SH. Lipids and secondary prevention of ischaemic heart disease (editorial). *BMJ* 1996; 313: 1273–1274.

19. Durrington P. Dyslipidaemia (seminar). *Lancet* 2003; 362:717–731.

## Chapter 28 The Scottish paradox and the actions of statins

1. Shepherd J, Cobbe SM, Ford I, *et al.*, for the West of Scotland Coronary Prevention Study Group. Prevention of coronary heart disease with pravastatin in men with hypercholesterolaemia. *N Engl J Med* 1995; 333: 1301–1307.

2. West of Scotland Coronary Prevention Group. Influence of pravastatin and plasma lipids on clinical events in the west of Scotland coronary prevention study (WOSCOPS). *Circulation* 1998; 97: 1440–1445.

3. Freeman DJ, Norrie J, Sattar N, *et al.* Pravastatin and the development of diabetes mellitus; evidence for a protective treatment effect in the west of Scotland coronary prevention study. *Circulation* 2001; 103: 357–362.

4. Smilde TJ, van Wissen S, Wollersheim H, *et al.* Effect of aggressive versus conventional lipid lowering on atherosclerosis progression in familial hypercholesterolaemia (ASAP): a prospective, randomised, double-blind trial. *Lancet* 2001; 357: 557–581.

5.  Aronow HD, Topol EJ, Roe MT, *et al*. Effect of lipid-lowering therapy on early mortality after acute coronary syndromes: an observational study. *Lancet* 2001; 357: 1063–1068.

6.  Schwartz GG, Olsson AG, Ezekowitz, *et al*., for the Myocardial Ischaemia Reduction with Aggressive Cholesterol Lowering (MIRACL) Study Investigators. Effects of atorvastatin on early recurrent ischemic events in acute coronary syndromes. *JAMA* 2001; 285: 1711–1718.

7.  Vaughan CJ, Murphy MB, Buckley BM. Statins do more than just lower cholesterol. *Lancet* 1996; 348: 1079–1082.

8.  Heeschen C, Hamm CW, Laufs U, *et al*., on behalf of the Platelet Receptor Inhibition in Ischaemic Syndrome Management (PRISM) Investigators. Withdrawal of statins increases event rates in patients with acute coronary syndromes. *Circulation* 2002; 105: 1446–1452.

9.  Mundy G, Garrett R, Harris S *et al*. Stimulation of bone formation *in vitro* and in rodents by statins. *Science* 1999; 286: 1946–1949.

10. Edwards CJ, Hart DJ, Spector TD. Oral statins and increased bone-mineral density in postmenopausal women. *Lancet* 2000; 355: 2218–2219.

11. Kobashigawa JA, Katznelson S, Laks H, *et al*. Effect of pravastatin on outcomes after cardiac transplantation. *N Engl J Med* 1995; 333: 621–627.

12. Katznelson S, Wang XM, Chia D, *et al*. The inhibitory effects of pravastatin on natural killer cell activity *in vivo* and on cytotoxic T lymphocyte activity *in vitro*. *J Heart Lung Transplant* 1998; 17: 335–340.

13. Katznelson S, Wilkinson AH, Kobashigawa JA, *et al*. The effect of pravastatin on acute rejection after kidney transplantation: a pilot study. *Transplantation* 1996; 61: 1469–1474.

14. McCarey DW, McInnes IB, Madhok R, *et al*. Trial of atorvastatin in rheumatoid arthritis (TARA): double-blind, randomised placebo-controlled trial. *Lancet* 2004; 363: 2015–2021.

15. Vollmer T, Keys L, Durkalski V, *et al*. Oral simvastatin in relapsing–remitting multiple sclerosis. *Lancet* 2004; 363: 1607–1608.

16. Bayer Corporation quoted by Bacol, USA. http://www.baycol-rhabdomyolysis.com/baycol_recall/.

17. Wagstaffe LR, Mitton MW, Arvick BM, Doraiswamy PM. Statin-associated memory loss: an analysis of 60 case reports and review of the literature. *Pharmacotherapy* 2003; 23: 871–880.

18. King DS, Wilburn AJ, Wofford MR, *et al*. Cognitive impairment associated with atorvastatin and simvastatin. *Pharmacotherapy* 2003; 23: 1663–1667.

19. Green RC. Alzheimer's disease and other dementias. Conference coverage of the 54th Annual Meeting of the American Academy of Neurology. *Medscape Neurol Neurosurg* 2002.
20. Canty J. *Statins may stimulate stem cells for heart repair.* Press release. University of Buffalo: Buffalo 2005.

## Chapter 29 The elderly paradox

1. Meador C. The last well person. *N Engl J Med* 1994; 330: 440–441.
2. McCormick J, Skrabanek P. Coronary heart disease is not preventable by population interventions. *Lancet* 1988; 332: 839–841.
3. Martin MJ, Hulley SB, Browner WS *et al.* Serum cholesterol, blood pressure, and mortality: implications from a cohort of 361,662 men. *Lancet* 1986; 328: 933–936.
4. Rose G, Shipley M. Plasma cholesterol concentration and death from coronary heart disease: 10 year results of the Whitehall study. *BMJ* 1986; 293: 306–307.
5. Anderson KM, Castelli WP, Levy D. Cholesterol and mortality: 30 years of follow-up from the Framingham study. *JAMA* 1987; 257: 2176–2180.
6. Forette B, Tortrat D, Wolmark Y. Cholesterol as risk factor for mortality in elderly women. *Lancet* 1989; 333: 868–870.
7. Dyer AR, Stamler J, Paul O *et al.* Serum cholesterol and risk of death from cancer and other causes in three Chicago epidemiological studies. *J Chronic Dis* 1981; 34: 249–260.
8. Krumholtz HM, Seeman TE, Merrill SS, *et al.* Lack of association between cholesterol and coronary heart disease mortality and morbidity and all-cause mortality in persons older than 70 years. *JAMA* 1994; 272; 1335–1340.
9. Schatz IJ, Masaki K, Yano K, *et al.* Cholesterol and all-cause mortality in elderly people from the Honolulu Heart Program: a cohort study. *Lancet* 2001; 358: 351–355.
10. Dyker AG, Weir CJ, Lees KR. Influence of cholesterol on survival after stroke: retrospective study. *BMJ* 1997; 314: 1584–1588.
11. Heart Protection Study Collaborative Group. MRC/BHF heart protection study of cholesterol lowering with simvastatin in 20,536 individuals: a randomised placebo-controlled trial. *Lancet* 2002; 360: 7–22.

## Chapter 30 The geography of cholesterol

1.  Keys A. *Seven Countries: a multivariate analysis of death and coronary heart disease.* Harvard University Press: Cambridge 1980.
2.  Kromhout D. *On the waves of the Seven Countries Study: a public health perspective on cholesterol.* ESC Lecture on Population Sciences. *Eur Heart J* 1999; 20: 796–802.

## Chapter 31 Burnley, Colne and Nelson

1.  Barker DJP, Osmond C. Inequalities in health in Britain: specific explanations in three Lancashire towns. *BMJ* 1987; 294: 749–752.

## Chapter 32 Geography of coronary heart disease in the UK

1.  Cade JE, Barker DJP, Margetts BM, Morris JA. Diet and inequalities in health in three English towns. *BMJ* 1988; 296: 1359–1362.
2.  UK Department of Health. *Health Statistics Quarterly 11. Autumn 2001.* The Stationery Office: London 2001. www.doh.gov.uk/healthinequalities.
3.  Keys A. *Seven Countries: a multivariate analysis of death and coronary heart disease.* Harvard University Press: Cambridge 1980.
4.  British Heart Foundation. *Coronary Heart Disease Statistics.* British Heart Foundation: London 1999.
5.  Public Health Laboratory Service. Surveillance of influenza, England, Wales and Scotland 1999/00. *Public Health Laboratory Service Activity Update* 2000; 12: 1–4.
6.  Cousens S, Smith PG, Ward H, *et al.* Geographical distribution of variant Creutzfeldt–Jakob disease in Great Britain, 1994–2000. *Lancet* 2001; 357: 1002–1007.
7.  National Statistical Office. *Age-Standardised Mortality Rates: by Cause and Sex, 2001.* Regional Trends 38. National Statistical Office: London 2001.
8.  Elford J, Phillips AN, Thomson AG, Shaper AG. Migration and geographic variations in ischaemic heart disease in Great Britain. *Lancet* 1989; 333: 343–346.

## Chapter 33 Geography of coronary heart disease in Europe

1.  Keys A. *Seven Countries: a multivariate analysis of death and coronary heart disease.* Harvard University Press: Cambridge 1980.
2.  World Health Organization. *World Health Statistics Annual.* World Health Organization: Geneva 1986.

3. Levi F, Lucchini F, Negri E, La Vecchia C. Trends in mortality from cardiovascular and cerebrovascular diseases in Europe and other areas of the world. *Heart* 2002; 88: 119–124.
4. Bobak M, Marmot M. East–west mortality divide and its potential explanations: proposed research agenda. *BMJ* 1996; 312: 421–425.
5. Goossens H, Ferech M, Stichele RV, Elseviers M, for the ESAC project group. Outpatient antibiotic use in Europe and association with resistance: a cross-sectional database study. *Lancet* 2005; 365: 579–587.

## Chapter 34 The geography of coronary heart disease in the USA

1. Hechter HH, Borhani NO. Mortality and geographic distribution of arteriosclerotic heart disease: recent changes 1950–60. *Pub Health Rep* 1965; 80: 11–24.
2. Fabsitz R, Feinleib M. Geographical patterns in county mortality rates from cardiovascular diseases. *Am J Epidemiol* 1980; 111: 315–328.
3. Voors AW, Johnson WD. Altitude and arteriosclerotic heart disease mortality of white residents of 99 of the 100 largest cities in the United States. *J Chronic Dis* 1979; 32: 157–162.
4. Mortimer EA, Monson RR, MacMahon B. Reduction in mortality from coronary heart disease in men residing at high altitude. *N Engl J Med* 1977; 296: 581–585.

## Chapter 35 The Northern Ireland paradox

1. Evans AE, Ruidavets J-B, McCrum EE, *et al.* Autres pays, autres coeurs! Dietary patterns, risk factors and ischaemic heart disease in Belfast and Toulouse. *QJM* 1995; 88: 469–477.
2. The PRIME study group (prepared by JWG Yarnell). The PRIME study: classical risk factors do not explain the several-fold differences in risk of coronary heart disease between France and Northern Ireland. *QJM* 1998; 91: 667–676.

## Chapter 36 The French paradox and the effect of alcohol

1. Renaud S, De Lorgeril M. Wine, alcohol, platelets, and the French paradox for coronary heart disease. *Lancet* 1992; 339: 1523–1526.
2. Masiá R, Pella A, Marrugat J, *et al.*, and the REGICOR investigators. High prevalence of cardiovascular risk factors in Gerona, Spain, a province with low myocardial infarction incidence. *J Epidem Public Health* 1998; 52: 707–715.

3.    Ferrières J. The French Paradox: lessons for other countries. *Heart* 2004: 90: 107–111.

4.    BBC News. French winegrowers grapes of wrath. *BBC News* 4 March 2004; 09:01 GMT.

5.    Muminovic M. Hospital prescribes wine to heart attack survivors. *Student BMJ* 2003; 11: 263.

6.    Bradley KA, Merrill JO. Doctor, is wine good for my heart? *Lancet* 1999; 353: 1815–1816.

7.    Marmot MG, Rose G, Shipley MJ, Thomas BJ. Alcohol and mortality: a U-shaped curve. *Lancet* 1981; 317: 580–583.

8.    Berkel J, de Waard F. Mortality patterns and life expectancy for Seventh Day Adventists in the Netherlands. *Int J Epidem* 1983; 12: 455–459.

9.    Lutgendorf SK, Russell D, Ullrich P, *et al.* Religious participation, interleukin-6, and mortality in older adults. *Health Psychol* 2004; 23: 465–475.

10.   Berger K, Ajani UA, Kase CS, *et al.* Light-to-moderate alcohol consumption and the risk of stroke among US male physicians. *N Engl J Med* 1999; 341: 1557–1564.

11.   Hart CL, Davey Smith G, Hole DJ, Hawsthorne VM. Alcohol consumption and mortality from all causes, coronary heart disease, and stroke: results from a prospective cohort study of Scottish men with 21 years of follow up. *BMJ* 1999; 318: 1725–1729.

12.   The PRIME study group (prepared by JWG Yarnell). The PRIME study: classical risk factors do not explain the several-fold differences in risk of coronary heart disease between France and Northern Ireland. *QJM* 1998; 91: 667–676.

13.   Evans AE, Ruidavets J-B, McCrum EE, *et al.* Autres pays, autres coeurs! Dietary patterns, risk factors and ischaemic heart disease in Belfast and Toulouse. *QJM* 1995; 88: 469–477.

## Chapter 37 The geography of agriculture in Europe

1.    Minerva. *BMJ* 2004; 328: 176.

2.    Keys A. *Seven Countries: a multivariate analysis of death and coronary heart disease.* Harvard University Press: Cambridge 1980.

3.    World Health Organization. *World Health Statistics Annual.* World Health Organization: Geneva 1986.

4.    Eurostat Agriculture and Fisheries. *Agricultural Statistics Quarterly Bulletin 1.* European Commission: Brussels 2004.

5.    National Statistical Office. *Age-Standardised Mortality Rates: by Cause and Sex, 2001.* Regional Trends 38. National Statistical Office: London 2001.

# Chapter 38 Socio-economic deprivation and disease

1. Department of Health and Social Security. *Inequalities in Health: report of a research working group.* Department of Health and Social Security: London 1980.
2. Townsend P. Inequality and the health service. *Lancet* 1974; 303: 1179–1190.
3. McKeown T. *The Role of Medicine: dream, mirage or nemesis?* Nuffield Provincial Hospitals Trust: London 1976.
4. Forsdahl A. Are poor living conditions in childhood and adolescence an important risk factor for arteriosclerotic heart disease? *Br J Prevent Social Med* 1977; 31: 91–95.
5. Barker DJP, Osmond C. Infant mortality, childhood nutrition, and ischaemic heart disease in England and Wales. *Lancet* 1986; 327: 1077–1081.
6. Marmot MG, Shipley MJ, Rose G. Inequalities in death: specific explanations of a general pattern? *Lancet* 1984; 323: 1003–1006.
7. Marmot MG, McDowall ME. Mortality decline and widening social inequalities. *Lancet* 1986; 328: 274–276.
8. Rosengren A, Wedel H, Wilhelmsen L. Coronary heart disease and mortality in middle aged men from different occupational classes in Sweden. *BMJ* 1988; 297: 1497–1500.
9. Vagero D, Lundberg O. Health inequalities in Britain and Sweden. *Lancet* 1989; 334: 35–36.
10. Balarajan R. Inequalities in health within the health sector. *BMJ* 1989; 299: 822–825.
11. Kaplan GA, Salonen JT. Socioeconomic conditions in childhood and ischaemic heart disease during middle age. *BMJ* 1990; 301: 1121–1123.
12. Carvel J. Wealth brings 17 more years of health. *The Guardian* 2005; 24 February (based on Office for National Statistics press release 23 February 2005).
13. Tallis R. *Hippocratic Oaths.* Atlantic Books: London 2004.
14. UK Department of Health. *Health Survey for England: cardiovascular disease 1998.* The Stationery Office: London 1998.
15. Phillimore P, Beattie A, Townsend P. Widening inequality in health in northern England, 1981–91. *BMJ* 1994; 308: 1125–1128.
16. Pell JP, Pell ACH, Norrie H, *et al.* Effect of socioeconomic deprivation on waiting time for cardiac surgery: retrospective cohort study. *BMJ* 2000; 320: 15–19.
17. Hart JT. The inverse care law. *Lancet* 1971; 297: 405–412.

18. Macintyre K, Stewart S, Chalmers J, *et al.* Relation between socioeconomic deprivation and death from a first myocardial infarction in Scotland: population based analysis. *BMJ* 2001; 322: 1152–1153.
19. Barakat K, Stevenson S, Wilkinson P, *et al.* Socioeconomic differentials in recurrent ischaemia and mortality after acute myocardial infarction. *Heart* 2001; 85: 390–394.
20. Chalmers J, Capewell S. Deprivation, disease and death in Scotland: graphical display of survival of a cohort. *BMJ* 201; 323: 967–968.
21. UK Department of Health. *Annual Report of the Chief Medical Officer 2001.* The Stationery Office: London 2001.
22. Raphael D. Public health responses to health inequalities. *Can J Public Health* 1998; 89: 380–381.
23. Heberden W. *Observations on the Increase and Decrease of Different Diseases.* T. Payne: London 1801.
24. Hein HO, Suadicani P, Gyntelberg F. Lung cancer risk and social class. The Copenhagan Male Study: 17 year follow up. *Dan Med Bull* 1992; 39:173–176.
25. Tröhler U. *To Improve the Evidence of Medicine. The 18th century British origins of a critical approach.* Royal College of Physicians of Edinburgh: Edinburgh: 2000.
26. McAlister FA, Murphy NE, Simpson CR, *et al.* Influence of socioeconomic deprivation on the primary care burden and treatment of patients with a diagnosis of heart failure in general practice in Scotland: population based study. *BMJ* 2004: 328: 1110–1113.
27. Zittermann A, Schleithoff SS, Tenderich G, *et al.* Low vitamin D status: a contributing factor in the pathogenesis of congestive heart failure. *J Am Coll Cardiol* 2003; 41: 105–112.
28. Ismail AA, Beeching NJ, Gill GV, Bellis MA. Capture–recapture–adjusted prevalence rates of type 2 diabetes are related to social deprivation. *QJM* 1999; 92: 707–710.
29. Cowley AJ. Ischaemic heart disease. *Update Postgraduate Centre Series* 1990: 24–27.
30. Henley Centre. *Media Fitness.* Henley Centre: London 1993.
31. Hancox RJ, Milne BJ, Poulton R. Association between child and adolescent television viewing and adult health: a longitudinal birth cohort study. *Lancet* 2004; 364: 257–262.
32. East Lancashire Health Authority. *Annual Public Report.* East Lancashire Health Authority: Burnley 2004.
33. Percival T. *Observations on the State of the Population of Manchester and Other Adjacent Places.* Manchester 1773.

34. Marmot M. *Status Syndrome: how your social standing directly affects your health and life expectancy.* Bloomsbury Publishing: London 2004.

35. Department of Health and Social Security/Medical Research Council. *Research on Obesity.* HMSO: London 1976.

36. Doran T, Drever F, Whitehead M. Is there a north–south divide in social class inequalities in health in Great Britain? Cross-sectional study using data from the 2001 census. *BMJ* 2004; 328: 1043–1045.

37. Huxley A. *Doors of Perception.* Penguin Books: London 1959; 51.

## Chapter 39 Two Albanian paradoxes

1. Gjonça A, Bobak M. Albanian paradox, another example of protective effect of Mediterranean lifestyle? *Lancet* 1997; 350: 1815–1817.

## Chapter 40 The Greek paradox: smoking and coronary heart disease

1. Editorial. How does smoking harm the heart? *BMJ* 1980; 2: 573–574.

2. Eurostat. *Yearbook.* Eurostat: Luxembourg 2002.

3. Keys A. *Seven Countries: a multivariate analysis of death and coronary heart disease.* Harvard University Press: Cambridge 1980.

4. UK Department of Health. *Annual Report of the Chief Medical Officer 2001.* The Stationery Office: London 2001.

5. West RR. Smoking: its influence on survival and cause of death. *J R Coll Phys Lond* 1992; 26: 357–366.

6. Doll R, Hill AB. Mortality in relation to smoking: ten years' observations of British doctors. *BMJ* 1964; 1: 1399–1410.

7. Yarnell JWG. Smoking and cardiovascular disease. *QJM* 1996; 89: 493–498.

## Chapter 41 Respiratory disease and coronary heart disease

1. Jousilahti P, Vartiainen E, Tuomilehto J, Puska P. Symptoms of chronic bronchitis and the risk of coronary disease. *Lancet* 1996; 348: 567–572.

2. World Health Organization. *World Health Statistics Annual.* World Health Organization: Geneva 1992,1993.

3. Hole DJ, Watt GC, Davey Smith G, *et al.* Impaired lung function and mortality risk in men and women: findings from the Renfrew and Paisley prospective population study. *BMJ* 1996; 313: 711–715.

4. Littlejohns P, Macdonald LD. The relationship between severe asthma and social class. *Resp Med* 1993; 87: 139–143.

5. Nuorti JP, Butler JC, Farley MM, *et al.*, and the Active Bacterial Core Surveillance Team. Cigarette smoking and invasive pneumococcal disease. *N Engl J Med* 2000; 342: 681–689.

## Chapter 42 Inflammation and coronary heart disease

1. Mann DL. Inflammatory mediators in heart failure: homogeneity through heterogeneity. *Lancet* 1999; 353: 1812–1813.

2. Tipping PG, Maliaros J, Holdsworth SR. Procoagulant activity expression by macrophages from atheromatous vascular plaques. *Atherosclerosis* 1989; 79: 237–243.

3. Liuzzo G, Biasucci LM, Gallimore JR, *et al.* The prognostic significance of C-reactive protein and serum amyloid A protein in severe unstable angina. *N Engl J Med* 1994; 331: 417–424.

4. Mendall MA, Patel P, Ballam L, *et al.* C Reactive protein and its relation to cardiovascular risk factors: a population based cross sectional study. *BMJ* 1996; 312: 1061–1065.

5. Haverkate F, Thompson SG, Pyke SDM, *et al.*, for the European Concerted Action on Thrombosis and Disabilities Angina Pectoris Study Group. Production of C-reactive protein and risk of coronary events in stable and unstable angina. *Lancet* 1997; 349: 462–466.

6. Tataru MC, Heinrich J, Junker R, *et al.* C-reactive protein and the severity of atherosclerosis in myocardial infarction patients with stable angina pectoris. *Eur Heart J* 2000; 21: 1000–1008.

7. Buffon A, Biassucci LM, Liuzzo G, *et al.* Widespread coronary inflammation in unstable angina. *N Engl J Med* 2002; 347: 5–12.

8. Imhof A, Froehlich M, Brenner H, *et al.* Effect of alcohol consumption on systemic markers of inflammation. *Lancet* 2001; 357: 763–767.

9. Ridker PM, Rifai N, Rose L, *et al.* Comparison of C-reactive protein and low-density lipoprotein cholesterol levels in the prediction of first cardiovascular events. *N Engl J Med* 2002; 347: 1557–1565.

10. Sakkinen P, Abbott RD, Curb JD, *et al.* C-reactive protein and myocardial infarction. *J Clin Epidemiol* 2002; 55: 445–451.

11. Ridker PM, Glynn RJ, Hennekens CH. C-Reactive protein adds to the predictive value of total cholesterol and HDL cholesterol in determining risk of first myocardial infarction. *Circulation* 1998; 97: 2007–2011.

12. Hirschfield GM, Pepys MB. C-reactive protein and cardiovascular disease: new insights from an old molecule. *QJM* 2003; 96: 793–807.

13. Timms PM, Mannan N, Hitman GA, *et al.* Circulating MMP9, vitamin D and variation in the TIMP-1 response with VDR genotype: mechanisms for inflammatory damage in chronic disorders? *QJM* 2002; 95: 787–796.

## Chapter 43 Cholesterol and inflammation

1. Martin MJ, Hulley SB, Browner WS *et al.* Serum cholesterol, blood pressure, and mortality: implications from a cohort of 361,662 men. *Lancet* 1986; 328: 933–936.
2. Rose G, Shipley M. Plasma cholesterol concentration and death from coronary heart disease: 10 year results of the Whitehall study. *BMJ* 1986; 293: 306–307.
3. Sijbrands EJG, Westendorp RGJ, Defesche JC, *et al.* Mortality over two centuries in a large pedigree with familial hypercholesterolaemia: family tree mortality study. *BMJ* 2001; 322: 119–123.
4. Abramson J. *Overdosed America: the broken promise of American medicine.* HarperCollins: London and New York 2004.
5. Ravnskov U. High cholesterol may protect against infections and atherosclerosis. *QJM* 2003; 96: 927–934.
6. Bhakdi S, Tranum-Jensen J, Uttermann G, Füssle R. Binding and partial inactivation of *Staphylococcus aureus* α-toxin by human plasma low density lipoprotein. *J Biol Chem* 1983; 258: 5899–5904.
7. Jacobs D, Blackburn H, Higgins M, *et al.* Report on the conference on low blood cholesterol: mortality associations. *Circulation* 1992; 86: 1046–1060.
8. Iribarren C, Jacobs DR Jr, Sidney S, *et al.* Cohort study of serum total cholesterol and in-hospital incidence of infectious diseases. *Epidemiol Infect* 1998; 121: 335–347.
9. Iribarren C, Jacobs DR Jr, Sidney S, *et al.* Serum total cholesterol and risk of hospitalization, and death from respiratory disease. *Int J Epidemiol* 1997; 26: 1191–1202.
10. Claxton AJ, Jacobs DR Jr, Iribarren C, *et al.* Association between serum total cholesterol and HIV infection in a high-risk cohort of young men. *J Acquired Immuno Synd Human Retrovirol* 1998; 17: 51–57.
11. Pacelli F, Doglietto GB, Alfieri S, *et al.* Prognosis in intra-abdominal infections. Multivariate analysis on 604 patients. *Arch Surg* 1996; 131: 641–645.
12. Shepherd J, Cobbe SM, Ford I, *et al.*, for the West of Scotland Coronary Prevention Study Group. Prevention of coronary heart disease with pravastatin in men with hypercholesterolaemia. *N Engl J Med* 1995; 333: 1301–1307.

## Chapter 44 Could coronary heart disease be due to a microbe?

1. Benditt EP, McDougall JK. Viruses and vascular disease. *Cardiol Prac* 1989; 7: 34–39.
2. Nicholls AC, Thomas M. Coxsackie virus infection in acute myocardial infarction. *Lancet* 1977; 309: 883–884.
3. Editorial. Virus, immunology and the heart. *Lancet* 1979; 314: 1111–1113.
4. Griffiths PD, Hannington G, Booth JC. Coxsackie B virus infections and myocardial infarction. *Lancet* 1980; 315: 1387–1389.
5. Adam E, Melnick JL, Probtsfield JL, *et al.* High levels of cytomegalovirus antibody in patients requiring vascular surgery for atherosclerosis. *Lancet* 1987; 330: 291–293.
6. McDonald K, Rector TS, Braunlin EA, *et al.* Association of coronary artery disease in cardiac transplant recipients with cytomegalovirus infection. *Am J Cardiol* 1989; 64: 359–362.
7. Cunningham MJ, Pasternak RC. The potential of viruses in the pathogenesis of atherosclerosis. *Circulation* 1988; 77: 964–966.
8. Syrjänen J, Valtonen V, Iivavainen M, *et al.* Preceding infection as an important risk factor for ischaemic brain infarction in young and middle aged patients. *BMJ* 1988; 296: 1156–1160.
9. Meier CR, Derby LE, Jick SS, *et al.* Antibiotics and risk of subsequent first-time acute myocardial infarction. *JAMA* 1999; 281: 427–431.
10. Folsom AR. Antibiotics for prevention of myocardial infarction? Not yet! *JAMA* 1999; 281: 461–462.
11. Mendall MA. Inflammatory responses and coronary heart disease. The 'dirty chicken' hypothesis of cardiovascular risk factors (editorial). *BMJ* 1998; 316: 953–954.

## Chapter 45 *Chlamydia pneumoniae*

1. Saikku P, Leinonen M, Mattila K, *et al.* Serological evidence of an association of a novel *Chlamydia*, TWAR, with chronic coronary heart disease and myocardial infarction. *Lancet* 1988; 332: 983–985.
2. Gupta S, Leatham EW, Carrington D, *et al.* Elevated *Chlamydia pneumoniae* antibodies, cardiovascular events, and azithromycin in male survivors of myocardial infarction. *Circulation* 1997; 96: 404–407.
3. Gurfinkel E, Bozowich G, Daroca A, *et al.*, for the ROXIS study group. Randomised trial of roxithromycin in non-q-wave coronary syndromes: ROXIS pilot study. *Lancet* 1997; 350: 404–407.

4.  Cercek B, Shah PK, Noc M, *et al.*, for AZACS investigators. Effect of short-term treatment with azithromycin on recurrent ischaemic events of patients with acute coronary syndrome in the Azithromycin in Acute Coronary Syndrome (AZACS) trial: a randomised controlled trial. *Lancet* 2003; 361: 809–813.
5.  Neumann F-J, Katrati A, Miethke T, *et al.* Treatment of *Chlamydia pneumoniae* infection with roxithromycin and effect on neointima proliferation after coronary stent placement (ISAR-3): a randomised, double-blind, placebo-controlled trial. *Lancet* 2001; 357: 2085–2089.
6.  Kuo C, Shor A, Campbell LA, *et al.* Demonstration of *Chlamydia pneumoniae* in atherosclerotic lesions of coronary arteries. *J Infect Dis* 1993; 167: 841–849.
7.  Taylor-Robinson D, Thomas BJ. *Chlamydia pneumoniae* in arteries: the facts, their interpretation, and future studies. *J Clin Path* 1998; 51: 793–797.

## Chapter 46 *Helicobacter pylori*

1.  Marshall BJ, Warren JR. Unidentified curved bacilli in the stomach of patients with gastritis and peptic ulceration. *Lancet* 1984; 324: 1311–1314.
2.  Malcolm CA, MacKay WG, Shepherd A, Weaver LT. *Helicobacter pylori* in children is strongly associated with poverty. *Scott Med J* 2002; 49: 136–138.
3.  Editorial. Cardiovascular disease and peptic ulcer. *BMJ* 1974; 2: 760–761.
4.  Mendall MA, Goggin PM, Molineaux N, *et al.* Relation of *Helicobacter pylori* infection and coronary heart disease. *Br Heart J* 1994; 71: 437–439.
5.  Wald NJ, Law MR, Morris JK, Bagnall AM. *Helicobacter pylori* infection and mortality from ischaemic heart disease: negative results from a large, prospective study. *BMJ* 1997; 315: 1199–1201.
6.  Danesh J, Youngman L, Clark S, *et al.*, for the International Studies of Infarct Survival (ISIS) Collaborative Group. *Helicobacter pylori* infection and early onset myocardial infarction: case-control and sibling pairs study. *BMJ* 1999; 319: 1157–1162.
7.  Stone AFM, Mendall MA, Kaski J-S, *et al.* Effect of treatment for *Chlamydia pneumoniae* and *Helicobacter pylori* on markers of inflammation and cardiac events in patients with acute coronary syndromes. *Circulation* 2002; 106: 1219–1223.

8. Ameriso SF, Fridman EA, Leiguarda RC, Sevlever GE. Detection of *Helicobacter pylori* in human carotid atherosclerotic plaques. *Stroke* 2001; 32: 385–391.

9. Montenero AS, Mollichelli N, Zumbo F, *et al. Helicobacter pylori* and atrial fibrillation: a possible pathogenic link. *Heart* 2005; 91: 986–961.

## Chapter 47 Dental health and coronary heart disease

1. Jenkins GN. Recent changes in dental caries (editorial). *BMJ* 1985; 291: 1297–1298.

2. Office for National Statistics. *Adult Dental Health Survey.* The Stationery Office: London 1998

3. British Heart Foundation Statistics Database. *Coronary Heart Disease Statistics.* British Heart Foundation: London 1999.

4. Shaw JH. Causes and control of dental caries. *N Engl J Med* 1987; 317: 996–1004.

5. Desai HG, Gill HH, Shankaran K, *et al.* Dental plaque: a permanent reservoir of *Helicobacter pylori? Scand J Gastroenterol* 1991; 26: 1205–1208.

6. Mattila K, Nieminen MS, Valtonen VV, *et al.* Association between dental health and acute myocardial infarction. *BMJ* 1989; 298: 779–782.

7. DeStefano F, Anda RF, Khan HS, *et al.* Dental disease and risk of coronary heart disease and mortality. *BMJ* 1993; 306: 688–691.

8. Janket S-J, Qvarmstrom M, Meurmim JH, *et al.* Asymptomatic dental score and prevalent coronary heart disease. *Circulation* 2004; 109: 1095–1100.

9. Hujoel PP, Drangsholt M, Spiekerman C, Derouen TA. Examining the link between coronary heart disease and the elimination of chronic dental infections. *J Am Dental Assoc* 2001; 132: 883–889.

## Chapter 48 Infections of the heart

1. Kawasaki T. Acute febrile mucocutaneous lymph node syndrome (in Japanese). *Allergy* 1967; 16: 178–222.

2. Burns JC, Glodé MP. Kawasaki syndrome. *Lancet* 2004; 362: 533–544.

3. Kato H, Inoue O, Kawasaki T, *et al.* Adult coronary artery disease probably due to childhood Kawasaki disease. *Lancet* 1992; 340: 1127–1129.

## Chapter 49 Koch's postulates and the concept of proof

1.  Lewis B, Rose G. Prevention of coronary heart disease: putting theory into practice. *J R Coll Physicians Lond* 1991; 25: 21–26.
2.  Hill AB. *A Short Textbook of Medical Statistics*. Hodder & Stoughton: London 1977.
3.  Fredricks DN, Relman DA. Sequence-based evidence of microbial disease causation: when Koch's postulates don't fit. *J NIH Res* 1996; 8: 39–44.

## Chapter 50 Science works by paradigms

1.  Khun T. *The Structure of Scientific Revolutions*. University of Chicago Press: Chicago1996.
2.  Marmot M. *Status Syndrome: how your social standing directly affects your health and life expectancy*. Bloomsbury Publishing: London 2004.
3.  Cross M. Truth is out there. *New Scientist* 19 February 2000; Supple 128 Inside Science (Philosophy): 1–4.
4.  Buchanan M. *Ubiquity*. Weidenfeld & Nicolson: London 2000.
5.  Skrabanek P. Non-census consensus. *Lancet* 1990; 335: 1446–1447.
6.  Sheldon TA, Davey Smith G. Consensus conferences and drug promotion. *Lancet* 1993; 341: 100–102.
7.  HEART UK. Diet and heart health symposium 11. *Br J Cardiol* 2004; 11 Supple 1.
8.  Hill AB. *A Short Textbook of Medical Statistics*. Hodder & Stoughton: London 1977.
9.  Mendall MA. Inflammatory responses and coronary heart disease. The 'dirty chicken' hypothesis of cardiovascular risk factors (editorial). *BMJ* 1998; 316: 953–954.

## Chapter 51 South Asian ethnicity and coronary heart disease

1.  Finch PJ, Millard FJC, Maxwell JD. Risk of tuberculosis in immigrant Asians: culturally acquired immunodeficiency? *Thorax* 1991; 46: 1–5.
2.  Marmot MG, Adelstein AM, Balusu L. *Immigrant Mortality in England and Wales 1970–78*. OPCS Studies of Medical and Population Subjects No. 47. HMSO: London 1984.
3.  McKeigue PM, Marmot MG. Mortality from coronary heart disease in Asian communities in London. *BMJ* 1988; 297: 903.

4. Hughes LO, Raval U, Raftery EB. First myocardial infarction in Asians and white men. *BMJ* 1989; 298: 1345–1350.
5. Balarajan R. Ethnic differences in mortality from ischaemic heart disease and cerebrovascular disease in England and Wales. *BMJ* 1991; 302: 560–564.
6. Haskey J, Huxstep S. *Population Projections by Ethnic Group*. National Statistics Studies on Medical and Population Subjects. HMSO: London 2002.
7. Maxwell JD, Strachan DP. Risk of coronary heart disease in Hindus and Muslims from Indian subcontinent is similar. *BMJ* 1996; 313; 563.
8. Bhopal R. Epidemic of cardiovascular disease in South Asians. Prevention must start in childhood. *BMJ* 2002; 324; 625–626.
9. UK Department of Health. *The National Service Framework for Coronary Heart Disease: winning the war on heart disease*. The Stationery Office: London 2004.
10. Ball S, Lloyd J, Cairns T, *et al*. Why is there so much end-stage renal failure of undetermined cause in UK Indo-Asians? *QJM* 2001; 94: 187–193.
11. Balarajan R, Raleigh VS. Patterns of mortality among Bangladeshis in England and Wales. *Ethnicity Health* 1997; 2: 5–12.

## Chapter 52 The spleen and coronary heart disease

1. King H, Shumacker HB. Splenic studies. I. Susceptibility to infection after splenectomy performed in infancy. *Ann Surg* 1952; 136: 239–242.
2. Editorial. Splenectomy: a long-term risk of infection. *Lancet* 1985; 326 928–929.
3. Davies JM, Barnes R, Milligan D. Updates of guidelines for the prevention and treatment of infection in patients with an absent or dysfunctional spleen. *Clin Med* 2002; 2: 440–443.
4. Robinette CD, Fraumeni JF. Splenectomy and subsequent mortality in veterans of the 1939–45 war. *Lancet* 1977; 310: 127–129.
5. Schilling RF. Spherocytosis, splenectomy, stokes, and heart attacks. *Lancet* 1997: 350: 1677–1678.

## Chapter 53 Sex and coronary heart disease

1. Stamler J. The marked decline in coronary heart disease mortality rates in the United States, 1968–1981; summary of findings and possible explanations. *Cardiology* 1985; 72: 11–22.

2.     UK Department of Health. *The National Service Framework for Coronary Heart Disease: winning the war on heart disease.* The Stationery Office: London: 2004.

3.     Lawlor DA, Ebrahim S, Davey Smith G. Sex matters: secular and geographical trends in sex differences in coronary heart disease mortality. *BMJ* 2001; 323: 541–545.

4.     Schalk G, Forbes MR. Male biases in parasitism of mammals: effects of study type, host age, and parasite taxon. *Oikos* 1997; 78: 67–74.

5.     Ananthaswamy A. The inner strength that keeps women going. *New Scientist* 2001; 15 September: 14.

6.     Aspinall R, Pido-Lopez J. Both age and gender affect thymic output: more recent thymic migrants in females than males as they age. *Clin Exp Immunol* 2001; 125: 409–413.

7.     Schuurs AHWM, Verheul HAM. Effects of gender and sex steroids on the immune response. *J Steroid Biochem* 1990; 35: 157–172.

8.     Barratt-Connor E, Grady D. Hormone replacement therapy, heart disease, and other considerations. *Annu Rev Public Health* 1998; 19: 55–72.

9.     Grodstein F, Stampfer MJ, Colditz GA, *et al.* Postmenopausal hormone replacement therapy and mortality. *N Engl J Med* 1997; 336: 1769–1775.

10.   The ESPRIT team. Oestrogen therapy for prevention of re-infarction in postmenopausal women: a randomised placebo controlled trial. *Lancet* 2002; 360: 2001–2008.

11.   Herrington DM, Reboussin DM, Brosnihan KB, *et al.* Effects of estrogen replacement on the progression of coronary–artery atherosclerosis. *N Engl J Med* 2000; 343: 522–529.

## Chapter 54 Immune-suppression and coronary heart disease

1.     Uretsky BF, Murali S, Reddy PS, *et al.* Development of coronary artery disease in cardiac transplant patients receiving immunosuppressive therapy with cyclosporin and prednisone. *Circulation* 1987; 76: 827–834.

2.     Coleman MP, Rachet B, Woods LM *et al.* Trends in socio-economic inequalities in cancer survival in England and Wales up to 2001. *Br J Cancer* 2004; 90: 1367–1373.

3.     Huddart RA, Norman A, Shahidi M, *et al.* Cardiovascular disease as a long-term complication of testicular cancer. *J Clin Oncol* 2003; 21: 1513–1523.

4.     Kobashigawa JA, Katznelson S, Laks H, *et al.* Effect of pravastatin on outcomes after cardiac transplant. *N Engl J Med* 1995; 333: 621–627.

5. Lezner J. Unreported cholesterol drug data released by companies show drug is ineffective. *BMJ* 2008; 336: 180–181.
6. DAD, Data Collection on Adverse Events of anti-HIV Drugs Study Group. Combination retroviral therapy and the risk of myocardial infarction. *N Engl J Med* 2003; 349: 1993–2003.

## Chapter 55 Chronic renal failure, vitamin D and coronary heart disease

1. Department of Health and Social Security. *Inequalities in Health: report of a research working group.* Department of Health and Social Security: London 1980.
2. Feehally J. Ethnicity and renal disease: questions and challenges. *Clin Med* 2003; 3: 578–582.
3. Raleigh VS, Kiri V, Balarajan R. Variations in mortality from diabetes, hypertension and renal disease in England and Wales by country of birth. *Health Trends* 1996; 28: 122–127.
4. Holmes B. Fanning the flames. *New Scientist* 2004; 22 May: 41–43.
5. Baigent C, Burbury K, Wheeler D. Premature cardiovascular disease in chronic renal failure. *Lancet* 2000; 356: 147–152.
6. Go AS, Chertow GM, Fan D, *et al.* Chronic kidney disease and the risks of death, cardiovascular events and hospitalization. *N Engl J Med* 2004; 351: 1296–1305.
7. Anavekar NS, McMurray JJV, Velaquez EJ, *et al.* Relation between renal dysfunction and cardiovascular outcomes after myocardial infarction. *N Engl J Med* 2004; 351: 1285–1295.

## Chapter 56 Diabetes and vitamin D

1. Gillespie KM, Bain SC, Barnett AH, *et al.* The rising incidence of childhood type 1 diabetes and reduced contribution of high-risk HLA haplotypes. *Lancet* 2004; 364: 1699–1700.
2. Devendra D, Liu E, Eisenbarth GS . Type 1 diabetes: recent developments. *BMJ* 2004; 328: 750–753.
3. Onkamo P, Väänänen S, Karvonen M, Tuomilehto J. Worldwide increase in incidence of type I diabetes: the analysis of the data and published incidence trends. *Diabetologia* 1999; 42: 1395–1403.
4. Matthews DR, Spivey RS, Kennedy I. Coffee consumption as trigger for diabetes in childhood. *BMJ* 1990; 300: 1012.
5. EURODIAB ACE Study Group. Variation and trends in incidence of childhood diabetes in Europe. *Lancet* 2000; 355: 873–76.

6. Bodansky HJ, Staines A, Stephenson C, *et al.* Evidence for an environmental effect in the aetiology of insulin dependent diabetes in a transmigratory population. *BMJ* 1992; 304: 1020–1022.

7. Nazroo J. *The Health of Britain's Ethnic Minorities: findings from a national survey.* Policy Studies Institute: London 1997.

8. Bjork S, Kapur A, Kelkar S, *et al.* Aspects of diabetes in India: a nationwide survey. *Res Clin Forums* 2003; 25.

9. Hutchison HS, Shah SJ. The aetiology of rickets, early and late. *QJM* 1922; 15: 167–195.

10. Stene LC, Ulriksen J, Magnus P, Joner G. Use of cod liver oil during pregnancy associated with lower risk of type 1 diabetes in the offspring. *Diabetologia* 2000; 43: 1093–1451.

11. Hyppönen E, Läärä E, Reunanen A, *et al.* Intake of vitamin D and risk of type 1 diabetes: a birth-cohort study. *Lancet* 2001; 2001: 1500–1503.

12. Stene LC, Joner G, Norwegian Childhood Diabetes Study Group. Use of cod liver oil during the first year of life is associated with lower risk of childhood-onset type 1 diabetes: a large population-based case-control trial. *Am J Clin Nutr* 2003; 78: 1128–1134.

## Chapter 57 The metabolic syndrome and insulin resistance

1. Bjork S, Kapur A, Kelkar S, *et al.* Aspects of diabetes in India: a nationwide survey. *Res Clin Forums* 2003; 25.

2. Fuller JH, Shipley MJ, Rose G, *et al.* Coronary heart disease risk and impaired glucose tolerance. The Whitehall study. *Lancet* 1980; 315: 1373–1376.

3. Salonen JT. Non-insulin dependent diabetes and ischaemic heart disease: related, but how? *BMJ* 1989; 298: 1050–1051.

4. Aguilar D, Solomon SD, Køber L, *et al.* Newly diagnosed and previously known diabetes mellitus and 1-year outcomes of acute myocardial infarction. *Circulation* 2004; 110: 1572–1578.

5. Lyon RLl. The early days of insulin use in Edinburgh. *BMJ* 1990; 301:1452–1454.

6. Yalow RS, Berson SA. Plasma insulin concentrations in nondiabetic and early diabetic subjects: determination by a new sensitive immune-assay technique. *Diabetes* 1960; 9: 254–260.

7. Karam JH, Grodsky GM, Forsham PH, McWilliams NB. Excessive insulin response to glucose in obese subjects as measured by immunochemical assay. *Diabetes* 1960; 12: 197–204.

8. Buchanan KD, McKiddie MT, Lindsay AC, Manderson WG. Carbohydrate metabolism in duodenal ulcer patients. *Gut* 1967; 8: 325–331.

9. Sloan JM, Mackay JS, Sheridan B. Glucose tolerance and insulin response in atherosclerosis. *BMJ* 1970; 4: 586–588.

10. Stout RW. Insulin and atheroma: an update. *Lancet* 1987; 329: 1077–1079.

11. Zavaroni I, Bonora E, Pagliara M, *et al.* Risk factors for coronary heart disease in healthy persons with hyperinsulinemia and normal glucose tolerance. *N Engl J Med* 1989; 320: 702–706.

12. Després J-P, Lamarche B, Mauriège P, *et al.* Hyperinsulinaemia as an independent risk factor for ischemic heart disease. *N Engl J Med* 1996; 334: 952–957.

13. Facchini FS, Hollenbeck CB, Jeppesen J, *et al.* Insulin resistance and cigarette smoking. *Lancet* 1992; 339: 1128–1130.

14. Grimes DS, Goddard J. The effect of cigarette smoking on gastric emptying. *BMJ* 1978; 2: 460–461.

15. Van Dam RM, Feskens EJM. Coffee consumption and risk of type 2 diabetes mellitus. *Lancet* 2002; 360: 1477–1478.

16. Reaven GM. Insulin resistance in noninsulin-dependent diabetes mellitus. Does it exist and can it be measured? *Am J Med* 1983; 74: 3–17.

17. Reaven GM. Role of insulin resistance in human disease. *Diabetes* 1988; 37: 1595–1607.

18. Himsworth HP, Kerr RB. Insulin-sensitive and insulin-insensitive types of diabetes mellitus. *Clin Sci* 1939; 4: 119–152.

19. Matthews DR, Hosker JP, Rudenski *et al.* Homeostasis model assessment: insulin resistance and □-cell function from fasting plasma glucose and insulin concentrations in man. *Diabetologia* 1985; 28: 412–418.

20. Cock T-A, Auwerx J. Leptin: cutting the fat off the bone. *Lancet* 2003; 362: 1572–1574.

21. Klein S, Fontana L, Young VL, *et al.* Absence of an effect of liposuction on insulin action and risk factors for coronary heart disease. *N Engl J Med* 2004; 350: 2549–2557.

22. Pajvani UB, Scherer PE. Apidonectin: systemic contributor to insulin sensitivity. *Curr Diabetes Rep* 2003; 3: 207–213.

23. Weiss R, Dziura J, Burgert TS, *et al.* Obesity and the metabolic syndrome in children and adolescents. *N Engl J Med* 2004; 350: 2362–2374.

24. Björntorp P. Thrifty genes and human obesity. Are we chasing ghosts? *Lancet* 2001; 358: 1006–1008.

25. McKeigue PM, Shah B, Marmot MG. Relation of central obesity and insulin resistance with high diabetes prevalence and cardiovascular risk in South Asians. *Lancet* 1991; 337: 382–386.

26. Baynes, Boucher BJ, Feskens EJM, Kromhout D. Vitamin D, glucose tolerance and insulinaemia in elderly men. *Diabetologia* 1997; 40: 344–347.
27. Boucher BJ. Inadequate vitamin D status: does it contribute to the disorders comprising syndrome X? *Br J Nutr*1998; 79: 315–327.
28. Boucher BJ, Mannan N, Noonan K, *et al.* Glucose intolerance and impairment of insulin secretion in relation to vitamin D deficiency in East London Asians. *Diabetologia* 1995; 38: 1239–1245.
29. Dandona P, Fonseka V, Menon RK. Vitamin D deficiency and the endocrine pancreas. *Diabetologia* 1986, 29; 268–469.
30. Whincup PH, Gilg JA, Papacosta O, *et al.* Early evidence of ethnic differences in cardiovascular risk: cross sectional comparison of British South Asian and white children. *BMJ* 2002; 324: 635–638.

## Chapter 58 The maternal factor and non-genetic inheritance

1. Forsdahl A. Are poor living conditions in childhood and adolescence an important risk factor for arteriosclerotic heart disease? *Br J Social Prev Med* 1977; 31: 91–95.
2. Barker DJP. The intrauterine origins of cardiovascular and obstructive lung disease in adult life. *J R Coll Physicians Lond* 1991; 25: 129–133.
3. Roseboom TJ, van der Meulin JH, Osmond C, *et al.* Coronary heart disease after prenatal exposure to the Dutch famine, 1944–45. *Heart* 2000; 84: 595–598.
4. Barker DJP, Hales CN, Fall CHD, *et al.* Type 2 (non-insulin dependent) diabetes mellitus, hypertension and hyperlipidaemia (syndrome X): relation to reduced foetal growth. *Diabetologia* 1993; 36: 62–67.
5. Barker DJP. Maternal and foetal origins of coronary heart disease. *J R Coll Physicians Lond* 1994; 28: 544–551.
6. Hofman PL, Regan F, Jackson WE, *et al.* Premature birth and later insulin resistance. *N Engl J Med* 2004; 351: 2179–2186.
7. Smith GCS, Pell, Walsh D. Pregnancy complications and maternal risk of ischaemic heart disease; a retrospective cohort study of 129,290 births. *Lancet* 2001; 357: 2002–2006.
8. Koupil I, Leon DA, Lithell HO. Length of gestation is associated with mortality from cerebrovascular disease. *J Epidemiol Comm Health* 2005; 59: 473–474.
9. Barker DJP, Forsén T, Uutela A, *et al.* Size at birth and resilience to effects of poor living conditions in adult life: a longitudinal study. *BMJ* 2001; 323: 1273–1276.

10. Richards M, Hardy R, Kuh D, Wadsworth MEJ. Birth weight and cognitive function in the British 1946 cohort: longitudinal population based study. *BMJ* 2001; 322: 199–203.
11. Brooke OG, Brown IRF, Bone CDM, *et al*. Vitamin D supplements in pregnant Asian women: effects on calcium status and fetal growth. *BMJ* 1980; 280: 751–754.
12. Prentice AM. Intrauterine factors, adiposity, and hyperinsulinaemia. Thin babies with excess body fat may explain later adiposity in Indians. *BMJ* 2003; 327: 880–881.
13. Olsen SF, Secher NJ. Low consumption of seafood in early pregnancy as a risk factor for preterm delivery: prospective cohort study. *BMJ* 2002; 324: 447–450.
14. Nowak R. Catch the rays. Sunshine before birth could be crucial for brain development. *New Scientist* 2002; 9 February: 7.
15. Davies G, Welham J, Chant D, *et al*. A systematic review and meta-analysis of northern hemisphere season of birth studies in schizophrenia. *Schizophr Bull* 2003; 29: 587–93.
16. Cui X, McGrath JJ, Burne THJ, *et al*. Maternal vitamin D depletion alters neurogenesis in the developing rat brain. *Int J Develop Neurosci* 2007; 25: 227–232.
17. Hyppönen E, Lääräe, Reunanen A, *et al*. Intake of vitamin D and risk of type 1 diabetes: a birth-cohort study. *Lancet* 2001; 358: 1500–1503.
18. Reaven GM. The fourth musketeer: from Alexander Dumas to Claude Bernard. *Diabetologia* 1995; 38: 3–13.
19. Rothwell PM, Staines A, Smail P, *et al*. Seasonality of birth of patients with childhood diabetes in Britain. *BMJ* 1996; 312:1456–1457.
20. Cagnacci A, Pansini FS, Bacchi-Modena A, *et al*. Season of birth influences timing of menopause. *Human Repro* 2005; 20: 2190–2193.

## Chapter 59 Hepatitis C virus, diabetes and the metabolic syndrome

1. Diehl AM, Li ZP, Lin HZ, Yang SQ. Cytokines and the pathogenesis of non-alcoholic steato-hepatitis. *Gut* 2005; 54: 303–306.
2. Sjöholm A, Nyström T. Endothelial inflammation in insulin resistance. *Lancet* 2005; 365: 610–612.
3. Knobler H, Schattner A. TNF-α, chronic hepatitis C and diabetes: a novel triad. *QJM* 2005; 98: 1–6.
4. Choo OL, Kuo G, Weiner AJ *et al*. Isolation of a cDNA clone derived from a blood-borne non-A, non-B viral hepatitis genome. *Science* 1989; 244: 359–362.

5.  Rocha M, Avenaud P, Ménard A, *et al.* Association of *Helicobacter* species with hepatitis C cirrhosis with or without hepatocellular carcinoma. *Gut* 2005; 54: 396–401.
6.  Mehta SH, Brancati FL, Sulkowski MS, *et al.* Prevalence of type 2 diabetes mellitus among persons with hepatitis C virus infection in the United States. *Ann Int Med* 2000; 133: 592–599.
7.  Mehta SH, Brancati FL, Strathdee SA, *et al.* Hepatitis C virus infection and incident type 2 diabetes. *Hepatology* 2003; 38: 50–56.
8.  Conn HO, Scheiber W, Elkington SG, Johnson TR. Cirrhosis and diabetes. *Am J Dig Dis* 1967; 14: 837–843.

## Chapter 60 Atmospheric pollution and the emergence of coronary heart disease in newly industrialising countries

1.  Felton DJC, Stone WD. Osteomalacia in Asian immigrants during pregnancy. *BMJ* 1966; 1; 1521–1522.
2.  Ford JA, Davidson DC, McIntosh W, *et al.* Neonatal rickets in Asian immigrant population. *BMJ* 1973; 2; 211–212.
3.  Hutchison HS, Shah SJ. The aetiology of rickets, early and late. *QJM* 1922; 15: 167–195.
4.  Ferguson M. *A Study of Social and Economic Factors in the Causation of Rickets, with introductory historical survey by Leonard Findlay.* Special Report Series No. 20. Medical Research Council: London 1918.
5.  Mathers CD, Sadana R, Salomon JA, *et al.* Healthy life expectancy in 191 countries, 1991 (World Health Report 2000). *Lancet* 2000; 357: 1685–1691.
6.  Singh RB, Verma SP, Niaz MA. Social class and coronary artery disease in India. *Lancet* 1999; 353: 154.
7.  Bobak M, Leon DA. Air pollution and infant mortality in the Czech Republic 1986–88. *Lancet* 1992; 340: 1010–1014.
8.  Dockery DW, Pope CA, Xu X, *et al.* An association between air pollution and mortality in six US cities. *N Engl J Med* 1993; 329: 1753–1759.
9.  Poloniecki JD, Atkinson RW, de Leon AP, Anderson HR. Daily time series for cardiovascular hospital admissions and previous day's air pollution in London, UK. *Occup Environ Med* 1997; 54: 535–540.
10. Katsouyanni K, Touloumi G, Spix C, *et al.* Short term effects of ambient sulphur dioxide and particulate matter on mortality in 12 European cities: results from time series data from the APHEA project. *BMJ* 1997; 314: 1658–1663.

11. Peters A, Döring A, Wichman E-H, Koenig W. Increased plasma viscosity during an air pollution episode: a link to mortality? *Lancet* 1997; 349: 1582–1587.
12. Samet JM, Dominici F, Curriero FC, *et al.* Fine particulate air pollution and mortality in 20 US cities 1987–94. *N Engl J Med* 2000; 343: 1742–1749.
13. Peters A, Dockery DW, Muller JE, Mittleman MA. Increased particulate air pollution and the triggering of myocardial infarction. *Circulation* 2001; 103: 2810–2815.
14. Clancy L, Goodman P, Sinclair H, Dockery DW. Effect of air-pollution on death rates in Dublin, Ireland: an intervention study. *Lancet* 2002; 360: 1210–1214.
15. Watts J. Toxic smog shrouds Beijing. *The Guardian* 2004; 11 October: 15.
16. Brown P. Welcome to Tirana, Europe's pollution capital. *The Guardian* 2004; 27 March: 15.

## Chapter 61 The climate of the British Isles

1. Kmietowicz Z. France heads WHO's health systems league table. *West Med J* 2000; 173: 154–155.
2. The PRIME study group (prepared by JWG Yarnell). The PRIME study: classical risk factors do not explain the several-fold differences in risk of coronary heart disease between France and Northern Ireland. *QJM* 1998; 91: 667–676.
3. Meteorological Office: Exeter (personal communication).
4. Paterson D. Did Tibet cool the world? *New Scientist* 1993; 3 July: 29–33.
5. Raymo ME, Ruddiman WF, Froelich PN. Influence of late Cenozoic mountain building on ocean geochemical cycles. *Geology* 1988; 16: 649–653.

## Chapter 63 Protection against cancer by vitamin D and sunlight

1. Apperly FL. The relationship of solar radiation to cancer mortality in North America. *Cancer Res* 1941; 1: 191–195.
2. Peller S. Carcinogenesis as a means of reducing cancer mortality. *Lancet* 1936; 2: 552–556.
3. Grant WB. An estimate of premature cancer mortality in the US due to inadequate doses of solar ultraviolet-B radiation. *Cancer* 2002; 94: 1867–1875.

4. Devesa SS, Grauman DJ, Blot WJ, *et al*. *Atlas of Cancer Mortality in the United States, 1950–1994*. Publication No. 99-4564. National Institutes of Health: Bethesda 1999. http://cancer.gov/atlas plus/new. html (accessed 22 October 2001).

5. NASA. *Total Ozone Mapping Spectrometer Data*. NASA. http:// jwocky.gsfc.nasa.gov/ (accessed 22 October 2001).

6. USDA. *UVB Radiation Monitoring Program*. USDA. http://uvb.nrel. colostate.edu/ (accessed 22 October 2001).

7. Hanchette CL, Schwartz GG. Geographical patterns of prostate cancer mortality. Evidence for a protective effect of ultraviolet radiation. *Cancer* 1992; 70: 2861–2869.

8. Luscombe CJ, Fryer AA, French ME, *et al*. Exposure to ultraviolet radiation: association with susceptibility and age at presentation with prostate cancer. *Lancet* 2001; 358: 641–642.

9. Silman AJ. Regional differences in cancer survival. *Hosp Update* 1985; October: 735–745.

10. Coleman MP, Babb P, Damiecki P, *et al*. Cancer survival trends in England and Wales, 1971–1995: deprivation and NHS region. Studies in Medical and Population Subjects No. 61. Office for National Statistics, The Stationery Office: London 1999.

11. Lieberman DA, Prindiville S, Weiss DG, Willett W. Risk actors for advanced colonic neoplasia and hyperplastic polyps in asymptomatic individuals. *JAMA* 2003; 290: 2959–2967.

12. Gatta G, Capocaccia R, Sant M, *et al*. Understanding variations in survival for colorectal cancer in Europe: a EUROCARE high resolution study. *Gut* 2000; 47: 533–538.

13. Kane KF, Langman MJS, Williams GR. Vitamin $D_3$ and retinoid X receptor mRNAs are expressed in human colorectal mucosa and neoplasms. *Gut* 1994; 35 Supple S2: Abstract W7.

14. Thomas MG, Tebbutt S, Williamson RCN. Vitamin D and its metabolites inhibit cell proliferation in human rectal mucosa and a colon cancer line. *Gut* 1992; 33: 1660–1663.

15. Reichel H, Koeffler HP, Norman AW. The role of the vitamin D endocrine system in health and disease. *N Engl J Med* 1989; 320: 980–991.

16. Misra N, Roberts L, Hardwick RH. Adenocarcinoma of the gastro-oesophageal junction in England and Wales: incidence and effect of accuracy of cancer registration. *Gut* 2004; 53, Supple III: A59 (Abstract 228).

17. Misra N, Hardwick RH. Oesophageal adenocarcinoma: a very British disease. *Gut* 2004; 53, Supple III; A60 (Abstract 229).

18. Parkin DM, Whelan SL, Felay J, *et al. Cancer Incidence in Five Continents*. International Agency for Research on Cancer: Lyon 2002.

19. Schernhammer ES, Laden F, Speizer FE, *et al.* Rotating night shifts and risk of breast cancer in women participating in the Nurses' Health Study. *J Natl Cancer Inst* 2001; 93: 1563–1568.

20. Schernhammer ES, Laden F, Speizer FE, *et al.* Night-shift work and risk of colorectal cancer in the Nurses' Health Study. *J Natl Cancer Inst* 2003; 95: 825–828.

21. Pauley SM. Lighting for the human circadian clock: recent research indicates that lighting has become a public health issue. *Med Hypoth* 2004; 63: 588–596.

22. Zhou W, Suk R, Liu G, *et al.* Vitamin D predicts overall survival in early stage non-small cell lung cancer patients. *Proc Am Assoc Cancer Res* 2005; 46: Abstract LB-231.

23. Isles CG, Hole DJ, Gillis CR, *et al.* Plasma cholesterol, coronary heart disease, and cancer in the Renfrew and Paisley survey. *BMJ* 1989; 298: 920–924.

24. Rose G, Blackburn H, Keys A, *et al.* Colon cancer and cholesterol. *Lancet* 1974; 1: 181–183.

25. World Health Organization. *World Health Statistics Annual 1969. Vol. 1. Vital statistics and causes of death.* World Health Organization: Geneva 1972.

26. Rose G, Shipley M. Plasma cholesterol concentration and death from coronary heart disease: 10 year results of the Whitehall study. *BMJ* 1986; 293: 306–307.

27. Keys A. *Seven Countries: a multivariate analysis of death and coronary heart disease.* Harvard University Press: Cambridge 1980.

28. Dawber TR, Kannel WB, Lyell LP. An approach to longitudinal studies in a community: the Framingham Study. *Ann NY Acad Sci* 1963; 107: 539–545.

29. Paul O, Lepper MH, Phelan WH, *et al.* A longitudinal study of coronary heart disease. *Circulation* 1963; 28: 20–31.

30. Stammler J, Berkson DM, Levinson M, *et al.* Coronary heart disease. Status of preventive efforts. *Archs Envir Hlth* 1966; 13: 322–341.

31. Keys A, Taylor HL, Blackburn H, *et al.* Mortality and coronary heart disease among men studied for 23 years. *Archs Intern Med* 1971; 128: 201–212.

32. Kuhn TS. *The Structure of Scientific Revolutions.* University of Chicago Press: Chicago 1996.

33. Balkwill F, Mantovani A. Inflammation and cancer: back to Virchow? *Lancet* 2001; 357: 539–545.

34. Mantovani A, Bottazzi B, Colotta F, *et al.* The origin and function of tumor-associated macrophages. *Immunol Today* 1992; 13: 265–270.

35. Dvorak HF. Tumors: wounds that do not heal. *N Engl J Med* 1986; 315: 1650–1659.

36. Lowndes CM, Gill ON. Cervical cancer, human papillomavirus, and vaccination. *BMJ* 2005; 331: 915–916.

37. Strandberg TE, Pyörälä K, Cook TJ, *et al.* for the 4S group. Mortality and incidence of cancer during 10-year follow-up of the Scandinavian Simvastatin Survival Study (4S). *Lancet* 2004; 364: 771–777.

38. Poytner JN, Gruber SB, Higgins PDR, *et al.* Statins and risk of colorectal cancer. *N Engl J Med* 2005; 352: 2184–2192.

39. Ogunwobi OO, Beales ILP. Simvastatin induces apoptosis and inhibits proliferation in adenocarcinoma cells by inhibiting activation of extracellular signal related kinase (ERK) and AKT. *Gut* 2006; 55 Supple II: A108 Abstract 417.

40. Boddy AP, Mehta S, Johnson IT *et al.* Dietary fish oil lowers mucosal PGE2 levels during oesophageal carcinogenesis. *Gut* 2006; 55 Supple II: A108 Abstract 418.

41. Szabo S, Haislip AM, Garry RF. Of mice, cats, and men: is human breast cancer a zoonosis? *Microsc Res Tech* 2005; 68: 197–208.

## Chapter 64 Crohn's disease

1. Banerjee AK, Peters TL. The history of Crohn's disease. *J R Coll Physicians Lond* 1989; 23: 121–124.

2. Crohn BB, Ginzberg L, Oppenheimer GD. Regional enteritis: a pathological and clinical entity. *JAMA* 1932; 99: 1323–1329.

3. Shanahan F. Crohn's disease. *Lancet* 2002; 359: 662–669.

4. Heaton KW, McCarthy CF, Horton RE, *et al.* Miliary Crohn's disease. *Gut* 1967; 8: 4–7.

5. Jayanthi V, Robinson RJ, Malathi S, *et al.* Does Crohn's disease need differentiation from tuberculosis? *J Gastroenterol Hepatol* 1996; 11: 183–186.

6. Sawczenko A, Sandhu BK, Logan RFA, *et al.* Prospective study of childhood inflammatory bowel disease in the British Isles. *Lancet* 2001; 357: 1093–1094.

7. Montgomery SM, Morris DL, Pounder RE, Wakefield AJ. Asian ethnic origin and the risk of inflammatory bowel disease. *Eur J Gastroenterol Hepatol* 1999; 11: 543–546.

8. Tsianos EV, Masalas CN, Merkouropoulos M, *et al.* Incidence of inflammatory bowel disease in north west Greece: rarity of Crohn's disease in an area where ulcerative colitis is common. *Gut* 1994; 35: 369–372.

9. Lapidus A, Bernell O, Hellers G, *et al.* Incidence of Crohn's disease in Stockholm County 1955–1989. *Gut* 1997; 41: 480–486.

10. Belluzzi A, Brignola C, Campieri M, *et al.* Effect of an enteric-coated fish-oil preparation on relapses in Crohn's disease. *N Engl J Med* 1996; 334: 1557–1560.

11. Wilkinson RJ, Llewelyn M, Toossi Z, *et al.* Influence of vitamin D deficiency and vitamin D receptor polymorphisms on tuberculosis among Gujarati Asians in west London. *Lancet* 2000; 355: 618–621.

12. Simmons JD, Mullighan C, Welsh KI, Jewell DP. Vitamin D receptor gene polymorphism: association with Crohn's disease susceptibility. *Gut* 2000; 47: 211–214.

13. Abreu MT, Kantorovich V, Vasilauskas EA, *et al.* Measurement of vitamin D levels in inflammatory bowel disease patients reveals a subset of Crohn's disease patients with elevated 1,25-dihydroxyvitamin D and low bone mineral density. *Gut* 2004; 53: 1129–1136.

14. Comes MC, Gower-Rousseau, Colombel JF, *et al.* Inflammatory bowel disease in married couples: 10 cases in Nord Pas de Calais region of France and Liège county of Belgium. *Gut* 1994; 35: 1316–1318.

15. Sanderson JD, Moss MT, Tizard MLV, Hermon-Taylor J. *Mycobacterium paratuberculosis* DNA in Crohn's disease tissue. *Gut* 1992; 33: 890–896.

16. Hermon-Taylor J, Barnes N, Clarke C, Finlayson C. *Mycobacterium paratuberculosis* cervical lymphadenitis, followed five years later by terminal ileitis similar to Crohn's disease. *BMJ* 1998; 316: 449–453.

17. Quirke P. *Mycobacterium avium* subspecies *paratuberculosis* as a cause of Crohn's disease. *Gut* 2001; 49: 757–760.

18. Kuhn TS. *The Structure of Scientific Revolutions.* University of Chicago Press: Chicago 1996.

19. Naser SA, Ghobrial G, Romero C, Valentine JF. Culture of *Mycobacterium avium* subspecies *paratuberculosis* from the blood of patients with Crohn's disease. *Lancet* 2004; 364: 1039–1044.

20. Grimes DS. *Mycobacterium avium* subspecies *paratuberculosis* as a cause of Crohn's disease. *Gut* 2002; 50: 155.

21. Fredricks DN, Relman DA. Sequence-based evidence of microbial disease causation: when Koch's postulates don't fit. *J NIH Res* 1996; 8: 39–44.
22. Morgan KL. Johne's and Crohns's. Chronic inflammatory bowel diseases of infectious aetiology? *Lancet* 1987; 329: 1017–1019.
23. Allen RN, Pease P, Ibbotson JP. Clustering of Crohn's disease in a Cotswold village. *QJM* 1986; 59: 473–478.
24. Zeng L, Anderson FH. Seasonal change in the exacerbations of Crohn's disease. *Scand J Gastroenterol* 1996; 31: 79–82.
25. Marks DJB, Harbord WM, MacAllister R, *et al.* Defective acute inflammation in Crohn's disease: a clinical investigation. *Lancet* 2006; 367: 668–678.
26. Mendall MA. Inflammatory responses and coronary heart disease. The "dirty chicken" hypothesis of cardiovascular risk factors (editorial). *BMJ* 1998; 316: 953-954.
27. Korzenik JR. Is Crohn's disease due to defective immunity? *Gut* 2007; 56: 2–5.

## Chapter 65 The sun, vitamin D and diseases of the central nervous system

1. Pulver AE, Liang KY, Brown CH, *et al.* Risk factors in schizophrenia. Season of birth, gender, and familial risk. *Br J Psychiatry* 1992; 160: 65–71.
2. Parker G, Mahendran R, Koh ES, Machin D. Season of birth in schizophrenia: no latitude at the equator. *Br J Psychiatry* 2000; 176: 68–71.
3. Sham PC, O'Callaghan E, Takei N, *et al.* Schizophrenia following pre-natal exposure to influenza epidemics between 1939 and 1960. *Br J Psychiatry* 1992; 160: 461–466.
4. Ravensholt RT, Foege WH. 1918 influenza, encephalitis lethargica, Parkinsonism. *Lancet* 1982; 320; 860–864.
5. Oxford J. On the trail of a killer. *New Scientist* 2003; 18 October: 35–37.
6. Mestel R. Mind-altering bugs. *New Scientist* 1997; 13 September: 42–45.
7. Chalmers RM, Thomas DRH, Salmon RL. Borna disease virus and the evidence for human pathogenicity: a systemic review. *QJM* 2006; 98: 255–274.
8. Timonen M, Laakso M, Jokelainen J, *et al.* Depression and insulin resistance. *BMJ* 2005; 330: 17–18.

9. Marlowe N, Dieter W, Bracewell MA, Samara M for the EPICure Study Group. Neurological and developmental disability at six years of age after extremely preterm birth. *N Engl J Med* 2005; 352: 9–19.

10. Kurtzke JF. A reassessment of the distribution of multiple sclerosis. *Acta Neurol Scand* 1975; 51: 137–157.

11. Jin Y, de Pedro-Cuesta J, Söderström M, *et al.* Seasonal patterns in optic neuritis and multiple sclerosis: a meta-analysis. *J Neurol Sci* 2000; 181: 56–64.

12. Killestein J, Rep MHG, Meilo JF, *et al.* Seasonal variation in immune measurements and MRI markers of disease activity in MS. *Neurology* 2002; 58: 1077–1080.

13. Oikonen M, Laaksonen M, Laippala P, *et al.* Ambient air quality and occurrence of multiple sclerosis relapse. *Neuroepidemiology* 2003; 22: 95–99.

14. Van der Mei IAF, Ponsonby AL, Dwyer T, *et al.* Past exposure to sun, skin phenotype, and risk of multiple sclerosis: case-control study. *BMJ* 2003; 327: 316–320.

15. Munger KL, Zhang SM, O'Reilly E, *et al.* Vitamin D intake and incidence of multiple sclerosis. *Neurology* 2004; 62: 60–65.

16. Munger KL, Levin LI, Hollis BW, *et al.* Serum 25-hydroxyvitamin D levels and risk of multiple sclerosis. *JAMA* 2006; 296: 2832–2838.

17. Willer CJ, Dyment DA, Sadovnick AD, *et al.* Timing of birth and risk of multiple sclerosis: population based study. *BMJ* 2005; 330: 120–123.

18. Torrey EF, Miller J, Rawlings R, Yolken RH. Seasonal birth patterns of neurological disorders. *Neuroepidemiology* 2000; 19: 177–185.

19. Ebers GC, Savodnick AD, Dyment DA, *et al.* Parent-of-origin effect in multiple sclerosis: observations in half-siblings. *Lancet* 2004; 363:1773–1774.

20. Giordano M, Momigliano-Richiardi P. Maternal effect in multiple sclerosis. *Lancet* 2004; 363: 1748–1749.

21. Kraytberg Y, Schwartz M, Brown TA, *et al.* Recombination of human mitochondrial DNA. *Science* 2004; 304: 981.

22. Scott K. Loch that could harbour a grim secret. *The Guardian* 2003; 7 June: 11.

23. Kutzke JF, Heltberg A. Multiple sclerosis in the Faroe Islands: an epitome. *J Clin Epidemiol* 2001; 54: 1–22.

24. Sriram S, Stratton CW, Yao S, *et al. Chlamydia pneumoniae* infection of the central nervous system in multiple sclerosis. *Ann Neurol* 1999; 46: 6–14.

25. Murray J. Infection as a cause of multiple sclerosis. *BMJ* 2002; 325: 1128.
26. Gay D, Dick G. Is multiple sclerosis caused by an oral spirochaete? *Lancet* 1986; 328: 75–77.
27. Dolei A, Serra C, Mameli G, *et al*. Multiple sclerosis-associated retrovirus (MSRV) in Sardinian MS patients. *Neurology* 2002; 59: 1071–1073.
28. Vollmer T, Key L, Durkalski V, *et al*. Oral simvastatin treatment in relapsing–remitting multiple sclerosis. *Lancet* 2004; 363: 1607–1608.

## Chapter 66 Rheumatic and auto-immune disorders

1. Silman AJ, Pearson JE. Epidemiology and genetics of rheumatoid arthritis. *Arth Res* 2002; 4, Supple 3: S265–S272.
2. Silman AJ. Has the incidence of rheumatoid arthritis declined in the United Kingdom? *Br J Rheumatol* 1988; 27: 77–78.
3. Rosenthal AK, McLaughli JK, Linet MS, Persson I. Scleroderma and malignancy: an epidemiological study. *Ann Rheum Dis* 1993; 52: 531–533.
4. Abu-Sharka M, Guillemin F, Lee P. Cancer in systemic sclerosis. *Arth Rhem* 1993; 36: 460–464.
5. Kröger H, Penttila IM, Alhava EM. Low serum vitamin D metabolites in women with rheumatoid arthritis. *Scand J Rheumatol* 1993; 22: 172–177.
6. Oelzner P, Franke S, Müller A, *et al*. Relationship between soluble markers of immune activation and bone turnover in post-menopausal women with rheumatoid arthritis. *Rheumatology* 1999; 38: 841–847.
7. Andjelovic Z, Vojinovic J, Pejnovic N, *et al*. Disease modifying and immunomodulatory effects of high dose 1α(OH) D3 in rheumatoid arthritis patients. *Clin Exp Rheumatol* 1999; 17: 452–456.
8. Cantorna MT, Mahon BD. Mounting evidence for vitamin D as an environmental factor affecting autoimmune disease prevalence. *Exp Biol Med* 2004; 229: 1136–1142.
9. Merlino LA, Curtis J, Mikuls TR, *et al*. Vitamin D intake is inversely associated with rheumatoid arthritis. *Arth Rheum* 2004; 50: 72–77.
10. Deluca HF, Cantorna MT. Vitamin D: its role and uses in immunology. *FASEB J* 2001; 15: 2579–2585.
11. Ponsonby A-L, McMichael A, van der Mei, I. Ultraviolet radiation and autoimmune disease: insights from epidemiological research. *Toxicology* 2002; 181–182: 71–78.

12. McCarey DW, McInnes IB, Madhok R, *et al.* Trial of atorvastatin in rheumatoid arthritis (TARA): double-blind, randomised placebo-controlled trial. *Lancet* 2004; 363: 2015–2021.

## Chapter 67 Is the sun dangerous?

1. UK Cancer Research Council. *Stay Safe.* UK Cancer Research Council: London 2006 http://info.cancerresearchuk.org/healthyliving/sunsmart/staysafe/shade/ (accessed 26 March 2008).
2. UK Cancer Research Council. *Reduce the Risk.* UK Cancer Research Council: London 2005. http://info.cancerresearchuk.org/images/pdfs/rtr_research_brochure.pdf (accessed 26 March 2008).
3. Hobday, R. *The Healing Sun: sunlight and health in the 21ˢᵗ century.* Findhorn Press: Forres 1999.
4. Peller S. Carcinogenesis as a means of reducing cancer mortality. *Lancet* 1936; 2: 552–556.
5. Peller S, Stephenson CS. Skin irritation and cancer in the United States Navy. *Am J Med Sc* 1937; 194: 326–333.
6. Office for National Statistics. *1995 Mortality Statistics, England and Wales.* Stationary Office: London 1997.
7. Ivry B, Ogle CA, Shim EK. Role of sun exposure in melanoma. *Dermatol Surg* 2006; 32: 481–92.
8. Coleman MP, Babb P, Damiecki P, *et al. Cancer Survival Trends in England and Wales, 1971–1995: deprivation and NHS region.* Studies in Medical and Population Subjects No. 61. Office for National Statistics, The Stationery Office: London 1999.
9. Elwood JM, Jopson J. Melanoma and sun exposure: an overview of published studies. *Int J Cancer* 1997; 73: 198–203.
10. Garland FC, White MR, Garland CF, *et al.* Occupational sunlight exposure and melanoma in the US Navy. *Arch Environ Health* 1990; 45: 261–267.
11. Ness AR, Frankel SJ, Gunnell DJ, Davey Smith G. Are we really dying for a tan? *BMJ* 1999; 319: 114–116.
12. Ness AR, Frankel SJ, Gunnell DJ, Davey Smith G. Are we still dying for a tan? *J Cosmetic Dermatol* 2002; 1: 43–46.
13. Moan J, Porojnicu AC, Dahlback A, Setlow RB. Addressing the health benefits and risks, involving vitamin D or skin cancer, of increased sun exposure. *PNAS* 2008; 105: 668–673.
14. Parkin DM, Whelan SL, Felay J, *et al. Cancer Incidence in Five Continents.* International Agency for Research on Cancer: Lyon 2002.

15. Grant WB. An estimate of premature cancer mortality in the US due to inadequate doses of solar ultraviolet-B radiation. *Cancer* 2002; 94: 1867–1875.
16. de Vries E, Steliarova-Foucher E, Spatz A, *et al*. Skin cancer incidence and survival in European children and adolescents (1978–1997). Report from the Automated Childhood Cancer Information System project. *Eur J Cancer* 2006; 42: 2170–2182.
17. Welch HG, Woloshin S, Schwartz LM. Skin biopsy rates and incidence of melanoma: population based ecology study. *BMJ* 2005; 331: 481–484.
18. Colston K, Colston MJ, Feldman D. 1,25-Dihydroxyvitamin D3 and malignant melanoma: the presence of receptors and inhibition of cell growth in culture. *Endocrinology* 1981; 108: 1086–1086.
19. Holick MF. Sunlight and vitamin D for bone health and prevention of autoimmune diseases, cancers, and cardiovascular disease. *Am J Clin Nutr* 2004; 80, Supple: 1678S–1688S.
20. Krone B, Kölmel KF, Henz BM, Grange JM. Protection against melanoma by vaccination with Bacille Calmette Guérin (BCG) and/or vaccinia: an epidemiology-based hypothesis on the nature of a melanoma risk factor and its immunological control. *Eur J Cancer* 2005; 41: 104–117.
21. Van der Mei IAF, Ponsonby AL, Dwyer T, *et al*. Past exposure to sun, skin phenotype, and risk of multiple sclerosis: case-control study. *BMJ* 2003; 327: 316–320.
22. Menter A., Griffiths CEM. Current and future management of psoriasis. *Lancet* 2007; 370: 272–284
23. Gillie O. *Sunlight Robbery: health benefits of sunlight are denied by current health policy in the UK*. Occasional Reports 1. Health Research Forum: London 2004.
24. Melamed ML, Michos ED, Post W, Astor B. 25-Hydroxyvitamin D levels and the risk of mortality in the general population. *Arch Int Med* 2008; 168: 1629–1637.

## Chapter 68 Epilogue: vitamin D and statins

1. Donaldson L. Meeting the need for vitamin D. *CMO Update* Summer 2005; 42: 6.
2. Tsoukas CD, Provvedini DM, Manolagas SC. 1,25-dihydroxyvitaminD3: a novel immunoregulatory hormone. *Science* 1984; 224: 1438–1440.
3. The RECORD Trial Group. Oral vitamin D3 and calcium for secondary prevention of low-trauma fractures in elderly people (Randomised Evaluation of Calcium Or vitamin D, RECORD): a randomised placebo-controlled trial. *Lancet* 2005; 365: 1621–1628.

4. Zittermann A. Vitamin D in preventive medicine: are we ignoring the evidence? *Br J Nutr* 2003; 89: 552–572.

5. Nagpal S, Lu J, Boehm MF. Vitamin D analogues: mechanism of action and therapeutic applications. *Curr Med Chem* 2001; 8: 1661–1679.

6. Edwards CJ, Hart DJ, Spector TD. Oral statins and increased bone-mineral density in postmenopausal women. *Lancet* 2000; 355: 2218–2219.

7. Canty J. *Statins may stimulate stem cells for heart repair*. Press release. University of Buffalo: Buffalo November 2005.

8. Zittermann A, Schleithoff SS, Tenderich G, *et al*. Low vitamin D status: a contributing factor in the pathogenesis of congestive heart failure. *J Am Coll Cardiol* 2003; 41: 105–112.

9. Sola S, Mir MQS, Lerakis S, *et al*. Atorvastatin improves left ventricular function and serum markers of inflammation in non-ischaemic heart failure. *J Am Coll Cardiol* 2006; 47: 332–337.

10. Go AS, Lee WY, Yang J, *et al*. Statin therapy and risks of death and hospitalization in chronic heart failure. *JAMA* 2006; 296: 2105–2111.

11. *New Scientist* 2005; 12 November.

12. Weidong LI, Cui Y, Kushner SA, *et al*. The HMG-CoA reductase inhibitor lovastatin reverses the learning and attention deficits in a mouse model of neurofibromatosis type 1. *Curr Biol* 2005; 15: 1961–1967.

13. Hackam DG, Mamdani M, Li P, Redelmeier DA. Statins and sepsis in patients with cardiovascular disease: a population-based cohort analysis. *Lancet* 2006; 367: 413–418.

14. Strazzullo P, Kerry SM, Barbato A, *et al*. Do statins reduce blood pressure? A meta-analysis of randomized, controlled trials. *Hypertension* 2007; 49: 792–798.

15. Brennan PJ, Greenburg G, Miall WE, Thompson SG. Seasonal variation in arterial blood pressure. *BMJ* 1982; 285: 919–923.

16. Strandberg TE, Pyörälä K, Cook TJ, *et al*., for the 4S group. Mortality and incidence of cancer during 10-year follow-up of the Scandinavian Simvastatin Survival Study (4S). *Lancet* 2004; 364: 771–777.

17. Poytner JN, Gruber SB, Higgins PDR, *et al*. Statins and risk of colorectal cancer. *N Engl J Med* 2005; 352: 2184–2192.

18. Lezner J. Unreported cholesterol drug data released by companies show drug is ineffective. *BMJ* 2008; 336: 180–181.

19. Le Fanu J. The case of the missing data. *BMJ* 2002; 325:1490–1493.

20. McMichael J. Dietetic factors in coronary disease. *Eur J Cardiol* 1977; 5/6: 447–452.